REDESIGNING SCHOOL HEALTH SERVICES

REDESIGNING
SCHOOL HEALTH SERVICES

Annette Lynch, M.D., D.P.H.

The Medical College of Pennsylvania
Philadelphia, Pennsylvania

Former director, Bureau of Children's Services
Department of Health, Commonwealth of Pennsylvania

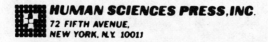
HUMAN SCIENCES PRESS, INC.
72 FIFTH AVENUE,
NEW YORK, N.Y. 10011

Printed in the United States of America
3456789 987654321

Library of Congress Cataloging in Publication Data

Lynch, Annette.
    Redesigning school health services.

    Includes bibliographical references and index.
    1. School hygiene. I. Title. [DNLM: 1. School health
services—Organization and administration.
WA 350 L987r]
LB3405.L93   1983   371.7   LC 82–12178
ISBN 0–89885–102–5

To My Parents

Mary Purcell and Raymond Lynch

Though nothing can bring back the hour
Of splendour in the grass, of glory in the flower;
We will grieve not, rather find
Strength in what remains behind;
In the primal sympathy
Which having been must ever be;
In the soothing thoughts that spring
Out of human suffering;
In the faith that looks through death,
In years that bring the philosophic mind.

—William Wordsworth
Ode: Intimations of Immortality

CONTENTS

FOREWORD

Can and should school health programs be revitalized? The answer given in this book is an emphatic yes. Dr. Lynch shows how this revitalization can occur without formation of new bureaucracies and without increase in expenditures beyond the current levels of investment.

The roots of school health are traced back to the Industrial Revolution and to the beginning of compulsory education. The parallel developments of public health and nursing are discussed. That discussion serves as a backdrop for a review of the history of school health. Evidence of early successes and eventual stagnation are documented.

With a focus on school-age children, not just children in school, the author reviews current diseases and conditions of this age-group. She describes how these diseases and conditions differ in variety and complexity from those of children in the early part of the century. Most school health programs, however, have remained essentially unchanged for the past several decades. The inadequacies of today's school health are highlighted in these unchanging programs. Schools now must adapt to the changing health needs of students. The assumption is made that society has an obligation to protect the health of children in areas beyond the capacity and responsibility of parents. Not only must the school reduce known health hazards in the school environment, but also it should provide students with the knowledge and skills to be informed and able managers of their own health.

Dr. Lynch shows that the major need of school health programs in the United States today is to free them from their past. The goal of developing a rational, purposive, and accountable school health program is established. Methods of organizational development, based on the Pennsylvania experience, are detailed. How to use these methods, to move from the old school health system to the new, is portrayed. The focus of the new goal-oriented system is children and their health. The new system is adaptable to the changing health needs of children. It is undergirded by three subsystems of health information, management, and services.

The heart of the new system is the school nurse practitioner, who is assisted by health aides. Physicians are available for consultation. The basic skills of the nursing profession include sensitive interviewing techniques, keen observation of individuals and environments, a caring attitude, an adeptness at developmental and family assessment, and a knowledge of community resources. The school nurse has these basic skills and, building on them adds practitioner skills through state-funded training programs. The new roles of the nurse practitioner, school physicians, and health aides are defined. Strong support from the school administration and the community is elicited at the onset. This support is sustained during the early phases of implementation.

The author, with a historical approach, focuses on innovative state leadership in the use of state funds. She describes a practical approach to organization development. She challenges health and education professionals and their communities to redesign school health programs. It can be done. It should be done. We have less than 20 years to have the new system in place by the end of this century.

Vince L. Hutchins, M.D., M.P.H.
Director, Office for Maternal and Child Health
Bureau of Community Health Services
U.S. Department of Health and Human Services
Rockville, Md.

PREFACE

The purpose of this book is to explore the problems and paradoxes presented by currently operating school health services, to discuss their increasing inability to deal with the health problems of today's schoolchildren, and to present a model of a quiet internal revolution that can restore for today's children and ensure for tomorrow's school health services that preserve and promote the health of student-workers in their unique place of occupation—the school.

School health services operate in all states of the Union and in most countries of the world; yet, despite this potential for diversity, they all adhere to the same model of care, which, although well designed for the health needs of schoolchildren at the end of the nineteenth century, has not changed to meet the different health problems and conditions of the twentieth century. The basic reason is that current school health services are static input systems not possessing a capacity for change, and are thus doomed to increasing irrelevance.

This book reviews the history of school health to identify the conditions and factors that produced the current system and then analyzes that system with emphasis on those factors responsible for its static nature. The chief factor is the complete absence, in responsible public health agencies, of an epidemiologic approach to the health needs of the school student population. Lack of public health leadership has been camouflaged by legal mandates requiring an ancient set of services. Local mechanisms for delivery of school health services have strangled initiative: the lesser number of local health departments, through indifference, diminishing resources, and part-time

13

staff assignments; and the larger number of school districts, through grossly inefficient use of full-time staff and control of the system by nonhealth personnel for nonhealth purposes.

The revolution being executed in Pennsylvania is described in these pages. Its goal is the change of school health services from an input system of specific activities to an output system in which the school district is held accountable for measurable improvement in the health status of the population of school students served. The shift is from state to local control. The new system at the school district level is conceptualized and described in terms of three necessary subsystems, services, information, and management, only one of which, services, currently exists. Each of the subsystems, the problems inherent in establishing each, and the features of the operating entity are described.

The discussions of the new subsystems and the review of the health needs of the school student population reveal the extent of our ignorance. We know little and do less. But these facts can be used positively. Those in the field of school health need to indicate where lack of knowledge is impeding their efforts. Their complaints should fall upon the ears of academicians, researchers, supporters of research, clinicians, educators, professional schools, legislators, administrators, advocate groups, parents, and all who influence the priorities governing the development of knowledge.

Experience in Pennsylvania indicates that adoption of the new school health system provides the means for a school district (or an individual school or a total state) to make continuing progress in development of an operating model that can tolerate lack of knowledge while preserving the ability to incorporate new understandings as they become available. The steps used in Pennsylvania have been expansion of the role of school nurse to school nurse practitioner with a consequent change of the school physician to consultant in pediatric matters. These changes improve efficiency while increasing the range and competence of the services subsystem. Services, with greater abilities in assessment and management of the health problems of students, produce new health information, which in turn stimulates the management subsystem. The new system requires health professionals to use epidemiologic skills and to design needed preventive services.

The change described—concentration on measurably improving the health of students and change in the locus of control from central to local agencies—is not fast, but could be accomplished so that by the twenty-first century the system of school health services could more rationally deal with any of the health problems the future holds in store for those to be born only 12 years from now. I hope this book provides some view of how such a new school health system can operate and the general processes to be used to accomplish the change.

ACKNOWLEDGMENTS

How can one start or finish thanking those who have contributed to a work that arises from one's experiences spanning nearly two decades? The world may not be peopled with giants, but wherever I turned I encountered others who have found and seized upon some aspect of truth: a perception, a dream, an experience. They have guarded the flame and shared its light and warmth with those who came looking.

Such marvelous human beings existed in the days that preceded ours, and their spirit and valued discoveries travel by their words and deeds across the years; some have been found in positions of power and many more in schoolhouses and nurses' offices and classrooms; others have unexpectedly revealed the riches they had to share from the bowels of the most recalcitrant profession or institution, or from the recesses of an apparently dull personality and seemingly undistinguished career.

This book is possible because, in the fashion of a pilgrim, I have been able to journey from person to person in order to learn. The numbers are countless, yet the debt so great that only the words of Stephen Spender seem to express that which I wish to acknowledge:

> I think continually of those who were truly great—
> The names of those who in their lives fought for life,
> Who wore at their hearts the fire's center.

In the actual production of this book it is a pleasure to thank:
Those who saw that school health had problems, set me loose to explore them, and encouraged my first writings on the subject:

Edward M. Sewell, M.D., Director of the Division of School Health, School District of Philadelphia, 1970–1974; Gordon W. Allan, M.D., Director of the Bureau of Children's Preventive and Restorative Services, Pennsylvania Department of Health, 1973–1975. To Gordon also belongs the distinction of being the first person to recognize the structural nature of the problems faced by school health.

Those who wanted, or who were willing to be talked into, demonstrations of things new: Rosalind Y. Ting, M.D., Margaret Rose Connor, R.N., P.N.P., and Muriel J. Mummau, R.N., P.N.P., of the Head Start program of the School District of Philadelphia, 1971–1973; Elmer J. Berkebile, Ed.D., Superintendent, and Judith Hughes Miller, R.N., S.N.P., Director of Health Services, Penn Manor School District; the late Daniel A. Rohrbach, Ed.D., Executive Director, Francis R. Dietrich, Ed.D., Assistant Executive Director, and Lynne A. Sarig, R.N., School Health Coordinator, Berks County Intermediate Unit, who caught some of their enthusiasm from Theodore (Ted) Rights, M.D., District Medical Director, Pennsylvania Department of Health, 1974–1975; Wilma M. Lentz, R.N., P.N.P., Nursing Supervisor of Health Services for the Pittsburgh Board of Education; Henry R. Hoerner, Ed.D., Superintendent, and Shirley H. Woolf, R.N., S.N.P., Coordinator of School Health Services, Lower Dauphin School District; Frederic B. Garner, M.D., and Glen S. Bartlett, M.D., Ph.D., successively directors of the Pediatric Ambulatory Care Program, Department of Pediatrics, Milton S. Hershey Medical Center, and providers of the first school nurse practitioner education program in Pennsylvania, in which effort Grace E. Laubach, R. N., associate professor of nursing of the Pennsylvania State University, was an early partner; Corinne M. Barnes, R.N., Ph.D., professor and Director of Graduate Programs in the Nursing Care of Children, School of Nursing, University of Pittsburgh; Rosalie W. Washington, R.N., President, Philadelphia School Nurse Association, Local 3838, affiliated with AFL-CIO.

Those who have guided change, guarded tender beginnings, goaded when necessary, and never given up: Bernice P. Baxter, R.N., Director, and "school health planners," Muriel J. Mummau, R.N., P.N.P., Eileen H. Moult, R.N. P.N.P., Division of School Health, Pennsylvania Department of Health, at whose urging this book was finally begun.

Completion of the book would not have been possible without earlier papers, articles, and reports in which ideas were developed and reactions sought. The two secretaries of my past years in school health, Ruth Levi and Rose Bowman, were workhorses in those projects; they supported and encouraged and forebore beyond the call of duty or friendship. Without the patient typing, proofreading, and warm support of my friend Iris Darlington, this manuscript would still be locked in indecipherable pages. I thank Norma Fox, Renee Kaplan, and Edith Lewis, copy editor, of Human Sciences Press for professional work performed with graciousness.

I am pleased to acknowledge the permission granted by Daniel Katz, Ph.D., and Jossey-Bass, Inc. to reproduce a modified version of the table "Hierarchical Levels & Leadership Patterns" from "Handbook of Political Psychology," ed. J. N. Knutson, 1973, (see table 9–1).

Finally, I thank the schoolchildren of Pennsylvania whom I have come to know through direct and indirect contact. In the pain and desolation of their ill health they have provided the experiences from which we have learned, and in their boundless life and future promise they have given meaning to our present.

Permission from the publishers to reproduce excerpts from the following selections is gratefully acknowledged.

Silver, H. K. The School nurse practitioner program: A new expanded role for the school nurse. *Journal American Medical Association*, 1971, *216*, 1332–1334. Copyright 1971, American Medical Association. Reprinted with permission from the author.

Malenbaum, W. Progress in health: What index of what progress? *Annals American Academy of Political and Social Science*, January 1971, *393*, 109–121.

Levey, S., & Loomba, N. P. *Health care administration: A Managerial perspective*, Philadelphia: J. B. Lippincott, Co., 1973.

Rogers, K. D. School Age Children. In M. Green & R. T. Haggerty, (Eds.), *Ambulatory Pediatrics*, Philadelphia: W. B. Saunders Company, 1968.

Byrd, O. E. *School health administration*. Philadelphia: W. B. Saunders Company, 1964.

Kane, R. L. Primary care: Contradictions and questions. Reprinted by permission of the *New England Journal of Medicine, 296*:1410–1411, 1977.

Smillie, W. G. *Public health and its promise for the future: A Chronicle of the development of public health in the United States, 1609–1914*. Copyright 1955, Macmillan Publishing Co., Inc. New York: Macmillan Publishing Co., Inc., 1955.

de Saint Exupéry, A. The Little Prince, Copyright, 1943, by Harcourt, Brace and World, Inc., New York. Reprinted with permission from Harcourt Brace Jovanovich, Inc.

Cornely, D. A. Health Services for Children. In *Preventive Medicine and Public Health*, Tenth edition, P. E. Sartwell (Ed.), New York: Appleton-Century-Crofts, 1973.

Piel, G. Improving the nation's health: Joint leverage for economic and social adjustment. In G. F. Rohrlich, (Ed.), Social Economics for the 1970s, New York: The Dunellen Publishing Co., 1970.

Caplan, G. *Principles of Preventive Psychiatry* New York: 1964 Basic Books, Inc., Reprinted by permission.

Brockington, C. F. *The Health of the community.* Third edition, London: J. & A. Churchill Ltd., 1965, Reprinted with permission from Churchill Livingstone.

Brockington, C. F. *A Short history of public health.* London: J. & A. Churchill Ltd., 1956. Reprinted with permission from Churchill Livingstone.

Silver, H. K. & McAtee, P. R. A descriptive definition of the scope and content of primary health care. *Pediatrics,* 1975, *56*:957–959, copyright American Academy of Pediatrics, 1975. Reprinted with permission from author.

Linder, F. E. Sources of data on health in the U.S. Chapter 5. In D. W. Clark, B. MacMahon (Eds.), *Preventive Medicine,* Boston: Little Brown and Company, 1967.

Trevelyan, G. M., Illustrated English social history: The Nineteenth century, Vol. IV., London: Longmans, Green, 1960. Reprinted with permission from Longman Group Limited.

Susser, M. *Causal thinking in the health sciences: Concepts and strategies of epidemiology.* New York: Oxford University Press, 1973.

Young, G. M. *Victorian England: Portrait of an age.* London: (c) Oxford University Press 1960, by permission of Oxford University Press.

Bremner, R. H. (Ed.) *Children and youth in America, Vol II,* Cambridge: Harvard University Press, 1971. Reprinted with permission from the American Public Health Association.

Schaefer, M. Current issues in health organization. *American Journal Public Health,* 1968, *58*:1192–1199. Reprinted with permission from the author.

Silver, G. A. Reprinted from *Child health: America's future* by permission of Aspen Systems Corporation, (c) 1978.

Birch, H. G. Malnutrition, Learning, and Intelligence. *American Journal Public Health,* 1972, *62*:773–784. Reprinted with permission from the author.

Katz D. Patterns of leadership, Chapter 8 In *Handbook of political psychology,* J. N. Knutson (Ed.), San Francisco: Jossey-Bass, Inc., 1973. Reprinted with permission from the author.

Bryan, D. S. *School nursing in transition.* St. Louis: C. V. Mosby & Co., 1973. Reprinted with permission from the author.

Sigerist, H. E. *The Great doctors: A Biographical history of medicine from the ancient world to the twentieth century.* New York: Doubleday Anchor Books, 1958. Reprinted with permission from George Allen and Unwin.

White, K. L. Contemporary epidemiology. *International Journal of Epidemiology,* 1974, *3*:395–403. Reprinted with permission from the author.

Chapter 1

VIEWS OF SCHOOL HEALTH SERVICES

"Curiouser and curiouser!" cried Alice.

—Lewis Carroll, *Alice in Wonderland*

There are many reasons for writing a book: to announce the discovery of a new subject, to add new knowledge to an already existing subject, or to suggest a new way of looking at an old subject. This book falls more into the last category. The general thesis is that school health services, developed for the needs of the nineteenth century, have continued with little change into the twentieth century. As the health needs of this century's school students have drifted further away from the needs of their counterparts of 100 years ago, it appears that a certain sense of incongruity has crept into the souls of those who assiduously continue to provide the traditional services.

An indication that something is wrong is manifest in definitions that are both vague and grandiose, in practices that are said to embrace all things but in reality perform little or something quite different from what is described, and in the sweeping generalizations made by all who touch upon the field when, in fact, each is feeling but one part of an elephant that, it turns out, is a kind of invisible subject never having been fully seen, described, or studied. In addition, some very new approaches are being tried as ways to find a solution to the incompletely understood problem.

19

Before turning to some of these views it is necessary to define *school health services*. The term, as used in this publication, describes those medical, nursing, and dental services provided to individual children in or through school; the term does not necessarily include health or physical education or regular curriculum items.

School health services find their origins in state laws "which seek to discover and correct physical defects through health examinations."[1] School health services implement their legislative mandates by employing physicians for medical examinations and dentists for dental examinations; arranging for physical inspection of pupils in the class by physician, nurse, or teacher; requiring screening tests, by teacher or nurse, for vision, hearing, growth; obtaining the services of nurses for the role of "school nurse," which consists of some or all of the following: assistance to the physician and dentist, record keeping, attention to illnesses and injuries occurring on the school premises, and actions to obtain "correction" of physical defects found by examinations and inspections.

The exact nature and extent of current school health services in the United States cannot be accurately described. The last-known federal official concerned with school health was active in the U.S. Department of Health, Education, and Welfare in the late 1950's.[2] The last-known federal publication regarding state trends in school health was published in 1941.[3] In 1976 the American School Health Association undertook a survey of state school health programs.[4] On repetition in 1979 the survey was published by the U.S. Department of Health, Education, and Welfare.[5]

Education data show that in 1969/70 forty-eight states provided expenditures for school health services. The national average was $5.79 per student in *average daily attendance*, with a range of $.92 to $15.65. The number of full-time school nurse equivalents documented by 40 states in 1969/70 totaled 15,791, or 1 per 2,655 students in average daily attendance for the nation.[6] The American School Health Association survey for 1979 received data on the actual number of school nurses from 35 states and an indication that school nurses were provided by local agencies in 11 states; no data were returned by 5 states.[5] Nurses are certified as "school nurses" in 32 states, as "school nurse teachers" in 2 states, and must be public health nurses or registered nurses in 4 states. Thirteen states were described as having no requirements. Interesting differences were found between state agencies regarding responsibility for school health services in surveys of the 50 states and District of Columbia conducted by the American School Health Association in 1977/78 and by the Kansas State Department of Health in 1964.[7] (see Table 1–1).

Health departments see themselves responsible in 90 percent of

Table 1–1.

Agency:	American School health Association	Kansas State Department of Health
Date of survey:	1977/78	1964
Date of publication:	1979	1965
Survey sent to:	State school health consultants or state commissioners of education or state health commissioners	State health departments
Question:	Agency responsible for school health services?	School health program responsibility?
Answers:		
Education	22	3
Health	20	46
Education and Health	3	—
No answer	6	2
Total	51	51

Sources: American School Health Association—Castile and Jerrick[5]; Kansas State Department of Health—Gendel.[7]

states and are seen by those from education to have responsibility in 39 percent of states. Neither view fits the common perception that "70 percent of school health services in the country are under control and direction of the State Education Departments (20 percent are under State Health Departments)."[8]

State requirements reported by educators were certain health services for students and/or employees upon entry to school: physical examination (24), screening tests (31), immunizations (50), periodic physical examinations (9), and athletic sports examinations (11). Departments of health reported more requirements for the above service categories: physical examinations (32), hearing screening (39), vision screening (37), and athletic examinations (28). They also reported environmental inspections and standards for school buildings (39), dental services (36), training of teachers in health (27), mental health planning in schools (22), and planning of health curriculum in schools (19).

State health departments are probably very accurate in their interpretation of the legal role of departments of health in school health. The strange thing is that hardly anyone looking at school health services shares the view or even understands that state health departments have a part to play. The facts were clearly set forth by the American Association of School Administrators in 1942: in the period 1880–1940 the legislatures in all 48 states adopted laws regarding school sanitation, health promotion, and physical efficiency. Most provided for school health services consisting of health instruction, formation of correct health habits by children, and correction of physical defects through physical examination (see note 1). Some requirements are set forth in health law and others in education law. Subsequent publications on school health[9] or general public health[10] have tended to completely ignore the legal foundations of school health. The reasons are not clear but may lie in a tendency to view the local implementing agency as representing the total school health operation, in part because of the scant attention and resources directed by state health departments to their job.

A variety of local patterns have emerged through which state requirements are met: health services provided by local school boards, health services provided by local health departments, health services provided by state health departments under contract to local boards of education, by a combination of agencies, or by others. A 1949 study found school medical services provided by official education agencies (45 percent), official health agencies (41 percent), education and health agencies (11 percent), and other agencies (3 percent).[11] These differences concerning whether school health services should be provided by health or education agencies have provided a fruitful source for nonproductive dissension over the years, while more difficult problems, for example, permissive versus mandatory legislation, lack of implementation and enforcement of legislation, and lack of state personnel to provide the most minimal administrative services, let alone program development or leadership, have been ignored. In these matters it is worth quoting Silver, a highly qualified public health observer: "Connecticut assigns school health services—undefined—to the state department of education, which has had no person in charge for years. A clerk in the department of health, paid by the department of education, collects data and writes memoranda to the school nurses."[12] Such a situation might be considered exceptional if not supported by personal experience. In the Pennsylvania health department, one clerk was the only staff person assigned to school health for a period of about 15 years until 1973, yet Pennsylvania has a highly structured state-mandated program with prime program responsibility and fiscal responsibility residing in the state department of health.[13]

It is interesting that Silver used the example of Connecticut because the first law requiring periodic health examinations for public school students was enacted in Connecticut in 1899. One wonders if the law changed in Connecticut or whether administrative neglect has obscured its existence. Either case would be worthy of further study.

Despite the comprehensive range of school health services described by the survey responders in state departments of health, there are health experts who are critical:

A leader in the field of maternal and child health:

> No other area of health service [for children] has been the subject of more debate than that associated with the elementary and secondary schools. The traditional focus on prevention with inadequate resources and programs for curative care, jurisdictional conflicts between the educational system and the health agency, the utilization of nurses in large numbers performing many functions of low or questionable worth in the presence of a community nursing shortage, and the seeming retention of inappropriate means toward stated goals—e.g., perfunctory physical examinations—are the principal points of contention.[15]

The most highly regarded pediatrician commentator on school health:

> Some [school health programs] have become established by tradition and regulation so that they continue without respect to their effectiveness or relevance to health improvement. . . . The principal activities of many school physicians and nurses in the United States today are concerned with control of communicable disease through inspection of pupils returning from absence, detection of health problems by periodic physical examination and screening tests, and first aid care for minor morbidity . . . many of these [activities] have little or no demonstrable effect on health.[16]

An eminent professor of public health:

> But school health services are minimally attended to. . . . True, most states have laws requiring that schools have part-time or full-time doctors and nurses, but the preventive aspects are slighted. Children are examined casually, hurriedly, and superficially, if at all. If defects are found, follow-up is desultory. Immunizations are given, sometimes not. . . . The lack of a comprehensive school health program in the United States is probably one of the key elements in the poor record of untreated handicaps among American adults.[12]

Practitioners in the field of school health see things differently. A definition prepared for the National School Health Conference in Minneapolis, Minnesota, May 1977, went as follows:

> School health is a combination of comprehensive health services, health education, and healthful environment which services not only children but also their parents, the school staff, and the community at large. School health should be carried out in schools, homes, and community facilities by a team of persons from the schools, the health care field, and family members. School health should be implemented primarily through educational activities with the intended outcome being one of maintenance and promotion of an optimal state of physical, mental and social well-being for each of its recipients.[17]

The definition is an example of vague grandiosity purporting, as it does, to serve "everybody, by everybody, and in all places." Further study reveals that it is concerned only with "educational activities" for the "maintenance . . . of . . . well-being." Such a definition has no place for "children whose education is compromised, thwarted or irrevocably damaged by childhood mortality and morbidity."[18] The claim for such a sweeping mandate becomes irrational when the claimants declare, virtually in the same breath, that the child's health is "the parent's responsibility."[19]

Over the years many educators have imposed an educational view on school health services. Some have wanted health education and have refused clinical services for the students.[20] Others have welcomed such health services but have used them, not as means to improve the health of students, but as methods in health education—rather like sophisticated instructional aids![21] Yet, these same educators are in daily contact with school nurses, who are the major practitioners of school health, and should see that their services involve more than maintenance of well-being.

Hawkins studied the school nurse role and reported that many health problems of children handled by nurses are "extremely complex." He mentioned the intricacies of cases of school phobia, problem families, child neglect, and legal requirements on school nurses to report cases of child abuse; the function of the nurse as "family health resource" to mothers uncertain about the nature of illness in their children; the nursing role in obtaining prosthetic appliances, medical assistance, and free lunches and in relating to family physicians, hospitals and clinics, welfare agencies, juvenile courts, health associations, civic organizations, youth groups, and state and local health authorities.[22] Such weighty content cannot be lightly dismissed by those believing that school health consists only of education; yet it was necessary, in the resolution generated by the participants at the 1977 National School Health Conference, to note that "whenever we are talking about school health we are talking both about the service component as well as the educational component."[23]

A well-known text on school health administration describes the school administrator as the most important person in the school health program because he or she represents the power of the institution and provides leadership within the school for "this part of the *educational* program" (emphasis added). The same writer goes on to describe the quality of this leadership: "Many school administrators are at least partially confused in respect to the proper function of a school nurse. . . . The most fundamental concept of the school nurse is remarkably simple. Her services in the school should be related to her professional training and should result in maximum good to the children she serves." The author then lists a set of school nurse functions, many of which bear little relation to nursing:

> Curriculum assistant
>
> Liaison with parents
>
> Assistant to school physician
>
> Researcher on public health problems
>
> School grounds sanitarian
>
> Administrative assistant on health problems to principal or superintendent[20]

To this list one must add the performance of first aid, primarily to provide mental relief for the school principal and not because this function needs a college-trained professional—a fact to which the portrayal of emergency technicians on television attests.

Hawkins seized on the point made by the above list, declaring that "the school nurse's role cannot be understood at all in terms of nursing function" because nurses perform a role in which others, who do not understand nursing, define their daily tasks so that nurses lose "in the process much of their potential for demonstrating the value of their services." The best that can be done in the circumstances "seems to consist of a hodgepodge of improvisations."[22]

In the midst of all this, nurses' views are ambivalent. One author pointed to the "notable attempt" made by the American Nurses' Association to define school nursing and then added: "These and other similar words have been stated over and over again by nurses, health educators, physicians, school personnel, and more recently by comprehensive health planners and health manpower commissioners, yet there is always the *lingering doubt* if this is really what is thought and felt about school nursing" (emphasis added).[24] The definition provided by the American Nurses' Association is worthy of attention. It begins by declaring the importance of school nursing (vague grandiosity) and states without evidence that such has been proven: "School nursing is a highly specialized service contributing to the process of education. That it is a socially commendable, economically practical, and scientifically sound service can be *well demonstrated*" (emphasis added). The definition then goes on to outline some of the general areas for which the nurse has knowledge and experience, although it is clear that basic nursing education does not necessarily impart such skills: "The professional nurse with her experience and knowledge of the changing growth and behavioral patterns of children is in a unique position in the school setting *to assist* the children in acquiring health knowledge, in developing attitudes conducive to healthful living, and in meeting their needs resulting from disease, accidents, congenital defects, or psychosocial maladjustments" (emphasis added).[25] It is interesting that the nurse, faced with the needs and possessing the requisite knowledge and experience, is expected by the nursing profession merely "to assist" children.

It is also interesting that a book on school nursing practice that opens with this ANA definition contains little on meeting "needs resulting from disease" and nothing at all on meeting needs resulting from "accidents, congenital defects, or psychosocial maladjustments." Most of this book is concerned with obtaining a few simple health facts, ensuring that children receive physical examinations from their own physicians, performing vision and hearing screening, and providing a minimum brand of first aid in which the nursing protocols (1) often call for "exclusion" of the sick child even for noncontagious conditions, (2) have a quaint, Victorian sound to them, (3) never stoop to simple medications, such as aspirin, and (4) send children home as soon as possible. For example:

Headache

1. Take temperature. If elevated, exclude child from school.
2. Rest in quiet room with fresh air.
3. Cold compresses on head may be used for comfort.
4. If severe and persistent, notify parent and refer to usual source of medical care.[24]

Little wonder that high school students give scant credit to this kind of "assistance" and school staff and parents wonder what the nurse does that reflects professional training and salary.

Without the state certification requirements for school nurses, it is certain that many school administrators would have replaced them with less expensive aides who might be more willing to provide certain services to children. Part of the problem is the tendency of school nurses to view themselves as restricted in their ability to practice nursing. When New Mexico school nurses were challenged on what they said they could not do, it was discovered "that there were no state laws relative to school nursing and that there were no local regulations involved in these cases. These seem to have been built up by force of habit over many years."[26] On the other hand, when school nurses have moved to take on new tasks well within nursing, such as intermittent catheterization of handicapped children,[27] many educational administrators have moved to block the way, sometimes by going as far as to declare such procedures beyond the scope of nursing and school nursing.

On the positive side of school nursing is the fact that it has become more widespread than required by state law, presumably as needs seen by parents and administrators have been met by local public health departments or visiting nurse associations. In Pennsylvania, for example, state law requires at least 1 nurse for each 1,500 students; in 1969/70 school districts supported 1 nurse per 946 students.[6]

In recent years a new role for the school nurse has emerged: as school nurse practitioner. The new role defines a set of "expanded" nursing skills and provides education for their acquisition. Nurses can describe more clearly the contribution they can make to school health. The role has generated much enthusiasm. In the 1977/78 survey conducted by the American School Health Association, 476 school nurses, 3 percent of the total, were classified as school nurse practitioners.[5] A prestigious national foundation, Robert Wood Johnson, has supported varied demonstrations of this new role and services in Galveston, Texas, and Hartford, Connecticut, and a recent five-state evaluation study.

In turning to the medical view of school health, one finds the subject unrepresented not only in health departments but also in pediatric departments, medical schools, and boards of medical specialties. No mention was made of school health in a 897-page book on preventive medicine[28] published in 1967 or in the fourth edition of a classic on public health and preventive medicine;[29] in a review of the State of the Child: New York City[30] considerable attention was given to the Early Periodic Screening Diagnosis and Treatment (EPSDT) program and child health stations but none to school health; similarly, a "child health plan" developed for North Carolina in no manner recognized any health activity in schools.[31] A similar lack of recognition of the existence of school health and its potential was feared by those who saw the workings of the Select Panel for Promotion of Child Health authorized by the U.S. Congress to formulate goals and a comprehensive national plan for promoting the health of children by August 1980.[32]

In 52 of 65 issues of the *American Journal of Public Health* published from January 1975 to May 1980, children of school age were the subject of 35 of 530 articles and briefs, 6.6 percent of the total. Schoolchildren comprise 20 percent of the population. Medical researchers and departments of health often view schools as convenient collections of persons for studies, for obtaining information, or for performing certain procedures for the good of society generally. Communicable disease personnel in departments of health seem particularly prone to see the schools as territory over which they can roam with impunity to obtain information on disease outbreaks, often in order to demonstrate a procedure, for example, a "finer" surveillance net,[33] which has no demonstrable health benefits. Recent years have seen health department immunization personnel use schools to obtain immunization of schoolchildren without cost to health departments (but without counting the cost to the schools or the students); such unimmunized children represent the failure of the public health system to ensure adequate immunization in the first year of life.

The medical profession's view of school health is, on the whole, uninterested. The challenges of prevention provide little motivation for those trained for curative medicine.[12,34] The American Academy of Pediatrics exhibited some interest and made a useful distinction between "health services in the school," in which the physician performs his/her usual functions (e.g., physical examinations) in the school setting, and "school health service," which was defined as "a specialized area of practice concerned with the prevention, identification, observation and management of health problems in the school setting." The academy went on to note that, in communities where large numbers of children do not receive adequate medical care, the school health program may need to include various medical services "until better sources of care are developed." The academy also believed that children who receive regular, personal medical care from a private physician also benefit from a school health program that "emphasizes health education, health promotion, disease prevention, and identification of health problems with psychosocial etiologies."[9]

The views of the American Academy of Pediatrics are helpful in sorting out the two roles of physicians in schools. The prime focus of the school health program is prevention with attention to the health status of the student group, the environment, and the health curriculum. Experienced school physicians[35,36] see the scope of the school health program expanding to encompass the "new morbidity" of school students whose unmet health needs include "dental, emotional and learning problems, making decisions about sexual behavior, problems associated with alcohol and drug use, and coping with chronic handicapping conditions." It is seen that the physician in the school health program, needing to become conversant with such other fields of school health as "sports medicine, health education, cognitive perceptual difficulties, nutrition, physical education, handicap education, behavioral dysfunctions, speech problems," will require "review, updating, and refinement of previous knowledge and acquisition of *new* knowledge in other school health disciplines."[8] Lampe discussed the importance of the mental health area by referring to the leading problem seen by schools as "emotionally disturbed children," to the incidence of drug abuse, and to the fact that "more adolescents die each year from suicide than from heart disease, or contagious disease, or malignancies" and then noted that "most school physicians are not specifically trained for work in mental health."[36]

The Academy of Pediatrics' views of the two types of health services needed by schoolchildren provided a point of departure for different views regarding the relationship between the two types of services and who should direct the second, or preventive service.

Nader and his colleagues in Galveston stressed the need for "primary medical care."[37–39] The major role for schools becomes that of a channel through which children flow to primary-care providers, who in addition deliver the preventive services that were described by the Academy of Pediatrics under the rubric of the school health program. Nader wrote: "By bridging the health care system and the educational system, school health could hold the potential for facilitating family involvement in programs aimed at the promotion of the health of family members. School health might then become the link to successful preventive medicine as practiced by primary health-care deliverers."[37] This view requires one to believe that (1) because primary-care physicians provide some preventive services, they should provide all; (2) those who provide preventive services to individuals possess the skills to provide services to groups.

An analogy may be drawn to the automobile. Automobiles, like people, enter this world with obsolescence built in. They require primary-care providers—neighborhood mechanics—to fix the constant run of minor problems, provide major care or surgery from time to time, and provide a limited amount of preventive attention to meet safety (inspection) and manufacturer's requirements and also promote longevity (oil change and car maintenance schedule). It would be pressing the preventive abilities of primary-care mechanics beyond their capabilities to insist that (1) without training they should care for all household appliances or (2) they should be able to prevent the nation's highway accidents.

In a completely different approach to schoolchildren without sources of primary care, Porter and his colleagues in Cambridge, Massachusetts, established, in schools, primary-care neighborhood health centers staffed by pediatric nurse practitioners and available to all children from birth to sixteen years of age.[40] Silver melded the efforts of Nader and Porter by developing the school nurse practitioner role: (1) to provide primary care in the schools to those needing it, and (2) to provide the preventive services of the school health program, in which role Silver saw the nurse as being best equipped. Silver wrote that the task of the nurse practitioner's primary care in the schools is to:

> "offer comprehensive well-child care" and to "identify and assess the factors that may operate to produce learning disorders, psychoeducational problems, perceptive-cognitive difficulties, and behavior problems as well as those causing physical disease." The school will serve as a principal setting for comprehensive primary and continuing health care and services since it is " the one place where children between the ages of 5 and 18 years are regularly and readily accessible."[41]

The second matter—the direction of preventive school health services—involves

> attention to nutritional needs . . . health education, sex education, family life education, and psychological guidance . . . environmental responsibilities, such as safety measures, sanitation, and sports . . . *little of this is the doctor's role.* Nurses trained and educated in school health needs, with strong organizational support from the departments of health and education, in-service training programs to maintain morale, and a bit of medical [physician] consultation, can probably manage school health programs (emphasis added).[12]

The American Academy of Pediatrics, not surprisingly, saw a physician as director of the school health program. The reason as stated: "The physician sets the 'tone' or 'quality' of services for the school child."[9] Such a tone may not be worth four times the expense of a school nurse or school nurse practitioner.

Others took issue with the assumption of preventive school health roles by primary-care pediatricians outside the school, noting that physicians are trained to deal with disease and not with the "normalcy" of the school population, that they tend to see the child and not the circumstances of the child's condition as the problem, that in busy practices the personal preventive care of "interactional investigation and anticipatory care" is given by nurses, that physicians can see the school behavior of problem children more clearly in the classroom, that teachers are fine observers of anatomy and physiology, that therapy can be better tailored to the child in school if the physician knows the school, that schools are excellent foci for data systems and are more appropriately placed in communities than doctors' offices. In short, "primary care professionals have the clear responsibility to redefine their role relative to the school. The school *is* the responsible treatment agent and other resource people will be helpful to children and the school to the degree that their input is seen as being consistent with what schools and society see as important for all children."[42]

A view of the changes that are overtaking school health and requiring responses of both the professions of medicine and nursing came from an official English committee on child health services. It saw the health problems of schoolchildren as requiring medical and nursing professions equipped with new knowledge and skills. It described each school as needing an identified school doctor and school nurse who have expertise in educational medicine and educational nursing. Educational medicine was defined as:

> the study and practice of child health and pediatrics in relation to the process of learning. It requires an understanding of child development, the educational environment, the child's response to school, the disorders which interfere with a child's capacity to learn, and the special needs of the handicapped. Its practitioners need to work cooperatively with the teachers, psychologists and others who may be involved with the child and to understand the influences of the family and social environment.[43]

Chapter 2

HISTORY OF SCHOOL HEALTH SERVICES

It is bad enough to be ignorant, for this cuts one off from the commerce of minds. It is perhaps worse to be poor, for this condemns to a life of stint and scheming in which there is no time for dreams and no respite from weariness. But what is surely worst is to be unwell, for then one can do little about either poverty or ignorance.

—G. H. T. Kimble *

Guided by the belief that knowledge of the past will illuminate the confused present and help in planning the future, I have been disappointed to find little or nothing written on the history of school health services.[1] Such a situation also means that there are few references and hardly one indicating a basic source. Although this state of affairs supports the characterization of school health services as Cinderella, it places the nonhistorian in a difficult situation: on the one hand, wanting to provide some awareness of the history of the subject,

*Paraphrase of quote attributed to G. H. T. Kimble, Department of Health, Commonwealth of Pennsylvania, "Policy Planning for Public Health," Report No. 1, Policy Planning Council to the Deputy Secretary for Public Health Programs, January, 1976.

while on the other hand, knowing that the effort would be at best limited and at worst erroneous. It is obvious from these pages that I have opted for the first course. I shall give my sources and attempt to indicate the information they contain. I fully realize the limitations that attend this exercise, particularly as, in the absence of scholarly research, I am forced to rely on sometimes unreliable sources who have written their own interpretation into the events they describe.

I quite openly admit that I have, from my reading, formed firm notions of the history of this period. I offer in this chapter an interpretive essay that provides some possible explanations of the past, present, and future states of school health services. All I can hope is that, although no readers will accept my conclusions without questioning, all will be stimulated to question, and possibly the historian this field lacks will see the beacon of obvious need and move towards it.

School health services were a modern development, coming into being around the end of the nineteenth century to the beginning of the twentieth century in Western Europe and the United States. The need for school health services derived from the Industrial Revolution and the social changes it wrought, including the drive for compulsory public education for all children and public health efforts to render the environment less hazardous. These two streams of nineteenth-century change contributed to the development of school health services: the public health movement defining the content of the service and the public education movement defining the population to be served.

The obvious importance of the school in defining the population group served by school health may be seen by comparing two classics in the historical development of occupational medicine: Ramazzini, in his *Diseases of Workers* (1713), did not mention school or students,[2] whereas Thackrah, in his book of 1832 on the effects of arts, trades, and professions on health, devoted a section to "schools, a subject not inferior in importance to any [occupation] which has been discussed."[3]

What follows is a brief history of the early development of school health services in England serving as a prelude to a discussion of events in the United States. England has been selected for a number of reasons: The Industrial Revolution in England, in the years 1750 to 1850, preceded that in the United States, which did not gain momentum until after the Civil War and then followed the English model;[4] developments in England are somewhat easier to follow, not involving the United States' complications of Civil War, immigration, westward expansion, and the variations among states and regions; English solutions to problems, particularly in health matters, provided the models for the United States. There is, for example, no doubt that the landmark "Shattuck Report," which in 1849 outlined the first general public health plan in the United States, "was based in large part on contemporary work by British pioneers in modern public health."[5]

THE INDUSTRIAL REVOLUTION

The remarkable episode called the Industrial Revolution changed the relative simplicity of a scattered agricultural society into the complexity of densely urbanized masses operating industrialized, technological processes. The effects on the physical landscape were easily seen: the devastating mortality of disease epidemics sweeping through the masses gathered in unhygienic cities "created the conditions which made the consideration of public health a major necessity";[6] more gradually were the effects upon individuals and families noted as formerly agricultural folk separated from their diverse rural resources became absolutely dependent upon employers for their wages, which, in cities, were their only means to obtain food and housing. The rapacious behavior of those who owned factories and mines, in demanding long hours of labor for menial wages and keeping adults out of work by employing children for lesser wages, does not need to be retold here except to note:

> While children were employed, male unemployment was high. In the English cotton industry in 1835, only 26 percent of the employees were men whereas 13 percent were children aged thirteen to eighteen.[7]
>
> The working conditions of children moved humane observers. Villermé, a member of the Académié de Médicine and a great student of the conditions of workers in France during the Industrial Revolution, gave the following account: "Among them are large numbers of women, pale, starving, wading barefoot through the mud . . . and young children, in greater numbers than the women, just as dirty, just as haggard, covered in rags, which are thick with the oil splashed over them as they toiled by the looms."[8]
>
> It was hard to educate children who worked. In addition, there were instances, in Philadelphia for example, where parents wished to withdraw children from employment for a short period to attend school but were threatened with dismissal of the whole family from employment.[9]

The drive for compulsory public education was led by those who wished to see children out of the work force and those who wished to see children educated. Among the former were humanitarians who believed that children were not benefitted by exposure to mines and factories and degradingly long hours of labor and those who saw abolition of child labor as the main solution to male unemployment. Advocates of education ranged from those who believed that it provided means for personal satisfaction and for a citizenry better able to participate in civic affairs to those who believed that the new industrial era required workers who could read instructions and perform simple calculations. The Industrial Revolution thus demanded that society take action to preserve itself and protect its citizens; and, moved by pressures that in varying degrees were selfish, utilitarian, and humanitarian, social leaders focused primarily on development of the administrative, organizational, and institutional capacities necessary to carry out the new activities and functions of the state.[10]

ENGLAND

Compulsory Education

The nineteenth century, which saw in England establishment of compulsory public education, opened with the few children of the well-to-do obtaining a lengthy education, some children briefly obtaining the rudiments in a church school, others working, and many roaming the streets. Young noted that the success of the British and Foreign School Society (which advocated study of the Bible) and the National Society for Promoting the Education of the Poor in the Principles of the Established Church in diffusing elementary education "was admitted, and the first intervention of the State in the education of the people took the shape of a grant in aid, in 1833, for school-building; of £11,000 to the National Society and £9,000 to the British and Foreign."[11]

The first Factory Act of 1833 forbade night work by children, prohibited employment of children under nine years of age, restricted work hours to 9 each day for those under eleven years of age and to 12 each day for children aged eleven to eighteen, and required those who worked to attend factory schools for at least two hours each day until the age of thirteen.[12] It can be seen that the act was also an education act, although "a very imperfect one, since for the purposes of the Act any cellar might be returned as a school and any decayed peddlar as a schoolmaster."[11] In the history of education and child welfare, the act was important for another reason: it began to limit child labor, a process that continued until the Education Act of 1879, which brought all children of elementary age into the school building from work, home, or street. Not all work performed by children was in factories: in 1840 chimney-sweeping children were brought under public protection, and in 1843, the reports of the Special Assistant Poor Law Commissioners on the Employment of Women and Children in Agriculture noted that agricultural work employed "organized gangs of children working under gang-masters who arranged for their employment, which sometimes meant long journeys to and from work, and much immorality. The children [some only six years old] could be harshly treated . . . some gang-masters made [the children] do short work, and then refused them payment."[12] The lives of these children were com- pletely changed by the law requiring compulsory school attendance.

The meager allowance provided to the two voluntary educational societies by the Factory Act of 1833 was renewed annually. "To distri- bute this pittance, an educational committee of the Privy Council was set up, with a permanent Secretary and a system of inspection of the State-aided schools. Such was the humble origin of the present Minis- try of Education."[10] Government inspection as a condition of a govern- ment grant was established as a principle. Yet, the educational task facing England in the early Nineteenth Century was enormous:

> A survey of elementary education in the thirties revealed to
> thoughtful contemporaries a profoundly disquieting picture.
> School-buildings were rarely good, often indifferent, sometimes
> thoroughly bad. The same might be said of the teachers. The
> average school-life was perhaps two years, perhaps eighteen
> months. The Society Schools, which represented the best practice
> of the time, were helped out by Sunday Schools which also gave a
> little instruction in reading and writing, sometimes in arithmetic,
> and by a mob of private ventures . . . In Liverpool less than half the
> child population under fifteen went to school at all, and the other
> half did not miss much. . . . It was much if the victims could write
> their names. From the marriage registers it would appear that in
> the thirties about one-third of the men and two-thirds of the
> women could not.[11]

Such ignorance was both frightening and useless to a country in which voting rights were being extended and cheap newspapers were becoming available. The problem lay in finding appropriate adminis- trative machinery for the task. The county, with its ancient functions of justice and highways, was not considered, and the only other link between central government and the people was the Poor Law Union. In 1843 the Radicals proposed dividing the country into school dis- tricts, levying an education tax, maintaining infant and elementary schools and training colleges for teachers, and making education com- pulsory. These proposals eventually found expression in the Educa- tion Act of 1870 but not before enormous sectarian controversy over the role of religious instruction took place. "No party would have dared to turn the Bible out of the schools, and no two parties could agree as to the terms upon which it should be admitted." Initially the government relied upon the voluntary schools. As voluntary teacher training colleges were established in the 1840's, the government encouraged them through additional pay for teachers who had been awarded a certificate upon completion of apprenticeship and training-college course requirements.[11]

Finally the Education Act of 1870 was passed.

> It doubled the State grant to the existing Church schools and to the Roman Catholic schools so as to enable them to become a permanent part of the new system, while it introduced publicly controlled schools to fill up the large gaps in the educational map of the country. These new schools, called Board Schools, were to be paid for out of the local rates, and they were to be governed by popularly elected school boards. . . . the Act prohibited the use, in the religious teaching, of catechism or formulary distinctive of any denomination.[10]

> The Education Act of 1870 was, for most English people, the first sensible impact of the administrative state on their lives . . . the School Board Man, the Attendance Officer . . . the School Board Elections . . . gave a novel interest in local government: to a smaller circle of women as well as men, their first experience of administration. Nor, in any history of the Victorian age, should the school-builders be forgotten. Those solid, large-windowed blocks, which still rise everywhere above the slate roofs of mean suburbs, meant for hundreds of thousands their first glimpse of a life of cleanliness and order, light and air.[11]

The Act of 1870 was concerned only with elementary education and did nothing for secondary or higher education. Another defect was the smallness of the school board areas; encompassing the affairs of a single town or village, they could have no broader educational outlook. These defects were remedied by the Education Act of 1902, which abolished the 2,500 school boards and replaced them by 328 elected county councils and borough councils. These worked under a central board of education, created in 1899, and provided primary and secondary education and a route to the universities. A unified system, based on local government, was achieved.[10,6]

Public Health

The concept of public health also made its appearance during the nineteenth century in England. The essence of public health lies in the belief that diseases have causes and, therefore, if the causes can be controlled, diseases can be prevented. The focus of public health is the population group. Clinical medicine is different from public health in that, to a large extent, efforts are directed to return the sick individual to health; the focus limits preventive action to that which can be accomplished by or for the individual. Public health will seek any methods necessary to control disease, particularly the power of government. Public health requires two items in order to function: first, it must have the means to measure the health and disease levels of the population (vital statistics) and to manipulate and study these data in order to show which factors associated with the disease are possible causes (epidemiology), and second, it must have an organizational structure or social machinery that will allow it to control the revealed causes of disease. (An example: Statistics on deaths and injuries occurring in motor vehicle accidents show strong associations between death and lack of seat belts and also between certain chest injuries and solid steering columns; the social machinery exists to enforce the provision, in cars, of collapsible steering columns and seat belts. The same data that describe the problems record that deaths and chest injuries decline following the institution of these preventive measures.) The nineteenth century was marked by development of the concept of public health, development and use of vital statistics, and evolution of the necessary governmental administrative machinery.

Johann Peter Frank (1754–1821), writing in Austria, saw the concept of public health quite clearly:

> I perceive that doctors are seldom able to obviate those causes of disease which either act in bulk upon the general population or operate independently of the will of individuals (however careful they may be). Yet assuredly many of these causes could be obviated by systematic action on the part of the authorities . . . the topic . . . would certainly be *medical*, and, . . . the carrying into effect of measures likely to promote the general health left to a country's . . . public executive authorities and administrative measures of various kinds.[13]

Frank's concept of public health may not have been known in England, but that country's public health pioneers were developing the statistical, epidemiologic, and administrative methodologies to prevail against the devastating mortalities in many of the country's localities. It was these episodes of disease, which were like mass slaughter in urban areas, which stimulated the interest of medical people in community health matters. John Graunt and William Petty in the seventeenth century, using the parish bills of mortality, had shown that towns suffered higher mortalities than the surrounding country. This difference, now multiplied and exaggerated, began to command attention everywhere.[6]

The ability to look at the health status of the country through collections of statistics on birth, and on causes of death, illness, or morbidity developed from the first census, in 1801, to the 1836 act for "the registration of births, marriages and deaths in England and Wales." Dr. William Farr, the first compiler of statistics in the Registrar General's office, said, in his first report to the Registrar General, dated May 6, 1839, "The registration of causes of death, besides contributing to practical medicine, will give greater precision to the principles of physic. Medicine, like the other natural sciences, is beginning to abandon vague conjecture where facts can be accurately determined by observation; and to substitute numerical expressions for uncertain assertions." Brockington has noted that "The accurate information of . . . mortality figures, no longer the subject of 'vague conjecture,' had profound effect upon [the] leaders of those days, as they were used to the greatest advantage by social . . . reformers."[6]

One was Edwin Chadwick, the father of public health in Britain, who, beginning with an interest in the poor and the poor laws, began to see that "pauperism was the result of ill-health and if the cause were treated, in the long run, money would be saved. He thus changed his ground gradually from an interest in the poor law to an emphasis on preventive medicine." Having secured the appointment of medical inspectors to guide the work of the poor law commissions, Chadwick used their reports of medical conditions in their areas to compile one of the great social surveys undertaken in Britain. *The Sanitary Conditions of the Working Population of Great Britain* was published in 1842. "The account addresses itself precisely throughout to the enormous possibilities of the prevention of disease and the high cost of its presence."[6]

Studies and reports followed throughout the nineteenth century. The nonegalitarian, nonrandom distribution of disease in society having been quantitatively demonstrated, and the apparent causal relationship between disease and certain conditions in the environment, such as unsanitary housing, having been demonstrated to general satisfaction, the problem became one of instituting social action to ameliorate the causes of disease. By 1843 it was generally recognized that legislation was needed;[6] what was lacking was an administrative base. This was only partially supplied by the Public Health Act of 1848, which created a central board of health with power to create local boards.

The act proved cumbersome and virtually unworkable. It did, however, provide opportunities for local initiative and scientific investigation to show that filth and horror could be controlled. As Young wrote: "Perhaps the first step towards dealing effectively with slums was to recognize them as slums and not as normal phenomena of urban existence."[11] Effective public health had to await the administrative machinery provided by the Local Government Acts, beginning in 1871, through which elected county councils and county borough councils provided local services under central enabling legislation, authority, and standards. It was this structure that made the great Public Health Act of 1875 operational; the act stipulated the sanitary code under which local medical officers of health and sanitary inspectors were to work so effectively in rendering hygienic water, air, food, housing, cemeteries, slaughterhouses, waste disposal, ports, institutions, schools—in fact, the whole environment in their local jurisdiction.

It was the same Local Government Acts that enabled education to be changed, in 1902, from an operation of local school boards to one based in the elected county and county borough councils. It is worth noting that, although education was well served by the local school boards, public health was but little advanced by local health boards. The major reason for the difference lies in the nature of the two enterprises: a society that decides on education as a course to follow uses the local school board as a tool for implemention and administration. A society that desires public health and sets up local health boards to accomplish that goal is asking for something far different: the board, whether elected or appointed, with or without paid professional staff, must, in order to practice public health, collect statistics on the state of health of the local population, determine where the causes of health problems reside, and then proceed to prevent the causes. More than likely the causes of disease are connected with other human beings, whose economic or other self-interests are contained in the offending disease sources; they may be the owner of an unhygienic slaughterhouse, the stockholder of a mill discharging toxic wastes into a town's water supply, the landlord of substandard housing, or the administrator of a filthy institution. A local board acting to enforce its own view of health is no match for the powers it is forced to oppose. Power for the task is granted by laws that, for example, transform the sale of contaminated milk from an unethical business practice, disapproved by the local board of health, to an illegal act against which the local health department, as the administrator of the public health law, is required to act.

Before considering the joining of compulsory education and public health to form school health, the development of the nursing profession, also important in the evolution of the concept of school health services, needs to be mentioned.

The Nursing Profession

The development of the nursing profession ran parallel to that of education and public health. The first training school for nurses was opened in 1836 by a German clergyman, Theodor Fliedner, in Kaiserworth on the Rhine. Inspired by this venture and following her experiences in the Crimean War (1854–1856), Florence Nightingale founded the first professional nursing school at St. Thomas' Hospital in London in 1860. From these beginnings sprang, in England, hospital nurses, district nurses who provided care for the sick in their own homes, and health visitors who advised mothers especially on measures to prevent illness. The last two roles were sometimes combined in other countries as "public health nurses."

In 1861 Florence Nightingale was asked by William Rathbone, a wealthy Liverpool merchant, for assistance in an embryonic operation to provide trained nurses to care for the sick poor in their own homes. A Training School and Home for Nurses was established in connection with the Royal Liverpool Infirmary.[5,14] Later Rathbone discovered the desperate plight of the sick paupers in the Liverpool workhouse, who were cared for by able-bodied paupers by day and locked up at night. In 1864 Rathbone asked Nightingale to send nurses. Permission was not granted until 1865; in the long battle, Nightingale wrote, "there had been as much diplomacy and as many treaties and as much of people working against each other, as if we had been going to occupy a Kingdom instead of a Workhouse."[14]

At this point it would be well to stop and consider something of the nature of nursing—partly because today the essence of this profession seems to be difficult for others to grasp[15] and partly because there is a need to know what the leaders of the profession were thinking in the latter half of the nineteenth century, as nursing became indispensible in the health care of the sick and the well.

Florence Nightingale opened her 1859 classic, *Notes on Nursing: What It Is and What It Is Not,* with these words:

> Shall we begin by taking it as a general principle—that all disease, at some period or other of its course, is more or less a reparative process, not necessarily accompanied with suffering: an effort of nature to remedy. . . .In watching disease, both in private houses and in public hospitals, the thing which strikes the experienced observer most forcibly is this, that the symptoms or the sufferings generally considered to be inevitable and incident to the disease are very often not symptoms of the disease at all, but of something quite different. . . . If a patient is cold, if a patient is feverish, if a patient is faint, if he is sick after taking food, if he has a bed sore, it is generally the fault not of the disease, but of the nursing.

I use the word nursing for want of a better. It has been limited to signify little more than the administration of medicine and the application of poultices. It ought to signify the proper use of fresh air, light, warmth, cleanliness, quiet, and the proper selection and administration of diet—all at least expense of vital power to the patient.[16]

Nightingale went on to describe a nurse as "any person in charge of the personal health of another." The skills required by assuming charge of another's health included knowledge of normal physiology, knowledge of pathological processes and the special physiologic needs produced by diseases, and the skills necessary to organize the environment around the patient so as to best serve the patient's physiological needs. Nightingale's genius saw that skilled nursing could encompass the personal health of the well in addition to assisting repair of the personal health of the sick. "The same laws of health or of nursing, for they are in reality the same, obtain among the well as among the sick."[16]

The preventive role of nursing in maintaining the health of the well, so clearly seen by Nightingale, was also apparent to others. Thomas Turner, surgeon to the Manchester Royal Infirmary, distressed by the continuous flow of wasted and fatally ill babies in his wards, had been the prime mover, in 1852, in the first home-visiting scheme to teach mothers the elements of child care.[6]

Nightingale recognized that such home health nursing required "different but not lower qualifications" than hospital nursing and set up the first special training program in 1892. By the end of the century the graduates were increasingly in evidence. They were particularly found in the new well-baby or infant welfare centers that, modeled upon the *goutte du lait* established by Budin in Paris in 1892, from 1898 in Britain developed quickly into consultation centers where the new health visitors gave advice and education on infant management to mothers.[17] These infant welfare centers became

one of the most effective forms of social service in Britain. . . . So deep and significant was the need which it met that within a few years it had extended throughout the whole country . . . and gathered together for advice and group discussions nearly three-quarters of the total population at risk. The infant welfare centre absorbed the "schools of mothercraft" . . . begun . . . in 1907; and also the special arrangements for feeding mothers of which the pioneer venture took place . . . in 1901. The infant welfare centre itself was later merged into the maternity and child welfare centre as the ideas of hygiene in pregnancy and infancy extended both to the mother and the toddler.[6]

The new work of the nurse gained ground rapidly. In 1903, speaking of the work of the first full-time health visitors in his county of Warwickshire, Dr. Bostock Hill said:

> The most memorable step taken by the County Councils to guard public health was undoubtedly the appointment of a health visitor during the year . . . she found ample field for her work. She was able to give advice in a very large number of instances as to the proper feeding of infants. . . . Her functions are those of a friend of the household to which she gains access. . . . In this new departure of carrying sanitation into the home, I believe we have not only an important, but almost the only means of further improving the health of the people. (Annual Report of County Medical Officer).[17]

School Health

By the latter half of the nineteenth century, school hygiene was not an entirely new idea. In 1783 in France, the suggestion had been made to the National Convention that a district health officer be entrusted with visiting schools to examine children and lay down rules for safeguarding their health. Chadwick, in 1861, said that a special sanitary service for schools was needed for correction of common evils of school construction and protection of the health of the children.

It seems clear that the emphasis in these early suggestions was on school sanitation and the general effect of the school environment—buildings and practices—on the health of students. Such is hardly unexpected in an age of gross lack of sanitation in all aspects of life, including the not-yet-public schools. Thackrah, in his occupational health classic of 1832, described how a highly aware physician would approach the performance of school health duties. He noted that the following would be among the concerns of the physician: overcrowding, ventilation, heating, fixed posture, lack of exercise; in boarding schools, diet, clothing, sleeping quarters; the spread of contagious diseases among crowded inmates, the lack of muscular exertion for girls, the release of nervous energy, the early detection of symptoms and the prevention of disease, and the special needs of the chronically ill.[3]

As schooling increased in extent during the nineteenth century and particularly after compulsory education brought all children into schools, it became apparent that the health status of many children was poor. Charles Booth had referred to the "puny, pale-faced, scantily clad and barely shod [children] sitting limp and still at the school benches in all the poorer parts of London,"[18] and Margaret MacMillan had talked of those in Bradford [in 1894]: "Children in every stage of illness, children with adenoids, children with curvature, children in every stage of neglect, dirt and suffering. The condition of the poor children was worse than anything described or painted; the half-timers slept exhausted at their desks and from the courts and alleys children attended school in all stages of physical misery."[19] Thirty years after the inauguration of a general system of education, people were asking, "What was the good if scholars were physically unfit to benefit?"[17]

Enlightened but sporadic efforts were made during that latter half of the nineteenth century to establish health services in schools. "Physicians were placed on public school staffs in Sweden in 1868, Germany in 1869, Russia in 1871, and Austria in 1873. In Brussels, Belgium, the first organized, regular medical inspection system was instituted in 1874. Every three months all schools were inspected by a physician."[20] "Paris developed a school medical service between 1879 and 1883. Frankfurt-on-the-Main appointed a school doctor in 1883, the London School Board in 1891 and that of Bradford . . . in 1893."[6]

A pragmatic need for a health service was introduced by the 1870 Education Act, which brought together all children, including the blind, deaf, handicapped, retarded, and sickly. Arrangements had to be made for the special health and educational needs of these groups. By 1893 local education authorities were given power "to establish schools for the blind and deaf and . . . [in] 1899 similar powers for epileptic children, cripples, and what were then known as feeble-minded."[6] Obviously, medical inspection of school students was needed in order to place them in appropriate diagnostic categories preparatory to assignment to special education.

In 1907, England surging beyond the phase of sporadic attempts by a few towns and established a complete school medical service for all elementary schools in England and Wales. The impetus for this remarkable event was the public outcry that followed the findings that a large proportion of the recruits in the Boer War (1898–1901) were physically unfit. The report of the Duke of Devonshire's Committee on Physical Deterioration (1904) and a further Committee of Medical Inspection and Feeding of Children in 1905, with the background of the Royal Commission on Physical Training (Scotland) of 1903, left no doubt about the need for a service to safeguard the health of the schoolchild.[6]

It should be noted that the Education (Administrative Provisions) Act of 1907 was a bold administrative stroke that implemented what was regarded as an exploratory program of school medical services. The act required every educational authority to appoint school doctors and nurses and a principal county school medical officer (usually the

county public health officer) responsible for running the service locally. The service began with simple objectives: to find out the nature and
extent of what was amiss.[6,17] It was fundamentally a service of inspection "regarded as a means to arrive at accurate information about the
state of school children's health." The board of education circular that
set out guiding principles for the local education authorities said:
"Medical inspection of school children is not only reasonable but necessary as a first practical step towards remedy. Without such inspection
we not only *lack data* but we fail to *begin at the beginning* in any measure
of reform" (emphasis added).[6] In the face of the obvious health needs
of schoolchildren and their families, and in light of the rapid rise of the
nursing profession and its profoundly recognized success, there is little
surprise that nurses were appointed to the school health service when it
was established in 1907. Nurses' skills would enable them to advise
school staff on the environment necessary both to maintain the health
of students and to improve the health and function of the sickly and
handicapped; to have charge of the personal health of students and
therefore advise on personal preventive measures, observe for deviations from normal, and ensure the taking of necessary remedial action;
to provide health advice to students and parents to prevent illness and
remedy disease; to provide health visiting and teaching to those
mothers and families in the community with the greatest need by
identifying the most needy school students—made easy by the captive
nature of the school population.

The school medical service expanded slowly. The school doctor
extended his interest to the whole environment of the school; collaboration with teachers developed; minor ailments were treated in
clinics; the school nurse, increasingly also the health visitor of the area,
pursued her inquiries to the home; parents, present more frequently at
school inspections, were helped to appreciate their responsibilities;
health education in schools began. In 1918 a further act required
educational authorities to provide treatment for (in addition to minor
ailments) defects of the eyes and teeth and chronic tonsillitis and
adenoid disease. Open-air schools for delicate children appeared in
many parts of the country, and special clinics were established for
crippled children.[6]

THE UNITED STATES—EARLY DEVELOPMENTS

The history of the Industrial Revolution and the subsequent
drives to restrict child labor, enforce education, and practice public
health in the United States occurred with similar content to that in

England but with at least fifty different twists. The search for organizational structures for the more complex tasks of an industrial society involved not only awakening states to the use of their sovereign powers but also invoking for the federal government constitutional authorities never before considered.

Child Labor

The census of 1860 showed that about one-sixth of the population was directly supported by manufacturing. Adding to this number all persons engaged in production of raw materials for manufacturing and in distribution of manufactured goods, the census reporters declared, "It is safe to assume, then, that one third of the whole population is supported, directly or indirectly, by manufacturing."[21]

Industrialization received new impetus in the North during the Civil War and began in the South after that conflict. The most significant trend after the war until 1910 was the advance of industry to first place in employment of labor and capital.[22] Meanwhile, the population grew from 31 million in 1860 to 76 million in 1900.[23]

Control of child labor began just after the first English restrictions, expressed in the 1833 Factory Act. State laws that were passed were due to the efforts of reformers who sought the education of working children rather than their protection from industrial hazards and exploitation.[24] Such a law was that of New York, which in 1849 specified that "no child shall be employed in any factory or workshop who shall not have attained the age of 10 years and be able to read and write."[25] Compulsory education of all children in primary subjects was increasingly passed into state law after 1860,[21] and gradually the requirement to be educated was matched by free or state-supported schools for all, after Michigan led the way in 1869[24] and the bitter disputes over religious control and content were worked out in other states.[26] Compulsory education laws competed with industrial employment for the child's time and were, together with child labor laws, one of the factors in the gradual rescue of American children from industry, often against the wishes of parents and the desires of employers.

How well or poorly, the laws performed for children could be measured in the statistics produced—in response to the demands of reformers—by state labor bureaus created after 1869 and by special census questions.[21] The nationwide extent of child labor was seen in the 1870 census, which showed 1 in 8 ten-to-fifteen-year-olds gainfully employed. By 1900 the proportion was 1 in 6: 60 percent in agriculture and 40 percent in industry; half were children of immigrant families.

Such a situation existed because by 1899 only 28 states had passed some legislation regulating child labor. Most laws applied only to manufacturing and set the minimum age at twelve. Truant officers, established to enforce state compulsory education laws, found great resistance to school attendance, particularly among immigrant families, because adult wages were low and the children's salaries were needed. Parents and employers often flagrantly ignored child labor and school attendance laws. In 1903 New York required working children to have certificates attesting to their legal age and good health; children under fourteen were not permitted to work during school hours.

In 1877 organized labor condemned child labor. A coalition of organizations founded the National Child Labor Committee in 1904. It devoted its activities to reform in the individual states, aiming at a minimum age of fourteen in manufacturing and sixteen in mining, documentary proof of age, a maximum 8-hour workday, and prohibition of night work. By 1914 each of these separate provisions was met by less than 75 percent of states and there were grave loopholes: agriculture, domestic service, and street trades were not covered; canneries obtained exclusion; children of widows and poor parents were exempt. The latter was particularly important in Southern states that attracted Northern cotton mills with their cheap labor and resisted both anti-child labor and compulsory school attendance laws. Mississippi was the last state to enact a compulsory education law, in 1918. It became clear that federal legislation was the best way to prevent "this contest in callousness among states."[27] But a heartbreaking struggle ensued.

The federal Keating-Owen Act prohibiting child labor was passed in 1916 but declared unconstitutional in 1918. A 1919 law imposing a federal surtax on employers of child labor was declared unconstitutional in 1922. The drive for a constitutional amendment began with congressional approval in 1924, but it was clear by 1925 that the amendment, opposed by powerful manufacturing and certain church forces, could not pass. Of the 28 states ratifying it before it was dropped in 1938, none was in Dixie proper. Finally the Fair Labor Standards Act of 1938 provided most of what the Child Labor Amendment of 1924 sought by barring the products of industrial child labor from interstate commerce.[27]

Compulsory Education

It was in this turbulent, changing, exploitative and also humane flood of events that compulsory education was born. By 1900, except in the South, compulsory elementary education was taken for granted. State laws established the local school board as the implementing, administering agency (whether based on a school district or county or township entity), provided for taxation by the board, fixed years for attendance and the number of weeks of schooling per year, established teacher-training schools, set qualifications for certification of teachers and other staff, set standards for buildings and minimal essentials of the curriculum, and instituted truant officers and licensing of private schools as means for ensuring compliance.[21]

The South lagged behind. Negro schools barely held on to the brief beginnings of Reconstruction.[27]

Local school boards operating as separate corporations often were created in the absence of any local government organization in the cities or towns in which they existed. Such school board structures, it is claimed, have preserved education from local politics. The school boards operate under the detailed specifications of the state constitution, state laws, school codes passed by the legislature, state court decisions, the regulations of the state board of education, and policies and directives of the state department of education.[26]

State financial support to education has been used to help equalize funds among school districts of the state. Federal financial support has more recently helped equalize resources among rich and poor states while also directing assistance to special groups: the first federal funds given to states for education were granted in 1917 for vocational education in secondary schools; school lunches for public and nonpublic schools were provided as an emergency measure in the Depression and made permanent in 1946; and in later years federal funds under the Elementary and Secondary Education Act (ESEA) of 1965 and the Right to Education for the Handicapped (P.L. 94-142) of 1975 have had a profound effect upon the quality and extent of education.[26]

A U.S. Office of Education was established in 1867. In 1939 it was moved from the Department of the Interior to the Federal Security Agency and in 1956 to the Department of Health, Education, and Welfare. In 1979 a cabinet-level Department of Education was created, fulfilling a proposal first made in the 1920's and demonstrating both the growth of the educational enterprise and the political influence of its practitioners.

Public Health

The Industrial Revolution found the United States without any organized structures for meeting public health needs. Large port cities, which periodically faced epidemics apparently brought into the country, had learned of quarantine and would practice it, as necessary, with temporary health committees or boards of health.[25] Permanent boards of health were established in a few large cities from 1793 and gradually became departments with some staff from 5 to 75 years later.[28] Without enabling legislation their scope of activity was severely limited.

With growing industrialization, immigration, and urbanization after 1830, waves of epidemics struck the population, in towns in particular, as in England and on the Continent. The American Medical Association (AMA) noted that "the United States may be considered as a country in which no legislation exists regarding its sanitary condition."[25] A strong movement emerged for establishment of local, state, and national sanitary and preventive health institutions.[22,29] The movement was aided by special reports on sanitary conditions, for example, that on 12 cities by the Committee on Sanitary Improvement of the AMA in 1848 and the sanitary survey of the whole state of Massachusetts conducted by Lemuel Shattuck in 1849. Shattuck wrote, "It is the duty of the State to extend its guardian care, that those who cannot or will not protect themselves, may nevertheless be protected; and that those who can and desire to do it, may have the means of doing it more easily."[30]

National Quarantine Conventions held between 1857 and 1860 did much to focus attention on urban sanitation, lack of uniformity in quarantine regulations, and the need for state and federal boards of health.[28,29] Action ceased during the Civil War but began immediately after, forced by the needs of an increasingly industrial society. Efforts (1879–1883) to establish a national board of health failed. Attention returned to the state and local levels.

Massachusetts organized the first state board of health, in 1869. Its powers were limited to investigation and advice, its budget small, and its personnel untrained. The board began with efforts to create local boards. Little could be accomplished without the state board itself having authority and funds. Eventually, in the wake of public reaction to failure to control a smallpox epidemic, Boston established an autonomous board of health in 1872. In 1876 the legislature authorized appointment of boards of health in townships with populations over 4,000, where the electorate voted to do so—but with a disappointingly poor response. Gradually the state board, through definition of need and leadership, assumed responsiblities and, in conjunction with appropriate laws, restrained slaughterhouses, prevented stream pollution, and began to regulate housing. After many political difficulties, including the submerging of the board of health in the board of health, lunacy, and charity, 1879–1886, a permanent board and department of health were established in 1886 with greater statutory authority.[31]

State departments of health were gradually established across the country, from California in 1870 to New Mexico in 1919.[28] Many experienced the same birth struggles as Massachusetts and in like manner were frustrated in efforts to develop local public health authorities. Pennsylvania, for example, established a state board of health in 1886 after a serious epidemic of typhoid fever in a town. Many studies were conducted and emergency work in epidemics coordinated, but the board had no legal authority to prevent disease causes. The first sanitary code for the state was drawn up in 1895, and in 1905 a department of health with authority to enforce statutes and promulgate legally binding regulations was created. Still, apart from Philadelphia, which had a health department dating back to colonial times, and a few local health boards, there were no local public health administrative entities in the state. After a critical study by the American Public Health Association in 1948, a law was passed in 1951 permitting establishment of county health departments, supported in part by local taxes following voter approval. In the intervening 29 years four counties of the eligible 66 have accepted the option at referenda.[32]

Public health, like education, struggled for its existence at the state level but was far less successful than education in establishing local structures for operational purposes. School districts were mandated and were given the authority and responsibility to raise their own taxes. By the 1940's most states and cities had public health programs. Rural areas were often dependent on states for all health functions or were poorly served by minimal operations. Poorer states and rural areas were the most lagging.[29] Public health relied upon the willingness of local structures (townships and/or counties, or parishes) to become involved and to find the additional revenue. Little wonder that referenda results were often negative, especially when some level of service was already provided by the state. Where local governmental structures, especially cities, had been forced to act before the advent of state health operations, they were often superb, and indeed the history of public health and of early school health is a history written in large part by the innovation and leadership of city health departments. But all were not good, and those that were good were subject to the demands of politics and, before civil service, to the employment of politically related nonprofessional staff.

Over the years the funding of education has remained primarily a local/state matter with a relatively small federal addition. Public health often has little local money, and now federal funds frequently outweigh those of the state. State education agencies have used their powers and funds to reduce local differences. State health agencies have come to rely on federal funds to provide a minimum set of basic services.

The federal health presence on which states now rely so heavily for public health matters has grown piecemeal and from two different roots: One representing the environmental and communicable disease interests of public health—especially the latter—was founded in the U. S. Public Health Service; the second root—provision of preventive services for vulnerable population groups, especially mothers and children—was based in the U. S. Children's Bureau. Finally the two agencies joined with other health activities of the federal government in the U. S. Department of Health, Education, and Welfare in 1956; the department was reconstituted in 1979 as the U.S. Department of Health and Human Services and a separate Department of Education was formed.

The story in somewhat greater detail is as follows: The U.S. Public Health Service began its life in 1792 as the Marine Hospital Service (MHS) to provide medical care to ill merchant seamen, who were not a particular responsibility of the cities or new states between which they plied their trade. It also provided technical assistance to states in epidemics and matters of quarantine and assisted interstate coordination. With the growth of the science of bacteriology and the rapid discovery of many bacterial causes of disease from 1875 to 1900, the interest of the MHS in infectious, communicable diseases continued and became a world-recognized research venture when in 1901, close to an immigration station, a bacteriology laboratory was established that later became the National Institutes of Health. The MHS was renamed the U.S. Public Health Service in 1912 and was given a mandate for broader areas of health investigation including environmental sanitation. In 1917 it obtained the first federal appropriation for grants to states for public health services, in that case for demonstrations in rural health; in 1918 it made the first federal grants to states for V.D. control. In the depression substantial grants-in-aid for general public health work were made to states, a practice that has continued.[28]

The second source of current federal public health activity is the anti-child labor movement of the turn of the century. One of its leaders, Lillian Wald, suggested a Children's Bureau to Theodore Roosevelt in 1906. It was established in 1912 with a small budget and a mandate to "investigate [and] report."[24] By skillful political work with Congress, excellent studies of infant and maternal mortality, and choice of those forces to whom to report, the bureau exerted enormous influence. In 1919 it organized the second, most successful, White House Conference on Children, and in 1921 grants-in-aid were made available to states for maternal and child health programs, particularly in rural areas (Sheppard-Towner Act). Prior to passage of the act, 32 states had established child hygiene operations. Within 2 years of its passage an additional 15 states developed programs.[28] The work was continued in the Social Security Act of 1935 and in today's appropriations under Title V of that act for maternal and child health (which includes some responsibility for school health services) and crippled children's services.

Since the Second World War the federal government has moved

into many more health areas, including vital statistics, hospital construction, health insurance for the elderly and poor, mental health and mental retardation, drug abuse, child abuse, and health planning.

Nursing

The compulsory education and public health movements occurred later in the United States than in England, but the new nursing profession immediately crossed the Atlantic to appear on the American scene relatively early. It grew with amazing rapidity, quickly moved into community roles of district and public health nursing, and, in touch with developments overseas, was often the focus of innovation in services in this country. Nurses frequently showed public health departments what services for certain groups should be. In particular, well-baby clinics (infant hygiene) and school health are indebted to the energy and expertise of the nurses of that day. The rapid acceptance of such nurses is a tribute to the obvious effectiveness of their work in improving health.

By the time of Florence Nightingale's nursing revolution in England, the United States had a long history, dating back to colonial times, of recognizing the need for community and hospital nursing services but failing to find a successful formula to bring them about. In 1873 the Bellevue Hospital was opened in New York as the first nurses'-training school "to be based definitely on Miss Nightingale's uncompromising doctrine which insisted on the need for full authority for the matron or superintendent of the school who must be a nurse, not a physician or layman."[33] As training schools proliferated, trained nurses were introduced to the work of district and public health nursing. In 1877 the New York City Mission employed trained nurses for the bedside care of the sick poor in their homes. District nurse associations (or visiting nurse societies) were organized in Boston and Philadelphia in 1886.[25,34]

In 1893 Lillian Wald, who had graduated from nursing school only 2 years before, established a nurses' settlement house on Henry Street on the Lower East Side of Manhattan. It became the headquarters of the Henry Street District Nursing Service. Encouraged by the New York City (N.Y.C.) Department of Health, its public health nursing activities grew to include the nation's first school nursing service (1902), first infant hygiene service (1908), and instructive home visiting for tuberculosis (1903).[24] Public health nursing grew rapidly nationally, was adopted by all health departments and the U.S. Public Health Service, and formed in 1912 the National Organization of Public Health Nursing.[28,34]

Nursing was not included in the initial organization of the state department of health in Pennsylvania in 1905. In a matter of months nurses were hired to provide bedside care in an epidemic of typhoid fever. Performing with distinction, they were kept on to provide nursing services in the state tuberculosis clinics. They responded to a continuous stream of disasters and of epidemics of typhoid, smallpox, scarlet fever, diphtheria, and influenza, with some loss of their own lives in the public course of such work. As epidemic work subsided it was the public health nurses who stimulated the department's first involvement in infant hygiene (1917), maternal health (1919), and well-baby clinics (1924).[32,34]

ESTABLISHMENT OF SCHOOL HEALTH SERVICES

Inspection of Schools

The nineteenth-century growth of schooling as an important feature in the lives of many children, culminating in compulsory attendance laws, took place in buildings that were, by many accounts, deficient in matters of sanitation and hygiene. It was this environmental health aspect of schooling that attracted the interest of the newly functioning departments of public health in the cities of the United States.

The first was New York City, which in 1871 appointed Dr. R. J. O'Sullivan as visiting physician to the board of education.[35] His duties were clarified in 1872 to include sanitary supervision of school buildings; "to this task he devoted his entire time during school hours, but apparently his vigorous criticism of the sanitary conditions in the schools aroused opposition. In any case his position was abolished in 1873."[25] A report on school buildings was made by two health inspectors in the *Third Annual Report of the Board of Health of the City of New York* in 1873. They found that a considerable number of buildings used as schoolhouses were old buildings or tenement houses, "reconstructed carelessly for the purpose of school accommodation," with overcrowding, lack of ventilation, and poor lighting; for example, the writers noted, "one of these basement-rooms, with over one hundred children, has only one window, and that opens into a space only eight feet in width, between the school building and a three-story brick building in the rear."[36] Other findings were offensive odors from improperly constructed urinals and privies set too close to the school, lack of traps in slop sinks, with escape of sewer gas into the classroom, lack of water supply, filthy walls and floors, peeling paint, falling plaster, and leaking roofs. The writers were concerned about the fate of the children in a fire. Their concern was shown to be realistic when in 1908, in

Collingwood, Ohio, a school fire killed 174 children and two teachers.[24]

In 1876 the New York Medico-Legal Society published the report of a Special Committee upon School Hygiene. They noted the relationship between overcrowding and the fact that schools were a "fruitful source of the propagation of contagious diseases"; however, they sympathized with school boards that, in obeying the new compulsory attendance laws with incomplete facilities, were forced to overcrowd classrooms before finally refusing admission to "several thousand children . . . owing . . . to insufficient school room."[37]

Considerable interest was generated in this new and increasingly pressing subject in the last decades of the nineteenth century. A symposium on "The Health of Pupils in the Public School" was held in Detroit in 1875 by the American Social Science Association, and an International Congress on Hygiene in Schools was held in Geneva in 1882. These meetings were reported in the literature and to the American Public Health Association.[25]

As state boards and departments of health were founded, they carried out work in the sanitation (Massachusetts, 1878)[38] and medical inspection (Pennsylvania, 1909) of schools. Part of the report by Pennsylvania school medical inspectors reads:

> The number of schools inspected in the Spring of 1909 was 11,094. The number having one or more unsanitary conditions was 10,730 leaving only 364 which could be pronounced in entirely satisfactory condition.
>
> The number inspected in the Autumn was 11,462. Of these 1,405 were found to be in all respects in good condition—showing a decided improvement. It is very evident however that the school directors are far from appreciating what constitutes a sanitary school house or indeed what are the requirements laid down by the school law in so many words, as many of the defective conditions noted are direct violations of its regulations.[39]

Progress in improving the school environment seems to have been made remarkably quickly, forced on the one side by compulsory attendance laws and on the other by the obvious presence of health departments, their inspectors, a growing number of new laws [e.g., the 1895 law requiring all schoolhouses in New York City to have an open-air playground][24] and the frightening specter of school fires, said to be about 100 per year in 1924.[40] A report on the situation in Cleveland in 1915 noted: "Ten years ago there was comparatively little concern about the safety of school buildings. Today the attitude of school officials has changed from indifference to active interest."[41]

Indeed the interest of departments of health in the school environment waned as that of school administrators increased, and the old problems began to disappear in the fine new school structures planned by school architects and built by school boards. That all the old problems did not completely disappear[42] and that there were, and are, other factors in the environment deleterious to health, warranting the continuing interest of departments of health, was not seen at the time. The point will be discussed later.

Inspection of Pupils

The early medical inspectors realized that appalling school buildings were deleterious to the health of children and sites for generation of disease. They also quickly saw that the children themselves were the source of many contagious diseases. The hapless Dr. O'Sullivan read a paper before the New York Academy of Medicine in 1873 in which he introduced the original idea that, in addition to supervision of the general sanitation of school buildings, a system of medical supervision of children should be instituted.[25]

Finally, urged by its chairman, Dr. Samuel Durgin, and threatened by a diphtheria epidemic, the Boston Board of Health established medical inspection of pupils in 1894. Fifty physicians were hired to examine children for early evidence of contagious disease, to exclude them in an attempt to reduce disease spread, and to insist on medical clearance before reentry.[24,25] Twenty years later it was written that prevention of epidemics was "still in the minds of most people the raison d'être of school inspection."[43]

Inspection of pupils was taken up with great fervor. In 1895 Chicago appointed its corps of school physicians, and in 1897 the New York Department of Health appointed 134 medical inspectors of schools.[25] Bolduan said that the work of the New York medical inspectors in regard to children

> consisted in visiting the public and other free schools of the Borough of Manhattan each morning before ten o'clock to examine all children sent to them by the principal or teachers as suspicious cases of contagious disease. Whenever a child was found to be suffering from a contagious disease, the inspector immediately excluded it from school attendance and it was not allowed to return until all danger of transmission of the infection had passed.[44]

Teachers welcomed the physicians' input. In Providence, Rhode Island, teachers were continually calling upon the health department for advice, for investigation of contagious diseases, or to visit and give an opinion on the physical condition of certain children. Hearing of the Boston medical inspectors, they worked with parents to raise funds in 1894 for their first school physician.[24]

The number of cities adopting school medical inspection rose from 4 in 1894 to 400 in 1910,[24] but the only course of management open to physicians was exclusion of sick pupils from school. As a result, large numbers of children were excluded from school, often for minor conditions not important enough for medical attention. There was no contact between parents and physicians, so parents must have had limited understanding of the medical conditions found by the physicians. Many of them, particularly immigrants, must have been baffled to find schools enforcing compulsory attendance laws on the one hand and excluding children, for unclear reasons, on the other. Without understanding and in the face of family poverty, many children were not medically treated, stayed out of school, and roamed their neighborhoods infecting others.[45] The new medical inspection "caused enforced absence from school, and not only interfered with the education of the children, but often made them habitual truants."[40] The absentee rate in the New York schools ran as high as 60 percent,[45] mostly because of disease.

To deal with this situation—that physicians could detect disease and exclude the children so affected, but were powerless to ensure treatment and the ultimate return of children to school—school nursing was created.

School Nursing

The case of a twelve-year-old boy excluded from school because of an untreated skin condition led Lillian Wald, founder of the Henry Street Visiting Nurse Service, to discuss the wastefulness of medical inspection without follow-up. Wald was familiar with some of the early work in schools performed by district nurses' associations in London.[46] A Henry Street nurse was offered for a 1-month demonstration in six schools in 1902.[45,46]

The nurse, Lina L. Rogers, wrote of the experiment in her book on school nursing, published in 1917.[45] All children with the "slightest indication of any contagious disease," who formerly would have been automatically excluded by the physician were sent to the nurse, who, in a small space under the stairs or in special room, treated the condition and if necessary visited the mother to give a practical demonstration of the type of treatment needed to be carried out at home.[47] Within a few weeks absenteeism was reduced by 50 percent.[45] As a result the N.Y.C. Department of Health in November 1902 hired 12 nurses to work in the schools; by the end of 1903 the number of nurses was 33. In addition, the obvious need for a health room in schools had been demonstrated.

In January 1903 the N.Y.C. Department of Health expanded the system of medical inspection by moving physicians into the classroom to examine all children for the presence of contagious disease.[40,48] It is important to understand what was meant by *medical inspection*. Lina Rogers wrote: "The routine inspection is made once a week by the doctor, who goes into the classroom, stands with his back to a window, and as the children pass before him he looks at the eyes, throat, hands and hair of each individually."[47]

An enormous amount of contagious diseases was found. Rogers recorded that, in early 1903 in 120 days of school, 135,854 treatments were given. Infectious conditions of the eyes headed the list (leading to the opening of a municipal hospital for trachoma in 1902),[48] followed by pediculosis, ringworm, eczema, and scabies.[47] Nurses administered treatment for pediculosis, conjunctivities, ringworm, impetigo, favus, molluscum contagiousum, scabies.[48] In some instances, such as pediculosis infection, the child would be excluded, the nurse would visit the home with the appropriate solutions, instruct the mother in their use,[47] and keep the case under observation until the child returned to school. Home visits were made by nursing and medical staff to absent children where the school suspected sickness. A large number of cases of contagious disease were found and treated.[48]

The N.Y.C. Department of Health reported in 1903 that the system of observation and treatment reduced "the necessary exclusions 98 percent by comparison with the number when the present Medical School Inspection System was first instituted," decreased contagious diseases needing nurse treatment because of "the cleaner state of the children," and diminished the incidence and prevalence of trachoma.[48] Others reported that infected eyes and heads and also ringworm were "practically stamped out" by constant nursing supervision.[49]

The physicians' review of *all* children in the classroom revealed to a skilled observer for the first time that there were in the population a substantial number of physical problems, other than contagious disease, of a nature so gross that they were apparent in the fully clothed state. The N.Y.C. Department of Health noted of the situation, "We are spending immense sums of money to educate our children; is it not worthwhile to spend at least a fraction of that sum to render them capable of assimilating that knowledge?"[50] So saying, in 1905 the department added a new service, the physical examination, to school health.

The object was a complete physical examination of every schoolchild, noting nutritional condition; enlarged glands; chorea; cardiac disease; deformities of spine, chest, or extremities; defective vision or hearing; problems with nasal breathing, teeth, palate, tonsils, posterior nasal growths; deficient mentality.[40] It was also noted if treatment was necessary, and a notice was sent to the parents advising them of the condition and the need for immediate medical care.[50] (The physical examination, sometimes called the *individual examination* to distinguish it from the classroom inspection, did not allow the physician to remove any clothing. Some cities went so far as to forbid the physician's touching a child during an examination. Much controversy occurred in medical ranks regarding the value of using a stethoscope over clothes. New York tested clothed versus unclothed examinations in 1939 and found little difference.)[51]

In the first quarter of 1906, of 24,000 children examined in New York City 18,000 (75 percent) were in need of treatment. Large numbers of children were found with defective eyesight and teeth, enlarged tonsils and adenoids, and nasal obstruction. It was noted that 87 percent of boys in a "truant school" were physically deficient.[51] In spite of the success of the physical examinations in uncovering disease, the new program succeeded in obtaining treatment for only 6 percent of the defective children. "The records soon amounted to little more than a mere compilation of statistical data, and very little to show for the work."[40]

Lina Rogers had developed an approach to school health[45] in which the school nurse took over control of contagious diseases in schools—the physician's former role—"leaving the medical inspector free to devote his entire time to making physical examinations of children."[40] The nurse took over classroom inspection of all children, treated minor problems, and referred children to the physician for confirmation of the diagnosis of major problems (which was followed by exclusion as necessary and home visits to ensure parental understanding and provision of care). The nurse used similar follow-up techniques and home visits to obtain care for the chronic and noncontagious diseases found by the physical examinations.[45]

In 1912 the N.Y.C. Department of Health introduced enough nurses to apply to chronic defects those follow-up techniques found so successful with acute contagious diseases. The department used the services of 74 medical inspectors and 179 nurses under staff supervisors. Significant improvements appear to have been made. With a school health history similar to New York's, Philadelphia recorded in the school year 1921/22 that treatment was obtained for 43 percent of "important defects" and 92 percent of "minor defects." By 1924 New York employed 211 school nurses, Philadelphia 98, and Chicago 50; 196 of 327 cities in the nation (58 percent) reported school nurses conducting or participating in health examinations of students.[40]

School nursing spread through the larger towns, often after a demonstration—similar to that of Lillian Wald—staged by a visiting nurse association or a Red Cross chapter. Sometimes the local board of education picked up the service, and somtimes it subsidized the visiting nurse association. This method of diffusion was built upon the school board structure already well in place, the phenomenal growth and apparent prestige of public health nursing, and the evidence that school health services were an effective addition to education.[34]

Philadelphia provides an interesting example of the process in which the local department of health played no part. In 1903 the Visiting Nurse Society (VNS) of Philadelphia offered the services of one nurse to the public schools; the offer was accepted, but the city made no move to appropriate funds for a school nursing service until 1907, when the VNS, with a certain amount of publicity, raised the number of nurses to four, whose services would end after a period of 3 months' demonstration. The board of education responded with an appropriation for a supervisor and five nurses.[34]

Additional Services

Other services were added to the basic core of physician-nurse services for the detection and care of contagious disease and chronic defects. Testing of vision was reported from Washington, D.C., (1893) and Baltimore (1896) and was enacted into state law in Connecticut in 1899 and in Vermont in 1903. Hearing testing was suggested in 1876 and mandated in Massachusetts in 1906. Compulsory vaccination of schoolchildren for smallpox was instituted in New York City in 1897. Dental examinations were conducted in Brookline, Massachusetts, in 1906. The success of a dental hygiene and clinic program was reported from Bridgeport, Connecticut, in 1919.[24,25] In Philadelphia a dental dispensary was orgainzed in 1910, and dental hygienists were employed by the 1920's. Prevention was stressed, although reparative work was also done: "Prevention, as applied to dental service in the school clinics, should carry with it the saving of the sixth-year molars by reparative work."[40]

Institutionalization of School Health Services

The value of school physicians and nurses in reducing the dirtiness and contagious diseases of schoolchildren, obtaining treatment for chronic conditions, and significantly reducing absenteeism due to illness had been seen in the large cities, where local departments of health had the understanding and energy necessary to see needs, establish demonstrations, and press for new appropriations. All agreed that the services had value, but how would they be carried to children in the smaller cities, townships, and counties where there were no local departments of health?

Massachusetts led the way in 1906 by showing that the school district structure could be used to extend desired health services to all school students in a state. School boards were required to appoint a physician for each school to examine children and "teachers, janitors and school buildings as in his opinion the protection of the health of the pupils may require." Children to be examined were specified as those showing signs of illness referred by a teacher, those returning from absence due to illness, and every child once a year to be tested and examined for "defective sight or hearing or from any other disability or defect tending to prevent his receiving the full benefit of his school work, or requiring a modification of the school work in order to prevent injury to the child or to secure the best educational results."[24]

By 1911 nine states had mandatory medical inspection laws. Ten others had permissive legislation. Pennsylvania law mandated medical inspection in first- and second-class school districts in 1911 and extended the mandate to districts of the third and fourth class in 1919.[34] These initial legislative requirements did not usually cover school nursing services, but they stimulated school districts to acquire the services of nurses. As West wrote of the history of nursing in Pennsylvania in about 1932: "Because school officials realize that failure on the part of parents to comply with the recommendations of the school physician is due to lack of understanding rather than indifference, school nurses have been employed to visit the homes and explain to parents the significance of health handicaps."[34]

Treatment Services

The gap between finding health conditions of schoolchildren and having those conditions appropriately treated has presented school health services with dilemmas from its earliest days. The dilemma of finding services, especially for children from financially less able families, has been compounded by opposition from the powerful forces of organized medicine.

The first suggestion that schools need to provide some medical services was made by the International Congress on Hygiene in Schools, held in Geneva in 1882, with the recommendation that "myopics be provided with glasses."[25] Dr. Lincoln of Boston noted in 1886 that in Europe medical treatment was given to a large number of children at school "beyond what is likely to be thought advisable in America at present."[21] Dr. Chapin reviewed medical inspection in Providence in 1909 and noted two classes of problems revolving around defective eyesight. The first, the problem of getting the child to care, involved lack of parental understanding and lack of financial resources; the second was lack of quality in the care that was received. The second matter is usually not described so openly. The organized medical profession usually ignores or denies it; public health personnel recognize it but consider it too explosive to bring into the open. Therefore, it is worthwhile considering Chapin's words:

> A hindrance to successful school inspection is the inability of a considerable proportion of the practising physicians to properly treat the children that are sent to them by the school inspectors. Before we employed our oculist we were greatly annoyed by parents consulting cheap and incompetent physicians or mere opticians. We have found that the average family physician in the majority of instances cannot cure scabies, and frequently makes slow progress with ring-worm. We send most of our cases of scabies to the hospital, and the school inspectors treat the ring-worm, the city furnishing the necessary ointment.[52]

When one considers the times, it is no wonder the schools had such difficulties:

1. It is estimated that about 1910 the medical profession had gained sufficient knowledge to ensure for any patient a slightly better than 50 percent chance of benefitting from an encounter with it.[53]
2. Many physicians in practice were products of the medical degree mills that flourished in the latter half of the nineteenth century. Medical education was reformed from the 1910 Flexner Report onward.
3. Even physicians of quality lacked much knowledge of children. In 1891 the new American Pediatric Society maintained that it was "no exaggeration to state a large number of sick infants and young children . . . are suffering from the vigorous treatment of their zealous medical attendants, rather than from the disease with which they started."[54,55]

When in 1906 Massachusetts required that all school boards conduct physical examinations, it also required that they correct physical defects found. The latter aroused great opposition,[25] and its fate is not clear. Faced with a dearth of treatment facilities for children, the N.Y.C. Department of Health, in 1912, began conducting dental clinics in school buildings and providing other free clinics for eye, ear, and orthopedic defects, skin problems, removal of tonsils and adenoids, and general medical care.[25,56] These activities, although predating the

1918 addition of treatment to English school health services, ceased in 1915 as a result of pressure from the medical society.[56]

Despite activity in its first year (1847) supporting public health statistics and later (1848) conducting sanitary surveys of towns, the American Medical Association and its state and county branches generally have been hostile to public health. They have opposed public health programs for the control of tuberculosis and veneral disease, public health centers, immunization activities that might lose them fees, and services to any but the impoverished which could cut into their market. At the national level the AMA opposed federal grants to states for maternal and child health services under both the Sheppard-Towner Act of 1921 and the Social Security Act of 1935[57] and was successful in blocking Medicare health insurance under social security for 20 years between 1945 and 1965.[58]

Its opposition to repassage of the Sheppard-Towner Act in 1929 was vehement. In 1930 the House of Delegates of the AMA condemned the act as "unsound in policy, wasteful and extravagant, unproductive of results and tending to promote communism."[55] The Pediatric Section of AMA, however, was in favor of the act. When the House of Delegates ruled it could not publish its views independently, section members withdrew and organized the separate American Academy of Pediatrics—"for the welfare of children." The academy has since played a distinguished role in establishing standards of child health care, child health studies, pediatric education,[55] and the recent experiments in developing the successful role of the pediatric nurse practitioner and the school nurse practitioner.

The AMA—NEA Alliance

The previous history is important in order to understand the role played by the American Medical Association in the Joint Committee on Health Problems in Education of the National Education Association (NEA) and the American Medical Association. The two organizations joined forces in 1911; the Joint Committee was formed in 1921 and still functions to the present day.

Gradually the Joint Committee evolved a philosophy that has successfully permeated the whole atmosphere of school health. The philosophy makes sense if its aims are to ensure that school health services do not interfere with the private practice of medicine or pry into the workings of the school. The NEA-AMA decided:

Schoolchildren are basically healthy and do not need health services.

Some health assessment is needed for such hidden conditions as problems with eyesight and hearing but primarily it is a device for education.

All children have family doctors who can treat all conditions found by the school.

Some children do not have family doctors and therefore need the services of the school health program, but such services shall not include treatment.

In the face of the diseases of children found by school health services, the 43 percent treatment rate, the low income of many families, the persistence of child labor, and the low quality of many school buildings in the first decades of this century, the above position has the same fairy-tale quality which the Joint Committee brought to health education. It would have a certain charm if it were not so callous. The full story of this misalliance is yet to be written.

Later Developments

It is hard to find historical accounts much beyond the first two decades of this century. There is no doubt that, compared with today's activities, school health has increased in size from these early beginnings. More states and school districts are involved and certainly many more school nurses. In the early 1930's, Pennsylvania boasted of 450 school nurses in the state. Currently it has about 2,500.[34] In 1946 4,400 full-time school nurses were identified in a national study. In 1955 the number of full-time school nurses had increased to 7,730. The ratio of school nurse to public school population was 1:4,291 in 1950, in 1960 it was 1:3,113. In the period 1937–1952 the proportion of public health nurses employed by school boards rose from 20 to 29 percent.[59]

Obviously, an increased number of nurses absorbed in school health means increased fiscal resources devoted to school health. No data are available that show the percentage of total educational resources consumed by school health and relative changes in the proportion over the years. Sources of funds for school health were initially local. Some state monies have been added over the years either directly, as the 1949 Pennsylvania law reimbursing school districts for performance of certain mandated services, or indirectly in a state educational formula for certified staff. Little federal money has found its way into school health, although some districts have used ESEA or other special grants to expand basic services.

Services have changed little over the years. Additions have been made in immunization requirements, such screening tests as tuberculosis, and more physical examinations for athletics, working papers, and driver education. The number of physical examinations in the general program has usually decreased from an annual requirement, which was beyond the capacity of any school district to do well,[60] to a more common three times in the child's school life. The quality of physical examinations increased with the relaxation of restrictions against undressing children; this was a legacy of the Second World War, in which many in the general population were educated to the procedure.[61]

There appear to have been certain stimuli to improvements in school health services, usually resulting in increases in numbers of staff, especially nurses, but not in much change in mandated services. One stimulus was the world wars, in which the large number of draftees rejected for health reasons (the main reason being flat feet) was taken as a sign that school health needed improvement. The Astoria study published in 1942, which demonstrated refinements in school health screening, record keeping, and nurse-teacher collaboration, resulted in increased hiring of school nurses.[62]

The type of staff providing school health services has remained the same over the years. Physicians and dentists are drawn from the general practitioners of the community for part-time work. Nurses and dental hygienists are usually full-time employees who in many states are required to be "certified" by the state department of education.

Health Education

A different stream of activities shaped that part of the school curriculum entitled "health education." Concern for the public health of the nation between 1850 and 1900 generated a great deal of interest in health matters, ranging from formation of public associations for improved sanitation of towns to the birth of health foods[25] and emphasis on physical activity.[26] At the same time education, bursting with increasing compulsory attendees, also brought forth new ideas. In that period more new textbooks were written on health education, in English, than on any other subject.[60] In keeping with these developments, many schools provided or required courses in physiology or hygiene.

Leadership was stolen by the Women's Christian Temperance Union, which was the first of many movements seeking to impose certain knowledge or ideas upon schools. It seized upon the hygiene portion of the curriculum as its vehicle and between 1880 and 1889, obtained laws requiring teaching of physiology and hygiene in 38 states. Instruction in the effects of alcohol and narcotics (and sometimes tobacco) was specifically required in most states. Such subjects were hardly likely to stimulate the interest of elementary students or the enthusiasm of teachers, and much that was available on the subject was unscientific opinion.[60]

At the same time health education was frequently linked with physical education because of the specific relationship seen at that time between physical activity and health. States began requiring physical education in the curriculum from 1892 (Ohio) into the 1920's. Many laws required health instruction as part of physical education.[25,60]

This relationship was strengthened after 1916, when the high level of rejection from the draft led to popular proposals to increase physical (and health) education. The collaboration proved disadvantageous to health education, particularly when physical education found competetive sports and forgot its own health roots and its sickly health "partner." As a consequence, health education is today passed like a deflated football to the new and/or lesser teachers in the school's physical education department.

Health education in the elementary schools was revived in 1918 from the almost lethal alcohol and narcotics requirements by the Child Health Organization of America, which developed numerous publications designed "to develop interest, initiative, and originality on the part of the teacher" and "wholesome change in health habits" on the part of the pupils. In this drive for process without content and habit without knowledge, such characters as "Cho Cho the Health Clown" were introduced, such practices as weighing of schoolchildren were promoted ("A Scale in Every School"), and "healthy rules" were promulgated which were without a scientific basis (drinking at least four glasses of water a day) or deleterious (having a bowel movement every morning).[60]

Health education without content or without specific objectives tended to fit the approach to teacher education of the time, however, it provided poor moorings for any kind of health education that had specific and measurable health objectives. A good example is safety education, which could not get its concerns regarding fire prevention and traffic safety into the health curriculum without legislative help in the 1930's[60] Today it sometimes exists as a separate department in a school district. Often it depends on such outside groups as police or the health department, and often its most visible section is a separate driver education program.

Chapter 3

HEALTH PROBLEMS OF SCHOOL STUDENTS

Illness is the night-side of life, a more onerous citizenship. Every-
one who is born holds dual citizenship, in the kingdom of the well
and in the kingdom of the sick.

—Susan Sontag, *Illness as Metaphor*

Schoolchildren are the "healthiest group in the population"![1] With this
truism all who look at the health of children of school age are invited to
turn aside and direct attention elsewhere. Why this is so is not clear. It is
apparent that schoolchildren die with less frequency than infants and
the elderly and are less physically disabled than the aged, but it is also
known that certain conditions, such as episodes of acute illness and
injuries, bear most heavily on children; that some classes of disasters,
such as abuse and neglect and delinquency, are confined to children;
that disruptions in childhood, such as pregnancy, adversely affect all
subsequent development; that chronic conditions in childhood present
to the immature person the specter of 60 years of disability compared
with one decade for the mature older person similarly afflicted; that
the immature organism is more susceptible to the physical, emotional,
and social hazards of the environment; that much disease of the young
and over half the deaths in the group are preventable; that the school

presents the only environment in which certain disease states, such as learning problems, are seen, yet which, because of its close, continuous, and developmentally appropriate role for children, offers an invaluable site for milieu therapy.

It appears that the health status of schoolchildren presents a situation unique in many respects: the population group, its health problems, the preventive possibilities, and the relationship with a social institution (the school); yet neither the excitement of the uniqueness nor the preventive potential has fired academic institutions or public health agencies. In 1973, from the perspective of a chairmanship in maternal and child health at the Johns Hopkins School of Hygiene and Public Health, Cornely could note that "the health needs of school-age children are not as succinctly established or accepted as in the younger age group,"[2] in spite of the fact that schoolchildren have been the recipients of organized public health services for most of this century, longer than any other population group. Few writers have had the courage of North to declare our abysmal ignorance in matters of school health: "We have very little data about most diseases. This can be amplified a number of times if we begin talking about the characteristics of a child which may be important for his functioning in school."[3] Most writers in describing the health of students mention the low mortality experience of school-age children, make passing reference to the preventable nature of the accidents that cause a large part of that mortality, note that communicable diseases are common in young children and problems associated with sexual maturity in the older child, and then refer to the special nature of handicapped children.

The approach taken in this chapter is different. The objectives are (1) to show that the health of schoolchildren now and in their future lives is compromised by multiple and complex conditions; (2) to demonstrate that we frequently lack the most elementary understanding of these conditions, falling short, in particular, in nosology,* statistics on incidence and prevalence, and the epidemiological studies necessary to understand causes, without which prevention is impossible; (3) to show the known or suspected role of the school in the etiology of many conditions affecting the health of students, because that knowledge endows the power of prevention.

The treatment given the subject is uneven in type and depth of analysis; for instance, not all diseases of children are mentioned. For this I do not apologize, if the reader is left with two impressions: (1) that

*Nosology (n.) (from Greek nosos, "disease"): (1) A systematic arrangement or classification of diseases. (2) That branch of medical science which treats of the classification of diseases. (Webster's New Universal Dictionary of the English Language, 2d ed., The Publishers Guild, New York, 1970.)

knowledge is already available, waiting to be used by those whose intent is to understand the health problems of students and to prevent and relieve their pain, misery, and distress; (2) that the problem is conceptual; it is necessary to understand that health is the result of interactions between the individual and the environment and that changes in health status can be achieved by manipulating or altering those interactions. Only then will the pooling of knowledge in the book that needs to be written result in any change in health services for school students.

THEORETICAL APPROACHES

Ecology, Epidemiology, and New Diseases

Many of the health problems of schoolchildren that are now being described are "new" in the sense that they were not noted in earlier generations or, if described previously, were ignored subsequently. For example, the American Social Science Association discussed "The Nervous System as Affected by School Life" in 1875,[4] yet the existence of psychiatric disturbances in children was not generally acknowledged until 1925.

The English 15-year longitudinal study of a cohort of children born in 1947 in Newcastle-upon-Tyne noted: "At fifteen not less than one in five had either physical handicap, recurrent illness, intellectual limitation, poor educational performance, or severe difficulties of emotional or social adaptation. This residual disability is the true measure of our failure to deal effectively with the physical and educational disorders of children."[5] Haggerty in his study of child health in New York noted that in the 1970's the "current major health problems . . . would have been barely mentioned a generation ago."[6] Problems included learning difficulties and school problems, behavioral disturbances, allergies, speech difficulties, visual problems, and the problems of adolescents in coping and adjusting, all of which constitute what has been called the "new morbidity."

Accurate description of these newly recognized health problems and development of an appropriate terminology have not occurred, partly because few have stopped to describe the problems, partly because clinicians faced with these problems are handicapped in describing what they see by their lack of knowledge and experience, and partly because the problems themselves are inherently complex.

McCormick noted this last point in discussing the pediatric evaluation of 21 children referred with school dysfunction, most of whom "had a mixture of social-environmental, physical, intellectual, academic, and developmental problems." He concluded that a multi-ple-category diagnostic schema was essential, with each category assessed independently and "then conclusions drawn about possible relationships."[7] Others, including the World Health Organization, have described child psychiatric disorders in terms of several parameters "which are logically and practically independent and separate." Thus there is seen to be no necessary association between intellectual level and emotional disorder or between a clinical "disorder and the type of etiological factor which is present."[8]

Such discussions are essentially concerned with the differences between the "manifestational" and "experiential" criteria of diseases, or disorders, with multiple causes. The causal factors interact in ways that are reciprocal and multiple before the given disease or disorder manifests itself through one or a number of presenting symptoms or signs. Susser described this situation as fitting an ecological model of disease, where ecology is understood as the interrelationships of all living things. For that "part of human ecology relating to states of health," epidemiology "describes the occurrence and evaluation of . . . disordered states of health and seeks to discover their causes and prevent them. For these purposes enumeration is an essential first step. The study of the relation of these states of disordered health to society and habitat follows as the next logical step."[10] In carrying out studies of the relationship between health and habitat, epidemiology has moved in the past century from a "simple sequential causal model" of disease occurrence, in which the environment served as a vehicle for a microorganism in its attack on a host, to a model of multiple causes engaged in reciprocal interactions.

Epidemiology, using the ecological model, has elucidated "how largely each factor influences the whole result" for the great complexities of malaria (waters, seasons, mosquito life cycle, density of mosquito vectors, parasite life cycle, human habitat, human habits)[11] and of coronary heart disease (genetics, culture, diet, occupation, exercise, smoking, obesity, socioeconomic status, hypertension). Only recently has attention begun to turn to the behavioral, emotional, and social end of the disease spectrum. In this slow turn of events the study of children has been slower and the existence of their new morbidity barely yet recognized as a subject for study and epidemiological analysis.[12]

Some support for this viewpoint can be found in a review of the subject matter studied and reported by epidemiologists in one of their major publications, *The American Journal of Epidemiology*. Sixty-three of the 65 issues from December 1974 to April 1980 were reviewed, and 591 "original contributions" were counted. Applicability to children of school age was confirmed for 46 contributions (7.8 percent) that used, in the title, the words *children* (17), *childhood* (7), *school* or *class* (9); that gave the age range of subjects (3); or that were on a subject assumed to include schoolchildren (10). The number of articles on children of school age averaged 7.2 per year and ranged from 2 to 10. The subjects covered in 46 articles are listed in Table 3–1. Trends noted during the period studied are shown in Table 3–2.

The infectious disease interest represents the traditional concern of epidemiologists. The studies of blood pressure and coronary artery disease may be viewed as attempts to understand the etiology and life history of diseases important to the adult population, and to the child population in time, but with little present benefit for the children studied. The recent articles on environmental subjects, which included air pollution and industrial cadmium emissions, seem to reflect the availability of the school population for study of a phenomenon applicable to the whole population rather than attempts to apply epidemiologic methods to disorders currently existing among schoolchildren. Of course epidemiologic studies are reported elsewhere, but it seems indicative of the problems faced by the field of child health today that so little interest has been provoked among the adherents of epidemiology to provide the definitions, measurements, and concepts through which we can grapple intelligently with the childhood disorders we can now perceive.

Table 3–1.

Infectious disease	35%
Blood pressure	26%
Coronary heart disease and risk factors	15%
Cancer and chronic disease	13%
Environmental factors	11%

Table 3–2.

	Number of articles on children	
Subject	*1975/76*	*1978/79*
Infectious disease	13	2
Blood pressure	3	4
Environmental factors	1	4

Models of the Impact on Health and Education of Disease and Health Services

Productivity. It is often stated that school health services exist to improve educational outcome; thus, it seems that the relationship between health and education has been clearly established. This is, in fact, not so; there are no hard data clearly establishing that children in better health advance in their ability to learn. This lack of data is due in part to the paucity of studies conducted on the health problems of school students and the consequences of those problems—a recurrent theme in this chapter.

In this instance, however, school health shares a deficiency in common with the rest of public health. One may be able to show that people live longer as a result of improved health, but do they function better? This question has been raised by economists in the case of underdeveloped countries, where the most effective use of investment resources is literally a matter of survival. Preliminary analyses suggest that changes in health status have positive effects upon labor productivity, that, in fact, a relationship exists between health and the function of the worker.[13]

Despite the suggestion of a relationship, "there seems to have been little effort to isolate the quantitative influence of health inputs on output or productivity in man."[13] This is not to say there are not many measures of health input. Data are available on number of programs, facilities, staff, and some data exist on the health consequences of such programs, that is, mortality, morbidity. It is also known that such measures are highly correlated with all measures of national progress.

The problems lie in data analysis. Usually data are aggregated for the nation or large areas, thereby concealing local inputs and outcomes; outcome data in aggregate form are hard to dissect to identify the varying influences of their many causes; health changes may affect the denominator (population) as well as the numerator (outcomes); time-sequenced relationships of input to output are often not seen, especially when local data are not analyzed. There appears to be growing recognition of the great variation in health observations within a country, thus pointing out the need for studying small areas in order to see any effect. Malenbaum reported regional data for agricultural production analyzed by health and education explanatory variables. "Health—and education, to a much smaller extent—revealed a more vigorous relationship to agricultural achievement than did labor and fertilizer, the more usual inputs of agricultural change."[13] Other accounts have shown the importance of medical and nursing personnel.

In what ways does improving health affect workers' productivity? The answer seems to have at least four parts:

Increasing the number of hours available for work by decreasing absence due to illness

Increasing output per hour by increasing vigor

Providing access to previously inaccessible resources

Developing new attitudes regarding ability to control one's environment and fate that may "engender a new motivation toward self-fulfillment and greater achievement"[13]

Economic growth theory has provided evidence that at least half the change in worker output is due to the quality, and not the quantity, of capital and labor inputs: improved machines, higher skills, more imaginative policies. In poorer countries where the need is for greater motivation, such quality enhancement is the key to economic expansion; in other words, "human aspects of the process become focal points." Usually efforts for quality enhancement directed to workers have been primarily educational. It is suggested that explicit consideration be "given to health elements as quality determinants.[13]

One might argue that school health services, in their early history, not only increased the time and energy children had available for education, but in improved sanitation of buildings and cleanliness and comfort of the children also engendered new attitudes regarding the ability to control one's fate and thus enhanced motivation to learn. It may be possible that such health outputs may still operate in the very poorest areas. The educational output generated would justify increased health inputs.

The basic formula linking health and education is as follows:

$$\begin{array}{cccc} \text{Input} & \text{Output} & \text{Input} & \text{Output} \\ \text{Health} & \rightarrow \text{Health} & \rightarrow \text{Education} & \rightarrow \text{Education} \end{array}$$

An example of the use of the formula for a school vision program is:

$$\begin{array}{cccc} \text{Input} & \text{Output} & \text{Input} & \text{Output} \\ \text{Vision} & \rightarrow \text{Visual} & \rightarrow \text{Reading} \rightarrow & \text{Education} \\ \text{Program} & \text{Acuity} & & \end{array}$$

A vision program in school health services may have as its objective detection of all children with abnormal vision and fitting of appropriate lenses for attainment of optimal visual acuity. It is thus a program that detects and corrects abnormality in function, namely, in the function of seeing. It is not concerned with prevention of the common underlying conditions that cause the diminished vision function; these conditions, primarily myopia (short sight), hypermetropia (long sight), and astigmatism, are due to alterations in the lens or cornea for which no known preventive or curative measures exist. Correction of vision function with appropriate glasses does prevent the consequences of these conditions, such as reduced ability to read and write, to be educated, to be employed, to be independent, to be an informed citizen and community member, and to engage in the pleasure and stimulation afforded by reading.

These relationships may be expressed in terms of work production functions derived from a modified Cobb-Douglas formula.[13]

$$\frac{\Delta EO}{EO} = \frac{\Delta Ll}{L} + \frac{\Delta Kk}{K} + \frac{\Delta Rr}{R} + \frac{\Delta Aa}{A} \qquad (1)$$

where
EO = education output
L = labor (number of workers)
K = capital value with technological level unchanged
R = reading productivity
A = factor productivity beyond labor, capital, and reading
l = coefficients for labor (L), capital (K), reading,(R), and other-
k = factor producitivity (A) with respect to output (O). $l + k + r +$
r = $a = 1$
a

Reading productivity is related to the level of visual acuity:

$$\frac{\Delta R}{R} = \frac{\Delta VAv}{VA} \qquad (2)$$

where
VA = visual acuity
v = coefficient of visual acuity with respect to reading

The health output of visual acuity is related to the health input of the vision program:

$$\frac{\Delta VA}{VA} = \frac{\Delta VP}{VP} p \qquad (3)$$

VP = vision program
p = coefficient of vision program with respect to visual acuity

Formula (1) can be rewritten in terms of visual acuity:

$$\frac{\Delta EO}{EO} = \frac{\Delta Ll}{L} + \frac{\Delta Kk}{K} + \frac{\Delta VAvr}{VA} + \frac{\Delta Aa}{A} \qquad (4)$$

or in terms of the vision program:

$$\frac{\Delta EO}{EO} = \frac{\Delta Ll}{L} + \frac{\Delta Kk}{K} + \frac{\Delta VPpvr}{VP} + \frac{\Delta Aa}{A} \qquad (5)$$

The formula is useful in that it provides a comprehensive analytical framework that specifies the dimensions of the relationship between health input and educational output. It fills a conceptual void in which those who would shrink and have shrunk from the task of relating health program input to worker productivity have blithely demanded that school health services show their positive effects upon educational productivity. It shows that health inputs must be carefully measured before any of their relationships to other measures of health or educational output will be revealed. This point is particularly valid for school health, whose services, or inputs, cannot be accurately described at the state or national level in the United States.

Cost/Benefit.   Cost/benefit analysis provides a model for expressing the value of public health programs. Basically, the costs of operating a certain program are compared with the costs of not operating it. All costs of running the program and all costs of the additional medical, educational, and institutional care, disability and loss of work productivity, and loss of life averted by the program are expressed in monetary terms.

Even though there is no agreement regarding the formula items used in such models,[14] an example (with hypothetical rates and data) illustrates the use of cost/benefit analysis. In a state with 1,000,000 children of school age it is calculated, based on the national prevalence rate of 0.5 percent, that 5,000 children, or 384 per grade, are classifiable as deaf or hard of hearing, according to specific criteria. The schools can account for 3,000 cases. A statewide hearing-screening program is instituted for all students in grades K,1,2,3,5,7,9. The screening program is successful in detecting those 40 percent of cases not known to the school. Detection results in earlier surgery and medical treatment for some, reducing future needs for medical care and hearing aids and referring children into earlier special education. The longer exposure to special education increases educational level, employment prospects, and overall work productivity. These benefits accrue for the lifetime of the individuals affected.

The following calculations are simplified and based on rough estimates only. They assume that the program has been running for some years and that each year 384 new cases enter the school student population group and 384 leave.

I. Program costs
   A. Screening
      1. Initial sweep screening of 538,461 students in the specified seven grades (plus permission forms, scheduling, explanation, records) × 2 min. per student × school nurse @ $12/h = $215,384.
      2. Threshold screening of 2% screening positives (10,770) × 10 min. per student × school nurse @ $12/h = $21,538.
   B. Referral
      1. 10% of threshold tested positive (1,077) are referred × 5 min. per student × school nurse @ $12/h = $1,077.
   C. Diagnosis
      1. 1,077 referrals tested by audiologist and otologist × $60 per student = $64,620 (identifies 384 cases and 693 "false positives").
   D. Treatment
      1. 10% of 384 require surgery ($500) and 3 days of hospitalization ($600) = $42,240.
      2. 20% of 384 require medical care of 4 visits × $20 and medication × $20 = $7,680.
      3. 30% of 384 require hearing aids × $300 each = $34,560.
   E. Special education
      1. 40% of 384 = 154 cases that would not otherwise be presented to special education. 10% are managed in regular class.
      2. 20% are managed in regular class with special itinerant teacher and other services × $1,000 above regular education costs = $76,800/year for average 10 years per student = $768,000.
      3. 10% are educated in special school × $2,500 above regular education costs = $96,000/year for average 12 grades per student $1,152,000.
   F. Maintenance
      1. 30% of 384 require maintenance services on hearing aids × $50 × 10 times in school and 12 times in adult life = $126,720.
   G. Total costs = 2,433,819.
II. Averted costs
   A. Treatment
      1. 10% of 384 × later, more costly surgery × $2,500 above program costs = $96,000.

10% of 384 not treated medically × later surgery × $1,100 each = $42,240. Total surgery costs = $138,240.
2. 10% of 384 × additional medical treatment × $300 = $11,520.
3. 35% of 384 need hearing aids × $300 = $40,320.
B. Special education
1. 40% of 384 = 154 cases are discovered by special education later. 10% are managed in regular class.
2. 5% are managed in regular class with itinerant and other services × $1,000 above regular education costs = $19,200 × 6 grades per student = $115,200.
3. 25% are managed in special school × $2,500 above regular education costs × 8 grades per student = $1,920,000.
C. Maintenance
1. 35% of 384 × maintenance services on hearing aids × $50 × 8 times in school and 12 times in adult life = $134,400.
D. Lost productivity
1. 40% of 384 = 154 cases receive special education services earlier leading to a 30% increase in level of education and overall productivity. Productivity expresses the overall economic value of human life and equates male and female lives with their different work histories; it disregards intangible costs such as pain and suffering. The per capita gross national product G.N.P./population, for 1976 was $7,950/year.[14] The loss in productivity occurs over the normal span of 44 work years for a 21 year old graduate from Special Education = $7,950 × 30% × (44 years × discount expressing lower value of future money) = $7,950 × 30% × 22 (estim.) = $52,470. For 154 cases the life time loss of productivity averted $52,470 × 154 = $8,080,380.
E. Total Averted Costs $10,440,060

The value of the cost/benefit model is that it demonstrates succinctly and in quantitative terms the relevance of a health program to the education and future life of children.[3]

Health Education Outcomes.   Health education may be viewed as a health service that influences education and/or the future life of children or may be seen as an educational service that influences health. Part of the problem in understanding health education is a confusion over "end points." Haggerty believed "that alterations in behavior rather than knowledge or attitudes should be the end result";[15] behavioral change is sought because it is believed to yield

Table 3–3.

Item	Program Costs or Costs of Program	Costs Averted or Costs Without Program
Screening		
Sweep	215,384	—
Threshold	21,538	—
Referral	1,077	—
Diagnosis	64,620	—
Treatment		
Surgery	42,240	138,240
Medical care	7,680	11,520
Hearing aids	34,560	40,320
Special education		
Regular class	—	—
Special services	768,000	115,200
Special school	1,152,000	1,920,000
Maintenance of hearing aids	126,720	134,400
Lost productivity	—	8,080,380
Total	$2,433,819	$10,440,060

improvement in health status. A model of the progressive steps in the effect of health education appears in Figure 3–1.

Health education has shown that it can increase knowledge.[15] This may be an objective in and of itself. Students should have sufficient knowledge of the human body and its functions, of the scientific process, and of the verification of information that they are able to deal with new information that emerges during their lifetime; as, for example, in the past two decades it has been necessary to deal with the facts of genetics, nutrition, and concepts of statistical risk from environmental pollutants. Health education has been less successful in efforts to change attitudes, although much work has been done on values clarification as a prelude to effective decision making or behavior.[16] However, when rigorous research criteria are applied, "few health education programs have shown much effect on bahavior"[15] let alone on actual health status.

The problem of the effectiveness of health education at the knowledge end point and its relatively unproven value at other end points is due to the untested assumptions often made about the connections between the end points:

MODEL OF HEALTH EDUCATION EFFECT

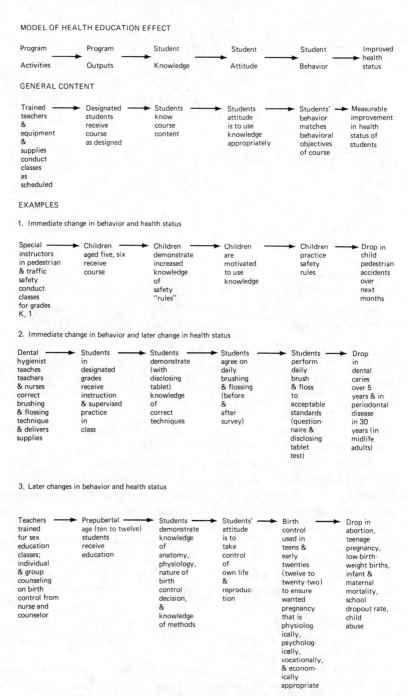

| Program Activities | → | Program Outputs | → | Student Knowledge | → | Student Attitude | → | Student Behavior | → | Improved health status |

GENERAL CONTENT

Trained teachers & equipment & supplies conduct classes as scheduled → Designated students receive course as designed → Students know course content → Students attitude is to use knowledge appropriately → Students' behavior matches behavioral objectives of course → Measurable improvement in health status of students

EXAMPLES

1. Immediate change in behavior and health status

Special instructors in pedestrian & traffic safety conduct classes for grades K, 1 → Children aged five, six receive course → Children demonstrate increased knowledge of safety "rules" → Children are motivated to use knowledge → Children practice safety rules → Drop in child pedestrian accidents over next months

2. Immediate change in behavior and later change in health status

Dental hygienist teaches teachers & nurses correct brushing & flossing technique & delivers supplies → Students in designated grades receive instruction & supervised practice in class → Students demonstrate (with disclosing tablet) knowledge of correct techniques → Students agree on daily brushing & flossing (before & after survey) → Students perform daily brush & floss to acceptable standards (question- naire & disclosing tablet test) → Drop in dental caries over 5 years & in periodontal disease in 30 years (in midlife adults)

3. Later changes in behavior and health status

Teachers trained for sex education classes; individual & group counseling on birth control from nurse and counselor → Prepubertal age (ten to twelve) students receive education → Students demonstrate knowledge of anatomy, physiology, nature of birth control decision, & knowledge of methods → Students' attitude is to take control of own life & reproduc- tion → Birth control used in teens & early twenties (twelve to twenty-two) to ensure wanted pregnancy that is physiolog- ically, psycholog- ically, vocationally, & econom- ically appropriate → Drop in abortion, teenage pregnancy, low-birth- weight births, infant & maternal mortality, school dropout rate, child abuse

Figure 3–1.   Model of Health Education Effect

1. It is assumed that direct relationships exist between knowledge, attitude, behavior, and health; yet, knowledge of birth control does not affect an attitude characterized by feelings of lack of personal control; a positive attitude to birth control may not alter unprotected sexual behavior; children's beliefs have been shown to be unrelated to health behavior in the use of the school nurse's office[17] and in acceptance of dental preventive activity;[18] antiobesity behavior may not prevent diabetes, and relaxation may not prevent mental disease.[19] Weisenberg et al. went so far as to suggest that "health beliefs and behavior might be parallel developments . . . that need not be causally related.[18]

2. It is assumed that no other variables operate to affect each of the end points. Yet it is known that antismoking education competes with cigarette advertising and government subsidies to tobacco growers; that children behaving in traffic according to rules of safety compete against and lose their lives because of poor urban design, poor traffic pattern planning, and their own developmental limitations in perception; and it is recognized that nutrition education goes for naught against lack of food and poverty.

Health education that aims to affect the health of children must be based upon studies of the etiologic connections between health, behavior, attitude, and knowledge plus the relative strength of these "causes" against other factors in the web of causation. To place responsibility for health solely on the individual[20] when most causes of disease lie in the environment is a case of "blaming the victim" and allowing the real culprits to escape. It is not in the tradition of public health, which recognizes that "real change in health must entail a difficult and protracted struggle."[18]

Developmental Models of Health and Disease. It has been noted above that a given event of mortality or morbidity in a child carries completely different import from the same event in an adult. Quantitatively, the number of years of life lost or afflicted is greater; qualitatively, the epigenetic nature of human development ensures that any interference with completion of a developmental task (biological, psychological, social) in one stage of life will be carried into all subsequent developmental stages as an incomplete foundation. We do not yet have ways to express these concepts in regard to a specific disease or to measure and compare the developmental impacts of a various disease entities at given ages.

The school is situated along the developmental track. It takes in children many of whose problems "have their origins in deeply rooted family and community situations"[21] as well as in the diseases of their prenatal environment and early childhood. In school other problems develop, some of which "have their origins in the school system itself."[20] Those with health problems in school appear to go on to have problems as adults.

An interesting example is afforded by one of the commonest criticisms of school health services, namely, the large number of rejections (15 to 21 percent)[21,22] for medical reasons from Selective Service examinations, which some observers view as lost opportunities for preventive services by the schools.[22] Rarely is it mentioned that 25 percent of babies born each year have a major or minor handicap that they bring to school with them. Strangely, few studies have been done of the actual reasons for Selective Service rejection. Densen et al., who conducted one of the few recent studies, noted that military rejection rates for "medical," "mental," or "administrative" classifications cannot, for procedural reasons, be used to determine population prevalence rates.[21] School health characteristics significantly associated with Selective Service rejection included uncorrected vision of 20/50 or worse, such eye ailments as strabismus, organic heart disease, asthma, and history of head injuries. The preventability of these conditions, except the last, is not high, and the optimal time for any such prevention would be well before school—during the mother's pregnancy or the pupil's early childhood.

Other conditions strongly associated with rejection were academic deficiency, behavioral problems, and absenteeism.[21] If failure on military examinations represents some measure of lack of optimal adult functioning, then identification of associated and preexisting conditions in the school population could begin to define those "at risk" in school as targets for preventive services and for reorientation of school health services.

Development is seen as the result of two processes, "the first being a response to the living and non-living environment, and the second the expression of inner capacities that lead the individual to explore and to change the world around him."[23] The model of the stages of human development and the transitional events between them (Figure 3–2) has been adapted and expanded from a 1972 report by the World Health Organization on *Human Development and Public Health*.[24] It is apparent that the choice of stages and transitional events is somewhat arbitrary although it attempts to cover significant physical-biological stages, changes in family relationships, and also relationships with such social institutions as school and work. It can be seen that the chosen developmental stages "fit," to a fair degree, Freud's stages of psychosexual development, Erikson's psychosocial stages, Piaget's cognitive development, and Jersild's affective changes.

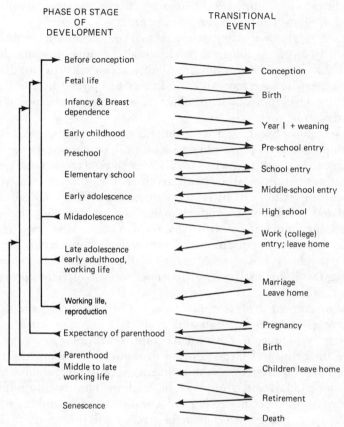

PHASE OR STAGE
OF
DEVELOPMENT

TRANSITIONAL
EVENT

Figure 3–2. Model of Stages of Human Development. Adapted from World Health Organization.[24]

The concept of stages and transitional events was applied to mental health by Caplan, who noted: "Personality development has long been described as a succession of differentiated phases, each qualitatively different from its predecessor. Between one phase and the next are periods of dedifferentiated behavior, transitional periods characterized by cognitive and affective upset. These periods have been called [by Erikson, 1959] 'developmental crises'."[25] The division of human life into developmental stages separated by transitional periods/events offers to the whole field of public health the possibility of measurements of health that go beyond the limits of mortality and morbidity rates.

Developmental Stage. Each stage is marked by certain *tasks* or work to be accomplished in the physical-biological, psychosocial, cognitive, and sociocultural spheres of life. Accomplishment of these tasks is a measure of optimal function and health. In order to accomplish certain tasks the person requires *supplies* in each of the four spheres of life. The provision of such supplies can be measured.

Each stage, by its very nature, is marked by certain predictable *hazards* of a physical-biological, psychosocial, cognitive, or sociocultural nature that may cause mortality, morbidity, accidents, crises, or disability or otherwise interfere with attainment of optimal health in that particular developmental stage. The incidence and prevalence of such hazards can be measured.

Transitional Event. Each transitional event presents a predictable "developmental crisis" of a physical-biological, psychosocial, cognitive, or sociocultural nature. A crisis may be viewed as "a transitional period presenting an individual both with an opportunity for personal growth and with the danger of increased vulnerability." Personal growth is stimulated by exposing individuals to situations of increasing challenge and helping them find constructive ways of mastering the stress. It is an approach known to education and with obvious implications for preventive psychiatry. "Resistance to mental disorder can be increased by helping the individual extend his repertoire of effective problem-solving skills."[25]

Management of developmental crises of transitional events is a measure of optimal function and health. To navigate crisis events successfully, people do better when equipped with *anticipatory guidance* before the crisis and *support* during the course of the crisis. Caplan defined support systems as "attachments among individuals, or between individuals and groups, or institutions that serve to improve adaptive competence in dealing with short-term crises and life transitions, as well as long-term challenges, stresses and privations."[26] They do this by cognitive guidance, feedback, and promotion of emotional mastery. The provision of anticipatory guidance and support to persons going through crises can be measured.

The above measures thus provide a system to quantify health as physical, mental, and social well-being by measuring the growth and development of individuals in terms of the outcome of stages and transitions, and by measuring also the process and content inputs to the above developmental outcomes, that is, supplies, hazards, anticipatory guidance, support.

The model, built on the epigenetic nature of human development, demonstrates the importance of supplies in one stage to prevention of problems in another; for example, services that ensure bonding between mothers and premature infants in the neonatal stage result in more optimal maternal psychosocial development with fewer episodes of child abuse or neglect; this optimal psychosocial environment also ensures more cognitive development in the child's next stage, as a school student, as evidenced by appropriate school progress and no learning or behavior problems.

It is clear that the family unit is the source of most supplies and supports for its members, especially children. Input to one family member has outcomes for others, as in the above examples, and particularly in the matter of maternal nutrition during pregnancy. Thus, the family-as-environment takes on new significance in prevention, and development of the family as a unit requires study and understanding if the growth and development of the child within it is to be fully comprehended and assisted as a school health undertaking.

Not only do human beings grow and develop. Diseases also have a life history. This situation is illustrated in Figure 3–3, in which there are two elements: a vertical line indicating disease progression and horizontal lines showing the mutual interaction, or ecological relationship, between the individual (in whom disease is at a given stage) and the environment.

With a specific genetic constitution and an evolving individual personality, the individual interacts with the physical-biological, psychosocial, and sociocultural elements in the surrounding environment provided by family, school or occupation, and community, drawing from them the "supplies" needed to accomplish the physical, mental, and social tasks of development and, in turn, being presented with specific hazards to optimal health. The environment also provides the anticipatory guidance and support systems needed to cope healthily with crises.

The first stage in the history of disease is that of no disease, just the unique interaction of a unique individual with the environment. This stage may progress to "predisposition," when disease will result unless the mutual interaction is changed on one or both sides; for example, a boy with a family history of early heart disease, living in a sociocultural environment that results in his obesity, lack of exercise, and cigarette smoking by age sixteen, is at high risk of heart disease and early death.

The second stage covers the early, silent, and therefore preclinical beginnings of the actual disease process. Initial precursor stages, such as alterations in fat metabolism or cellular dysfunction, precede slow structural alterations, such as fatty plaques in the walls of blood vessels or early cancer cells; if not turned back by defense mechanisms of the body or environment, these alter bodily integrity and function and eventually produce the earliest symptoms.

The third clinical stage extends from the time the presence of the disease or condition is first noted in the presentation of symptoms of discomfort or dysfunction. The impact of the condition on the present and future life of the individual depends on the destructiveness of the basic condition, the availability of curative or controlling measures, the relief of the discomfort and pain, and the degree to which physical-biological, psychosocial, and cultural dysfunction affects the environmental circles of family, school or occupation, and community. The

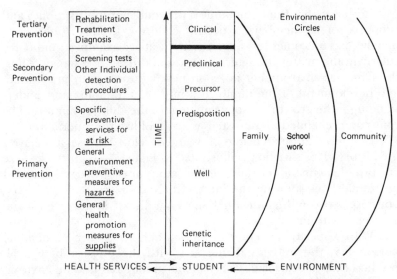

Figure 3–3.   Natural History of Disease—Ecological Relationships—Levels of Prevention.

model can be extended to show the preventive actions possible at each stage in the natural history of disease.

Primary preventive services aim to prevent development of disease by ensuring the provision of supplies for developmental tasks, reducing hazards, providing anticipatory guidance and crisis support, and providing specific preventive measures to those persons at risk of, or predisposed to, disease. Secondary preventive services aim to halt the progression of disease by early detection of the precursor and preclinical stages—usually through screening tests—followed by actions of known effectiveness to alter the individual or the environment. Tertiary preventive services aim to prevent physical deterioration, functional disabilities, and occupational and social-financial complications and to return individuals to optimal attainable function in all spheres of family, school or occupation, and community life.

Effects of Education on Health.   Education has enormous implications for health. Only 35 years ago the median number of school years completed was 8.6. Currently it is slightly over 12 years and 60 percent of the population has graduated from high school. The upward trend is continuing.[27]

Those with higher educational levels tend to have higher incomes and are thus better able to provide the basic supplies for health: shelter, food, clothing, stimulation; they have greater resources for a healthy psychosocial environment; they are healthier. With higher incomes and better health insurance, those with more education have more access to health services. They search for and use knowledge. Health education is more successfully directed to them. They use preventive services more.[27] In many studies the most important variable associated with increased health is educational level and not socioeconomic status. Increased life expectancy is associated with literacy. With literacy, knowledge and power over health actions have diffused from professionals to consumers. Richmond wrote: "A literate mother pushing her food cart through a supermarket is able to feed her infant better than her predecessor would have done with the prescribed pediatric dietary regimes of the twenties and thirties."[28]

It may be that, in terms of prevention of disease, compulsory education is the most important health measure enacted in the past or operating in the present. It is also a preventive measure that is enormously appealing to the population. In one study, 94 percent of parents favored compulsory education, and poor parents expressed a deep understanding of the implications of lost educational opportunities;[29] preschool children look forward to starting school;[30] and of a national sample of elementary students 75 percent expressed "like" or "love" of school.[31]

From the perspective of the better health that attends higher educational levels, school health services should concentrate attention on those failing in school or performing below capacity as a group at high risk of later health and social problems. Such an activity would aid the school in accomplishment of its role in serving society. As Mumford wrote: "The school deserves our best efforts and investments. It is a primary wedge for social change and a central medium for transmission of social patterns and basic premises that shape each successive generation."[32]

POPULATION

The school-age population may be defined as children within a certain age range, such as 4.7 to 18 years, or as children who attend school and those who should attend school. The latter definition, as found in the School Code of Pennsylvania,[33] recognizes the health needs of all children of compulsory school age and of all children, at any age who attend a school. Under this definition, health services rendered to children in parochial and nonpublic schools have been found constitutional as public health, not educational, services.[34]

The target population for school health services has more than doubled since the turn of the century, as schools have admitted more students. In the days of shorter compulsory education, high school students constituted a small portion of the total student body: 14 percent in Philadelphia in 1924.[35] By 1950, 85 percent of the pupils stayed on in high school nationwide,[36] and in Philadelphia 55 percent of the graduating class of 1978 went on to college.[37] At the other end of the age spectrum, the growth of kindergartens has meant that over 90 percent of five-year-olds are at school, as the age at which one may officially begin school has dropped below the compulsory entry age. Increasing numbers of children are found in preschool day care and Head Start programs operated by education authorities. Federal and state right-to-education laws for handicapped children enacted in the 1970's have brought into school handicapped children from preschool age to twenty-one; the laws also involve education authorities in finding, identifying, assessing, and referring for services handicapped children from birth to preschool age. These additions to the category of school-age children—youth, preschool, and the handicapped— bring with them specific health problems and needs for school health services beyond those originally designed for elementary school age children.

The broad age and disability categories of children currently attending school tend to obscure any recognition of those who "should attend school" but are not present. In 1974 the Children's Defense Fund published its report, *Children Out of School in America*,[29] in which most of the following categories are discussed:

1. The 1970 U. S. census revealed 2 million children between the ages of seven and seventeen *not enrolled* in school. This figure represents 4.8 percent of the total school-age population. Some states had higher rates of eligible children not enrolled: Mississippi the highest at 7.8 percent. Nonenrollment was generally higher in the sixteen-to-seventeen-year-old group, which was above 15 percent in eight states. The problem was greater in rural areas and among minority groups than in urban, nonminority populations.

2. Children *may never be registered* for school by their parents and thus may be unknown to the system, particularly if local school censuses are poorly done. This group used to include severely physically and mentally handicapped until the passage of P.L. 94–142; the number of handicapped still not served, although obviously smaller, is not known. Others in this group include migrant and immigrant children, whose additional health problems are well recognized.

3. Children registered for school but excluded because of *lack of placement or programs* include children in remote rural areas beyond reach of transportation and those who register too late. Children on waiting lists for special programs or those in jails represent groups with special and often untreated health problems. To this group must be added children

who are excluded from school entry because of lack of adequate immunization programs in their community.

4. Children, having successfully entered school, may be *forced out, partially excluded*, or *rejected*. Reasons with health connotations include:

    a. Pregnancy
    b. School-age motherhood
    c. Disabled and provided home instruction instead of school placement
    d. School phobias
    e. Truants ignored by attendance officers
    f. Children with few clothes, having no money for school activities, or ashamed of unhygienic clothes or lice
    g. Children unable to comply with special rules, such as to bring parent to school after suspension, obtain immunization,[38] obtain doctor's clearance after disease exclusion
    h. Hyperactive children until diagnosed or under treatment
    i. Compulsory attendance exemptions, for example, illness in family, need to work
    j. Children in mental institutions, training schools, and jails without adequate education or health services;[39] the 1960 census revealed over 101,000 children in correctional institutions: reform schools, prisons, jails, workhouses, detention homes, reformatories[40]
    k. Migrants
    l. Bilingual children
    m. "Troublemakers"
    n. Repeated suspensions

Some children are out of school for extensive periods of time. The Children's Defense Fund conducted a survey in a number of states and found that, of children out of school for 45 days or more 5.4 percent were aged six to seventeen and 19.6 percent were aged sixteen to seventeen.[29]

There are health factors associated with all classifications of students who are not in school. It is apparent that little attention has been devoted to health as a causal or associated factor in the etiology of school nonattendance and inadequate education. A study of dropouts from high school showed associations with low family socioeconomic level, large family, high parental punitiveness, low scores on IQ and academic achievement tests, poor classroom grades and being held back, high delinquency, lower self-esteem, but nothing on health status except that dropouts scored "higher than average in somatic symptoms."[41] A study of the health of adolescents enrolled in the Neighborhood Youth Corps revealed that "school dropouts had a greater percentage of obesity, significant hearing and visual defects, urinary abnormalities, and anemia than did those in school." In a number of instances a health problem had been the main factor "causing a youngster to become a dropout."[42]

CONDITIONS

Mortality

Mortality, although relatively low in the school-age population, provides an index of the overall health status of the group. It is of interest to review some of the changes in mortality experienced by children of school age during the history of the United States. Smillie collected data showing the proportion of deaths occurring in school-age children over a period of 156 years from 1789 (see Figure 3–4). Conditions were worse in 1850 than during colonial times and have greatly improved in association with compulsory schooling, improvement in public health, and general advances in the standard of living.[43]

During this century mortality in school-age children has continued to fall and in addition, infectious diseases, the leading causes of death in 1850, have virtually disappeared from among the major causes of death. The five leading causes of death for ages five to fifteen per 100,000 population are shown in Table 3–4. Kovar commented on the helpful distinction between deaths due to accidents and violence and deaths caused by diseases and conditions.[46] For the data on

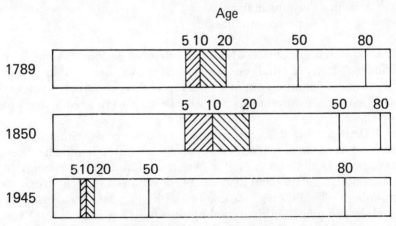

Figure 3–4.   **Proportion of Deaths by Age-Groups, Adapted from Smillie.**[43]

Table 3–4.

Cause of death	Rate per 100,000 population
1939–1941:	
Accidents	28.9
Infectious diseases	30.0
Influenza and pneumonia	9.5
Appendicitis	7.7
Rheumatic fever	7.1
Tuberculosis	5.7[44]
1974:	
Accidents	18.4
Malignant diseases	5.2
Congenital malformations	2.1
Homicides	1.5
Infectious diseases	1.3
Influenza and pneumonia	1.3[45]

the five-to-fifteen age-group, such a classification among the five leading causes of death would show rates per 100,000 population as in Table 3–5.

The distinction is greater in the twelve-to-seventeen-year-old group particularly because of the *increase* in deaths due to accidents, poisoning, and violence. Figure 3–5 shows the trends in these two classifications of death by sex from ages one to twenty-four. Death rates increase by single years of age throughout adolescence and are consistently higher for males than females. The great increase in accidents and violence for adolescent males continues to surge through the late teen years and into the early twenties. In the age-group fifteen-to-nineteen the death rate was 24 percent *higher* in 1969 than in 1960.[47] This extremely disturbing statistic appeared to have excited little interest in official public health circles—certainly nothing to match the interest created over the rising measles susceptibility of the same age-group.

The percentages of deaths in different categories reveal some of the causes within the accident and violence category (Table 3–6). The increases in the homicide and suicide rates with age are remarkable and will be discussed below. Both are related to behavior, are potentially preventable, yet neither has been subjected to epidemiologic

Table 3–5.

	1939–1941	1974
Accidents and violence	28.9	19.9
Diseases and conditions	30.0	8.6

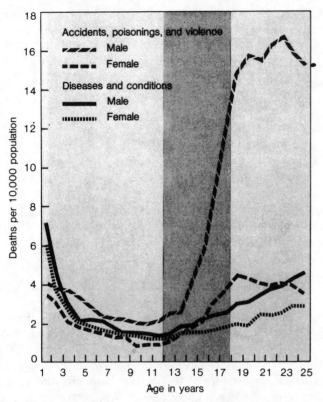

Figure 3–5.   Death Rates for Children and Young Adults Aged One to Twenty-Four, by Age, Sex, and Cause of Death, U.S., 1976, From National Center for Health Statistics. [47] *(Source:* **Kovar.)**

investigations to elucidate causes in which the school is studied as one in a number of etiologic factors. (Accidents are discussed further in another section.)

Table 3–6.

	Percentage of deaths, ages 12–15	*Percentage of deaths ages 16–17*
All causes	100.0	100.0
Accidents and violence	62.5	76.8
Accidents:	52.5	60.4
Motor vehicle	28.3	43.2
Fire and flames	2.2	1.0
Drowning	7.5	5.3
Suicide	4.0	6.7
Homicide	4.5	8.3

Source: Kovar.[46]

Homicide.   In Philadelphia deaths among school attenders recorded by school nurses (about one-third of total deaths in the age-group five to nineteen years) showed an increase in homicide and suicide deaths in the 10-year period from 1960 to 1969.[48] In 1960–1964 there were 8 deaths due to homicide and no suicides, whereas in 1965–1969 deaths by homicide had risen to 39 and suicides to 11. The death rate for homicides in the fifteen-to-nineteen-year-old group in the city in 1969, as calculated by the Philadelphia Department of Health, was 30 per 100,000[49] compared with a national rate of 4 per 100,000 in 1960.[50]

There were few comments on the increase in the adolescent homicide rate. There was an upsurge in violent youth gang activity at that time which was attributed by some to cutbacks in programs aimed at identifying and channeling gang leaders into positive activites and to a wider use of guns by more juvenile gangs.[51] In 1963 in New York City, 17 children were murdered, accounting for 1.5 percent of all child deaths. In 1973 there were 57 child murders, or 6.3 percent of all child deaths. 1972 appears to have been a peak year in the city. In that year 47 percent of *all* homicide victims were under sixteen years of age and of those 48 percent were black, 29 percent Hispanic, and 19 percent white.[52]

Homicide victims of school age are one problem. Children of school age who commit homicide are another. The two groups overlap, particularly in school and gang-related killings where both perpetrator and victim are children. Bender wrote that, for a child to commit homicide, a "certain combination of factors" must be present, including "a disturbed, poorly controlled, impulsive child, the victim as an irritant, and an appropriate or handy weapon coinciding with lack of protective supervision.[53] One study of murderous aggression by children and adolescents from socially acceptable "normal" families found a background of family psychopathology and a pattern whereby one or both parents had fostered and condoned murderous aggression.[54] A study of adult murderers found patterns of parental brutality directed at the murderer when a child.[55] Others have also noted the high prevalence of unfavorable home and life experiences and of personal experience with violent death in child and adolescent murderers, but also report organic brain damage and childhood schizophrenia, fire setting, school retardation, and reading disability.[53]

Suicide.   All observers agree that suicide attempts and actual suicides are underreported,[56] but the number of suicides has doubled in the fifteen-to-twenty-five-year-old group since 1960 and increased by 32 percent in the ten-to-fourteen-year-old category between 1972 and 1980. There is increasing recognition that suicide occurs in children below the age of ten even though such deaths are recorded as "accidental"—as indeed are many in the older age-groups—because it is believed that young children may want to die but do not comprehend the finality of the act.[57] The ratio of attempted to actual suicide is quoted as from 5:1 to 100:1.[58]

Despite the serious size of the problem and the trend upward, "there have been surprisingly few studies on suicidal attempts by children and adolescents."[59] One exception is that the Los Angeles Suicide Prevention Center has conducted systematic "psychological autopsies" on hundreds of cases, with findings of great importance to schools: "Fifty percent were diagnosed as having learning disabilities, were victims of dyslexia, hyperactive, suffered extreme loss of self-esteem . . . a hopeless feeling they could never catch up."[57] A Baltimore study showed 19 percent had failed one or more grades, 35 percent were dropouts or chronic truants, and 35 percent had behavior or discipline problems. On testing, 60 percent had results consistent with minimal brain dysfunction.[60]

Circumstances that are noted included pressure from parents to be successful; broken families, especially the occurrence of divorce;[57] parental ambivalence tending toward hostility and rejection;[61] inability to express overt aggression in an atmosphere of family hostility; unstable homes with excess of physical violence;[62] loss of a parent, particularly at an early age.[63] One study found that suicide attempters had more residential mobility, school changes, living with persons other than parents, and parent death or separation than control adolescents,[6] suggesting they had been subject to unexpected separations from meaningful relationships earlier in life.

Connell postulated that, in the face of the above, children with personality resources inadequate to deal with rejection and lack of family support show increasing emotional decompensation involving loss of self-esteem, shown by depressive symptomatology much of which is evident to teachers and school nurses:

Underfunctioning at school

Somatic symptoms (headache, abdominal pain)

Change in mood observed by others

Social withdrawal

"Compensatory symptoms": stealing, overeating

Thoughts of suicide communicated to others

Previous suicide attempts

Bouts of weeping

Sleep disturbances

Finally a trivial event acts as a trigger producing an impulsive act in which the child uses firearms or drugs available in the house, or a car.[62] More epidemiological work is required to sort out the causal and manifestational variables in this condition, as Gould wrote: "To understand the psychodynamic meaning of a suicide attempt one must realize that we are not dealing with a discrete, clinical entity, but rather a symptomatic act which may have multiple causes in varying combinations . . . the suicide attempt represents an effort to resolve several conflicts".[56]

Adolescents who attempted suicide expressed their liking for school as being due to its social life. "To be excluded from school was considered by these adolescents tantamount to exclusion from one of the key potential resources for establishing meaningful social relationships. This is even more true for the suicide attempter who has already been excluded from many of the resources still open to the average teenager."[64] Jacobs wrote of the preventive potential of schools for the suicidal adolescent who sees a complete breakdown of social relationships. Prevention of these suicides would require that schools recognize and attempt to achieve what adolescents see as the school's main virtue, to provide a place for them to meet and socialize with each other.[65]

The condition is serious, of significant size, and growing, and much of it detectable and preventable by schools. There would seem to be little reason why specific school-based suicide prevention programs should not be a feature of school health services.

Injuries

In the total population, injuries occurring as a result of accidents have shown two trends: (1) an increase in the injury rate, but (2) a decrease in overall fatalities from accidents (Tables 3–7 and 3–8). Some of the reduction in work injuries is due to the diminished proportion of blue-collar workers in the labor force and to enforcement of safety standards. Home injuries may be related to the number of home appliances and gadgets and the number of persons engaged in home repairs and projects. The increased death rate from motor vehicle accidents conceals the fact that deaths per 100 million vehicle-miles traveled dropped from 5.7 in 1966 to 4.2 in 1973, attributed to better road and car design, driver training, use of seat belts, and improved emergency medical care.[27]

Injury Mortality.   Accidents are the largest cause of death in children. Table 3–9 shows the distribution of accident deaths for five-to-fourteen-year-olds.

Table 3–7. Injuries from Accidents per 1,000 Population per Year

Place of accident	1962	1972
Motor vehicle	12	23
Work	47	39
Home	127	118
Other	105	145

Source: Cambridge Research Institute.[27]

Table 3–8. Deaths from Accidents per 1,000 Population per Year

Place of accident	1950	1972
Motor vehicle	.23	.27
Other	.37	.27

Source: Cambridge Research Institute.[27]

Motor vehicle deaths are of two types: (1) those in which the child is inside a vehicle involved in a crash; often seat belts are not worn although it has been shown that restrained children in the back seat have half the injury rate, in automobile crashes, of unrestrained children in the front seat;[67] (2) those where the child is a pedestrian. In one study, children aged five to nine accounted for 24 percent of all urban pedestrian accidents. Children of this age have developmental limitations in ability to perceive all traffic, especially that in front and behind them; these limitations, plus lack of impulse control, cause problems when children and traffic are mixed, such as when children travel to and from school and engage in after-school play in residential neighborhoods with few play facilities and little restriction on traffic flow. Improved lighting and one-way traffic are associated with a 20 percent reduction in pedestrian accidents.[68]

The death rate from drowning in ages five to fourteen—almost 5 per 100,000—is higher than for any other age-group.[68] These acci-

Table 3–9. Deaths from Accidents per 1,000 Population Aged 5–14, 1973

Motor vehicle accidents	.11
Drowning	.04
Fires, burns	.01
Other	.05
Total	.21

Source: National Safety Council.[66]

dents are unique in respect to their high mortality rate and because nonfatal incidents rarely cause injury. In a study of neardrowning accidents in Sweden, the proportion of fatal to nonfatal accidents was 45:1.5. Borderline cases with cardiac arrest may survive; in a Swedish series of 35 survivors of near drowning, severe brain damage was present in 6 percent.[69]

Preschool children often drown in shallow, unprotected water of ditches, ponds, pools. School-age children drown in lakes, pools, and the sea, in connection with bathing; often under "supervision" of parents or teachers who display ignorance of water safety measures and of the appropriate reaction to a drowning accident. The beneficial effects of swimming lessons and of safety fencing and screening of private pools and other water collections have been a decrease in mortality.[69]

Accidents are the leading cause of death in the adolescent age-group. Motor vehicles head the list, but other products related to home and recreational pursuits are constantly added: firearms, private planes, snowmobiles, minibikes, skateboards, motorcycles. There are cultural pressures for risk taking and aggressive competition among boys. Preventive measures, such as consumer product safety, seem to have little effect, and safety education programs appear slow to see the problem.[70]

Injury Morbidity.   Data collected on injuries sustained from accidents show that the rates in childhood and youth are almost double those occurring in the adult years (Table 3–10). Although the age ranges in which the data are published are broad, allowing only for gross generalizations regarding the characteristics of the population, some interesting features can be discerned. Children aged six to sixteen suffered their greatest number of injuries from falls, bumps, moving objects, cutting or piercing instruments, and twisting or stumbling. The five leading causes of injury for youth aged seventeen to twenty-four, many of whom are still in school, were motor vehicles, falls, bumps, cutting or piercing instruments, and moving objects.

Children aged six to sixteen had the highest injury rate in the population for accidents occurring outside moving motor vehicles (among which are school buses), for nonmotor vehicles in motion (which must include bicycles), cutting or piercing instruments, bumps into objects or persons, being struck by moving objects, handling or stepping on rough objects, and twisting or stumbling.

Youth aged seventeen to twenty-four had the highest rates for injuries incurred while inside a moving motor vehicle, from machinery in operation, and from foreign bodies in eye, windpipe, or other orifice.

Table 3–10. **Injuries per 1,000 Population per Year, Selected Causes, 1971–1972**

	All ages	Under 6	6–16	17–24	25–44	45–64	65+
Moving motor vehicle	23.2	7.0	19.8	56.1	26.3	16.0	9.7
Outside	2.2	1.6	3.0	2.7	2.4	1.0	1.9
Inside	20.7	5.4	16.5	52.7	23.9	14.6	6.8
Nonmotor vehicle in motion	5.9	10.4	17.5	2.1	2.0	0.5	1.2
Machinery in operation	6.2	—	2.0	13.4	9.6	7.4	1.8
Cutting or piercing instruments	20.6	14.9	34.6	26.6	17.3	13.6	9.7
Foreign body in eye, windpipe, or other orifice	7.2	10.9	6.1	12.0	8.5	3.9	2.9
Injury caused by animal or insect	13.2	25.2	18.5	7.6	10.9	9.0	10.7
Fall on stairs, steps, or from a height	21.7	52.8	27.7	15.6	16.1	13.5	14.4
All other falls	45.3	63.3	63.0	39.0	25.3	33.4	69.2
Bumped into object or person	27.8	24.0	50.8	36.8	21.9	14.8	9.0
Struck by moving object	20.2	23.5	38.1	24.8	15.6	8.5	5.7
Handling & stepping on rough object	11.4	15.7	18.5	13.2	9.2	6.0	4.7
Twisted or stumbled	14.2	0.9	24.7	19.4	14.5	10.3	5.0
Complications of medical, or surgical procedures	12.1	41.5	10.7	11.0	7.8	6.6	7.6
Total persons injured	311.9	393.6	391.8	386.2	289.2	209.7	211.8

Source: Adapted from National Center for Health Statistics.[71]

It should be noted that children aged six to sixteen carry on some of the injury patterns of the young-child population in their second highest population rates for falls and injuries from animals or insects. They also show a trend toward the patterns of older groups in the presence of injuries from machinery in operation—where it is not known, for example, what proportion of such injuries are sustained at home, in the school shop, or in actual work settings.

Injuries due to complications of medical and surgical procedures occur at higher rates in children and youth than in adults; the reasons are not apparent.

School Injuries.   A study of school accidents in the town of Greenwich, Connecticut, conducted by the Yale University School of Medicine in 1976–1978 underscored the extraordinary lack of data on this subject. The researchers wrote, "The body of literature relating to school accidents is extremely sparse."[72] The Index Medicus referred to accidents to school-age children but not to school accidents. Literature reviews on childhood accident prevention discuss primarily the preschool child. No information was available from large insurance companies or the Connecticut Department of Public Safety. The National Safety Council collects data from 32,000 school jurisdictions on accidents severe enough to cause the loss of one half-day or more of school time or of activity during school time. The data are published by grouped grade levels, such as seventh-to-ninth grades, and as accidents per 100,000 students days and are impossible to render as rates per student enrollment by grade level. The data indicated that grades 7 to 9 have the highest accident rates, with the greatest number of accidents occurring during physical education programs, followed by classroom and auditorium activities, interscholastic sports, time spent in corridors, vocational programs, and arts programs.[73]

The Greenwich study pointed out the paucity of data existing at the school level. This lack of information is due in part to laxity in completing forms, to the lack of understanding of injuries by those providing data, and to the fact that the accident-reporting system in schools is designed to record facts relevant to legal and financial liability and not to accident prevention and safety.[72] On special forms, data were collected over 2 years. The study showed the accident incidence rate per year and related data (see Table 3–11.)

Equipment caused 7.8 percent of accidents in the junior high school. Trips and excursions accounted for about 2 percent at all school levels. The greatest number of injuries occurred to the head; abrasions and bruises were more common at the elementary level and sprains in high school; factures accounted for 2.1 percent of injuries in elementary school, 3.2 percent in junior high, and 9.7 percent in senior high school; higher rates occurred in March, days earlier in the week, around midday recess in elementary school but at the beginning and

Table 3–11.

School Level	Accidents per 100 students per year	Percentage of accidents occurring in games & sports	Most frequent accident site, %	
Elementary	7.2	52	School grounds	42
Junior high	10.5	59	Gymnasium	34
Senior high	3.7	79	Gymnasium	45

Source: Grosso et al.[72]

end of the day in high school. "Malicious acts" were deemed the activity causing injury in 10 percent of elementary accidents, 7.2 percent of junior high school, and 2.4 percent of senior high school accidents.[72]

Investigators in Seattle, using the usual school accident reports, found that student aggressive behavior accounted for 9 to 15 percent of student injuries, with fighting being the main activity in high school and pushing in elementary school. The authors noted that "although aggression is accepted as a factor in auto accidents, it seems to be much more important as a factor in school accidents. The problem of aggressive behavior and conflict in schools invites further research."[74] Injuries incurred through aggressive acts occurred as shown in Table 3–12.

Product-Related Injuries. An additional way to look at injuries occurring in children is data from the National Electronic Injury Surveillance System, which gathers information on product-related trauma from 119 selected hospital emergency rooms in the United States.[68] The most common product sources of accidents in the five-to-fourteen age-group are bicycles (where five-to-fourteen-year-olds account for 61 percent of injuries), playground equipment, nails and carpet tacks, baseballs, swimming pools and related equipment, footballs, storage furniture, architectural glass and glass doors, beds, and liquid fuels (where five-to-fourteen-year-olds account for 24 to 59 percent of injuries.) Falls, often with head injuries, are the usual pattern in accidents involving bicycles, playground equipment, and beds.[68]

Epidemiology and Prevention. Understanding and prevention of accidents has been advanced by application of epidemiologic principles, enabling multiple causation to be addressed[75] while also providing a conceptual framework.[76] Collection of appropriate data has been and is a problem. Nonaccidents must be eliminated where possible; for example, it was estimated in one study that 16 percent of those admitted to a children's burn center were victims of child abuse.[77]

Table 3–12.

Injury	Elementary, %	Junior high, %	Senior high, %
Loss of teeth	22	9	5
Eye injuries	1	8	14
Fractures	11	2	18
Major site of aggression	Playground	Classroom	Corridor

Source: Johnson, Carter, Harlin, and Zoller.[74]

Injury, like disease, results from an unfavorable interaction between an etiologic agent (e.g., mechanical energy, thermal or electric energy, chemicals) and a susceptible host, occurring in a particular environment. The unfortunate tendency has been to see different accident or injury rates in different groups and proceed to "blame the victim" or educate him or her without looking for the underlying etiologic factors that increase the likelihood of the host meeting, for example, mechanical energy.[76] Teenagers have high injury rates because of the increase in quantity and quality of exposure as, for example, they become drivers of motor vehicles.[78] The concept of vehicle-miles allows for injury rates to be developed according to exposure.

The developmental level of children provides (1) hazard exposure, as when the toddler tries to manage stairs, the kindergartener goes further into traffic patterns, the junior high student works in shop class; and (2) the developmental lags or immaturities of that particular age (in young elementary school children, the lack of traffic perception already alluded to; the lack of cognitive abilities to understand risk; and the immaturity of psychosocial development needed to control impulses.) There appears to be a lack of knowledge among parents and child-minding adolescents of certain developmentally related safety practices.[79]

Sex differences reflect differences in exposure, such as more exposure of girls to household burns and of boys to moving vehicles. Those who are economically disadvantaged are more likely to be exposed to substandard housing and hazardous appliances. The higher drowning rate among blacks may be due in part to lack of swimming education.

There has been discussion in the past of the "accident-prone" individual as one with a certain personality characteristic.[80,81] What is being discussed is accident repetitiveness, which appears to be distributed normally in the population.[77] There is evidence that children who have repetitions of accidents tend to come from environments with increased exposure to inadequate play facilities and to poor and overcrowded housing where there is also marital disharmony, family separation, and illness.[80] Other researchers have documented that children undergoing stressful changes in their lives are more susceptible to accidents for limited periods of time and not as a lifetime personality characteristic.[81]

Approaches to prevention found successful in occupational settings but not tried in schools revolve around preventing or reducing the contact between the person (host) and the source of energy by:

Removing the energy source, such as flammable liquids, from premises

Removing the host from the energy source, such as removing children from traffic by a pedestrian bridge

Reducing the amount of energy, by, for example, making a street one-way to decrease number of cars

Erecting barriers to release of energy, for example, seat belts, electrical insulation, mechanical barriers

Erecting barriers to receipt of energy by host, for example, fire screen, fire doors

Modifying and dispersing the release of energy, as with automatic controls on hot water systems to reduce scalding and chemical fumes channeled away from operators in a fume cupboard

Modifying contact points between energy source and host, as by rounding of surfaces

Strengthening the host by, for example, athletic conditioning, swimming training, or perceptual aids

Reducing damage by increased response and ability of emergency systems and life-saving and rehabilitation services[76]

Various measures by which the environment may be modified probably have the greatest unrealized potential for prevention. To identify such methods of control is an epidemiologic function.[75] Little attention has been directed at the problem despite its magnitude. The National Academy of Sciences noted in 1965 how federal research grants were apportioned (see Table 3–13). In 1971 the following statement was given in testimony before a subcommittee of the U. S. House Committee of Appropriations:

Recently at a large children's hospital, the case of a young child was discussed who had retained a heart transplant for a month before dying. There was much enthusiasm expressed by the surgeons and immunologists who had accomplished this tremendous feat. They are all ready to try again. Not surprisingly, no mention was made of the heart donor. He happened to be a healthy youngster riding in

Table 3–13.

Condition	Cases	Research $ per case
Cancer	540,000	$220.00
Cardiovascular diseases	1,420,000	76.00
Disabilities due to accidents	10,000,000	0.50

Source: Schaplowsky.[82]

the back seat of a car traveling at 10 miles per hour when it was struck at an intersection. He was not in his seat belt. Both children should be alive—but consider the attention being devoted to cures versus the attention given to prevention.[83]

The Illness Experience

The overall experience of illness by the schoolchild population presents a different view from that of most of this chapter, which concentrates more on the expression of a certain type of disease condition within the schoolchild population. This section briefly examines a number of aspects of the experience of illness and disease reported in studies of representative samples of the nation's childhood population by the National Center for Health Statistics supplemented by the findings of others.

Conditions.

Acute Conditions. The outstanding characteristic of acute conditions among children is that the incidence rate is higher than in the rest of the population (see Table 3–14). This fact presents problems to parents who work, to schools, which are faced with potentially more absence due to acute illness than other occupational settings, and to the children involved, who suffer distress, discomfort, and loss of education.

Thus the average child of school age has just over 2.5 acute conditions per year. The major acute condition, respiratory illness, accounts for over half of the total.[84,85] Recent work which suggests that early diagnosis and home care reduce the length of absence from respiratory illness has important preventive implications for school health services and fiscal implications for school districts reimbursed by the state for days of attendance. Children with asthma have a significantly higher absentee rate (absent 8.4% of days) than do nonas-

Table 3–14.

Age-group	Number of acute conditions per 100 population per year, 1961
0–4	373
5–14	256
15–24	189
25–44	172
45–64	134
65+	119

Source: Schiffer and Hunt.[84]

thmatic children (absent 5.9% of days).[86] Injuries constituted 17 percent of the total acute conditions of children aged six to sixteen in 1973.[87]

Little attention has been given to the acute health conditions that children bring to school or that develop during the school day. These are of importance given the greater employment of mothers, busing, and the use of special education centers, all of which mean that the sick child and his or her parent are farther from each other. Contacting the parent is more complex and time-consuming, and the time it takes for the parent to get to the school is longer. Thus the school's role in providing direct care for the acutely ill child is increasing.

A similar problem has existed in day care centers, where there has always been a greater committment to care for the child until the end of the working day. Lakin et al. found the literature on the subject descriptive rather than analytic and discovered little data on the nature and incidence of minor illnesses. A minor illness inventory was developed as a standard tool for the needed research.[88]

Chronic Conditions. Accurate data on chronic conditions of children are difficult to obtain. The National Health Interview Survey provides the major source of information but, unfortunately, the method is rather inaccurate and the sample size too small to give reliable prevalence statistics on chronic conditions in children. The 1959–1961 survey revealed that almost one child in four under seventeen years of age had a chronic condition. The prevalence of conditions increased with age, from 169 per 1,000 children aged zero to four to 309 per 1,000 children aged fifteen to sixteen. Asthma, hay fever and other allergies, and respiratory conditions accounted for 48 percent, and paralysis and orthopedic problems for 12 percent of the total.[84]

Prevalence data on selected chronic conditions with particular importance for school attendance (asthma, chronic bronchitis) and school performance (heart conditions, hearing impairments, vision impairments) are given in Table 3–15. It appears that asthmatic children, possibly because they are confined indoors during the winter more than nonasthmatics, have an increased incidence of viral respiratory infections compared with their nonasthmatic siblings and that the rhino-virus involved in these respiratory illnesses is also important in precipitating attacks of asthma.[90]

Findings.

Health History.   The cumulative history of illness experience in the total lives of children can be seen in the health histories obtained from parents (Table 3–16). The number of children who have experienced severe trauma, hospitalization, and operations grows with age. Certain chronic conditions (running ears, trouble with talking, eye trouble) are more prevalent at younger ages and are apparently forgot-

Table 3–15.

Condition	Prevalence per 1,000 persons under 17
Asthma	31.1
Chronic bronchitis	38.9
Heart conditions	10.5
Hearing impairments	13.0
Vision impairments	9.4

Source: National Center for Health Statistics.[89]

ten in older age-groups as the condition clears or the correction, such as glasses, removes the problem. Other chronic conditions (asthma, hay fever, kidney and heart conditions, and trouble with walking) gradually accumulate more victims, a fact probably also reflected in the growing percentage of children taking medicine regularly (and needing to take it at school). Parents asked to evaluate the health of their children considered present health a problem in 19 percent of elementary-age children and 15 percent of high school children. Physicians, on physical examination, found three times more significant abnormalities in children whose health was rated poor by parents.[91]

Although families are not always accurate in their perception of the health status of their children, poor families worry more about the health of their children who, in fact, have a greater number of health problems than children of wealthier families.[92]

Physical Examination. Abnormalities found on physical examination vary by the definition of abnormality or defect, by the examining techniques used, and by the characteristics of the group of children examined. Lack of standardization of these aspects makes it impossible to compare findings in special studies or, unfortunately, to make much sense in terms of disease measures or trends of the findings from school physical examinations performed so regularly and widely over the past half century.

The National Health Examination Survey of a representative sample of the nation's children and the study of all children in the comunity of Bogalusa,[93] using similar methodologies, found that approximately 11 percent of children aged six to eleven had physical abnormalities, with boys having higher rates than girls. School physical examinations, which include more minor anomalies and deviations, found in the famous 1942 Astoria study, 57 percent with defects;[94] in the 1947–1953 Maine Program, 63 percent had "adverse conditions";[95] and in Philadelphia in 1970–1971, the examination of 69,275 students revealed 43 percent with defects.[96]

The leading conditions found and their prevalence in the Bogalusa community are indicated in Table 3–17. That relatively few types of

Table 3–16. Percentage of Children (1963–1965) and Youth (1966–1970) with Medical History of Selected Conditions and Experiences

	Age			
	6	9	12	15
Accidents				
Broken bones	5.5	7.3	16.4	19.3
Knocked unconscious	2.2	2.9	7.2	8.3
Allergies				
Asthma	4.2	5.5	5.0	6.0
Hay fever	3.5	5.8	7.1	9.6
Kidney conditions	3.9	4.2	3.3	5.6
Heart conditions	3.5	3.1	4.7	5.1
Sensory-neurologic conditions				
Convulsion	2.7	3.8	3.3	2.6
Eye trouble	6.4	16.1	6.6	6.2
Hearing trouble	3.7	4.8	3.0	4.4
Running ears	12.3	11.6	9.7	9.8
Trouble talking	12.9	7.1	4.9	4.0
Trouble walking	1.6	1.7	2.2	2.4
Operations	23.8	32.3	35.8	40.3
Hospitalized more than once	23.4	27.5	47.0	51.8
Taking medicine regularly	3.7	4.7	5.9	7.2

Source: National Center for Health Statistics.[91]

health problems are found on physical examination is immediately apparent from the table. Study of results obtained by school examinations reveals large numbers of minor findings, such as that 25 percent of the Astoria children were classified as having a "condition" of the tonsils,[94] 16 percent of the Maine group had "pronated feet"[95] and 4.6 percent of Philadelphia's children had wax in the ears.[97]

Table 3–17.

Condition	Number per 100 children
Obesity	2.9
Undernourished	2.4
Dental problems	2.6
Cardiovascular	1.5
Skin	1.2
Blood pressure	0.6

Source: Blonde et al.[93]

Functional Limitations.

Disability Days.   The volume of acute conditions in children of school age and the presence of chronic conditions are reflected in the large number of days on which children cannot engage in their usual activities and may be confined to bed.[84] Acute conditions account for the largest share of time lost from usual activity. The average child between the ages of six and sixteen in 1974/75 had just over 2.5 acute conditions per year leading to almost 4 days in bed, 8.6 days of restricted activity, and 4.5 days lost from school.[87] Girls have higher rates than boys, and urban rates are higher than rural.[85]

On the other hand, children with chronic conditions suffer a disproportionate burden of functional limitation. Six percent of children with asthma have 15 or more days in bed per year.[89] In 1969/1970, 3 percent of the noninstitutionalized childhood population under the age of seventeen were limited in their activity by a chronic condition. Over 50 percent of the group were unable to go to school or could engage in schooling only in a limited fashion.[92] Of particular interest are the higher rates for functional limitation due to illness in families with lower incomes. In 1973 children in families with incomes under $5,000 experienced an average 7.3 lost school days per year, whereas the rate for those in families with incomes of $15,000 and over was 4.6 days/year.[85]

Absenteeism.   Reduction of massive absenteeism was the outstanding contribution made to education by nurses when they were first introduced to schools at the begining of the twentieth century. The victory won was not only the result of improving the basic health of students but was also due to the assistance nurses gave parents in overcoming the school's administrative requirements in regard to infectious disease. The nurses clarified the notice from the school for parents, provided assistance in complying with requirements, and facilitated the flow of children back into school. The example is instructive in that it clearly shows that the phenomenon of absenteeism is complex and includes factors other than illness. Generally, the relationship between health, absence, and education is conceptualized as follows:

Decreased health status	→	Increased absenteeism	→	Decreased education

The relationship, derived from data presented below, may be closer to the schema of Figure 3–6.

The National Health Survey for 1971–1972 reported an average of 4.7 days of absence from school for children six to sixteen years old because of acute illness or injury.[92] Absences due to all causes, reported in a Pittsburgh high school in 1965, averaged 6 to 9 days and three to five episodes per student per year.[98] In five primary schools in Jerusalem, Israel, in 1969/70 the absentee pattern was remarkably similar: mean days of absence per child was 8.2 (standard deviation 7.2) and mean number of episodes of absence per child was 3.9 (standard deviation 3.2).[99] About 10 percent of a sample of Delaware students had perfect attendance, and 73.5 percent of the absence episodes lasted one day or less, yet at the other end of the scale of absentee experience was 40 separate episodes of absence and 140 days absent.[100]

Most researchers agree that school[101] and occupational[102] populations exhibit a high degree of consistency in their absence behavior and that similar consistency holds for individuals within the population.[98,101,102] This uneven distribution of absences within the population is interesting in light of the major immediate causes of absence—acute infectious illnesses—which would be expected to affect the population in a relatively random fashion.

Rogers and Reese classified immediate causes of absence of Pittsburgh high school students in a number of ways (Tables 3–18 and 3–19). About 75 percent to 80 percent of absences were due to illness. Respiratory disease (and respiratory disease manifested as general systemic illness) accounted for about 80 percent and gastrointestinal disease 15 to 20 percent. Trauma was associated with 4 percent of absences. About 60 percent of absences due to illness involved at least one day of bed disability. Rogers and Reese noted that these findings were in agreement with most morbidity surveys of children and young adults; "namely, that absenteeism due to illness or injury is common, that these illnesses and injuries are rarely serious from the standpoint

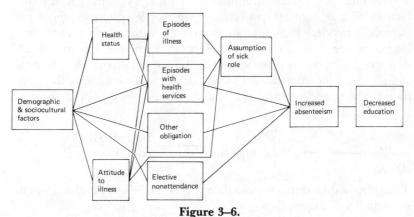

Figure 3–6.

Table 3–18.

Descriptive categories	Mean daily absence incidence per 1,000 students
Respiratory illness	6–11
General systemic illness	2–8
Gastrointestinal illness	2–5
Other illness	1–4
Health care	1–2
Not ill; legal absence	2–4
Not ill; illegal absence	1–5

Source: Rogers and Reese.[98]

Table 3–19.

Etiologic categories	Percentage of absences
Infection	41–51
Necessary obligation	9–16
Physiologic (female)	8
Elective	3–13
Trauma	2–7
Fatigue	2–6
Non-infectious noxious agent	2–5
Emotional	1–4
Combined etiology	1–3
Unknown and other	13–17

Source: Rogers and Reese.[98]

of death or permanent disability, and that certain persons consistently are absent more frequently than others." Study of the health of those children with high frequency of absences revealed no clues in absence pattern, absence cause, physical examination, or performance on standard fitness test.[98]

About 20 percent to 25 percent of absences reported by Rogers and Reese were for nonillness. In males half were "necessary" absences for such reasons as helping at home, job interviews, religious holidays, medical or dental care, visits to college for interview, and interscholastic events; the other half were "elective" absences and largely consisted of truancy.[98] Others have noted family crises, transportation and weather problems, and family health events.[101]

Characteristics of students with high absence frequency were overage for grade,[100] lower academic performance,[98,100] lower rates of participation in school activities, and higher rates for out-of-school work, dropping out,[98] and visits to the school nurse.[98,101] Environmental and demographic characteristics associated with high absence behavior have been shown to include female sex,[99] minority race, lower socioeconomic class, urban location, parental separation,[100] being eldest child, lower parental expectations for child's future education, and child's dislike of school.[101] It has also been shown that children with poorer diet have more absences, and that parents who are more sensitive to symptoms are more likely to keep children home.[101] This latter phenomenon probably explains the Israeli observation that absences for respiratory infections are higher in the higher socioeconomic groups.[99]

It is concluded that high absence behavior is not completely understood. It is "a highly complex phenomenon, dependent upon social, educational, and demographic variables".[100] High-risk groups would appear to be those with certain attitudes, family health characteristics, and types of stress. It is obvious that study of individual episodes of illness yields little insight.[102] Newer statistical probability models, such as the "absence liability level" that reveals differences in the form of absenteeism among various subgroups of the population,[103] provide tools for the needed epidemiologic study of absence behavior and influences upon it, for example, family-centered nursing intervention.[104]

Use of Resources.

Hospital Use and Experience.   In any given year about 5 percent of children under seventeen years of age are hospitalized once.[85] Seventy percent stay less than 6 days; the majority (90 percent) are admitted to general hospitals, where they constituted 17 percent of the patients in 1961; over one-half have surgery for removal of tonsils and adenoids, appendectomies, hernia repair, and reduction of fractures and dislocations.[84]

Low-income children are more likely to be admitted to hospital and stay longer once there: 5.2 days average length of stay in 1973 for those under fifteen years of age compared with a national average of 4.6 days.[105] These figures represent a distinct improvement from the mid-1960s. The number of hospitalizations of poor children has increased but length of stay has decreased, indicating that access to care has improved and severity of illness has been reduced. The main reason is found in government health insurance programs, such as medical assistance (See Table 3–20).

Table 3–20.

| | Children under 17 years of age | |
	Poor	Not poor
Number of discharges from hospital per 1,000		
1964	58	70
1973	96	63
Average length of stay in days		
1964	9.1	5.4
1973	6.4	5.3

Source: National Center for Health Statistics.[106]

Physician Visits. The average child under seventeen years of age makes about four visits to a physician per year. The number is greater for higher-income groups and those in metropolitan areas. During 1964 to 1973, with medical assistance, the number of visits to physicians made by poor children under seventeen years of age increased from 2.3 to 3.8 visits per child per year compared with 4.3 visits per nonpoor child. The percentage of children who see no physician for 2 years varies by income and minority status and has changed with time as shown in Table 3–21. The contact between child and physician is usually in the physician's office (64 percent) and by phone (20 percent) for white children and less often in the office (49 percent) and by phone (8 percent) for minority children, who get more care in hospital outpatient clinics (17 percent) and hospital emergency rooms (11 percent). Home visits account for less than 2 percent of the total.[85]

Mental Health Services. The 1977 national survey of children done by the Foundation for Child Development found that over 7 percent of children aged seven to eleven had an "emotional, behavior, mental or learning problem" so severe that parents felt or were told that the children needed professional help. About two-thirds of the total (or 5 percent of the population) received some sort of professional help during the year. 2.6 percent saw a psychologist or psychiatrist within the year.[31]

Table 3–21.

	Minority poor, %	White, not poor, %
1964	39	14
1973	22	11

Source: National Center for Health Statistics.[85]

There is evidence that the number of children seeing psychologists and psychiatrists increased 60 percent between 1966–1970 and 1977, indicating growing acceptance and availability of such services.[91,107] A random survey of households with children under fifteen in 12 counties in southwestern Pennsylvania found that 55 percent of parents with children with "learning, social or emotional" problems had sought counseling from school personnel and 70 percent had found the counseling very or moderately helpful.[108]

Psychosocial Disorders

Behavioral and Emotional Problems. There is little doubt that more emotional disturbance is recognized today than in 1932, when Isaacs wrote, "There seems reason to think that neurotic difficulties of many different types, and of varying grades of severity and persistence, are fairly common among children."[109] Isaacs noted many of the milder manifestations of normal development, and that whether a child will "grow out of" them or not depends on the degree to which environmental influences, such as the birth of a sibling, fit in with the dominant fantasies of the child at the time.

Long in 1941 studied the waxing and waning of undesirable behavior in 338 normal children, as reported by parents. Children averaged about five to nine behavior "tendencies" in each age-group. The three-to-four-year-olds exhibited behavior—capriciousness, bedwetting, temper tantrums—expected from their immature physiologic and psychologic states. The five-to-six-year-olds with whining and impudent talking were adjusting to the new school environment and its requirements and competitions, often without parental understanding of the transitional difficulties faced by the children. The seven-to-ten-year-old group, still inexperienced in socially acceptable ways of getting what they wanted, resorted to willful or stubborn behavior patterns. This group also had to orient themselve to growing school experiences and other demands, exhibited irritability and fears, and were easily discouraged. The eleven-to-fourteen-year-old group exhibited selfishness, shyness, and conflicts with parents over bedtime. In regard to schoolwork and other duties they were considered overly conscientious or avoiding responsibility or satisfied with efforts below their ability. More behavior problems were seen in lower socioeconomic classes, but Long concluded that "some parents in all classes are confronted with difficult behavior problems in their children" and that although some parents possessed superior ability many did not use methods of child training thought to be psychologically sound. "Successful parenthood . . . may be greatly facilitated by . . . understanding. . . the specifics of child development."[110]

Parents see and must cope with the behavioral problems of their children. Children who experience such "normal," developmentally determined difficulties may be pushed into deeper troubles if they are in a family that is unable to respond appropriately. Such children show deviant patterns as they enter school. Some are victims of "distorted and disturbed parental attitudes" that negatively affect the children's development, and in others their deviant growth and development are the result of "overwhelming social stresses within the family" where parental concentration on survival leaves little for the child's nurture.[111] Starting school may precipitate behavioral difficulties and make problems more noticeable than when the child was home.[32]

Teachers are exposed to large numbers of children with emotional problems and have had direct experience of children with severe problems. Teachers, not surprisingly, correctly identify emotional disorders among children at a much higher rate than the general public. The general public seems less able to identify paranoid behavior in a child, as indicative of mental illness, than in an adult.[112]

For the child whose home life has been less than successful, school can provide the second great chance. Schooling starts early; teachers, with their experience and their vantage point from which any individual child can be measured "against a normal range of bahavior in a single natural setting," can detect problems early; classwork can be a matter of "reassuring accomplishment and growth"; schooling socializes, "takes over status placement," lasts into adolescence, and "conditions occupational possibilities."[32]

Moreover, schools have been given the task of taking care of most of the emotionally disturbed children in society. Yet they can fail miserably. School can be "the scene of repeated defeat and humiliation, of confusion and distress," and teachers who ask for appropriate help for a child find a long time between request and receipt.[32] Asking for help may be "considered a sign of failure" in some schools.[113]

In 1960 it was written, "The present state of affairs in the relationship of the school to the emotionally handicapped child was found to resemble a negative spiral fed by reciprocal hostility, from which emerged a non-successful, bewildered or vengeful adolescent."[114] It is not known if the situation has measurably improved, although numbers of demonstrations have provided "evidence that delivering help through the schools is a promising direction."[32]

The Commission on Teacher Education of the American Council on Education published, in 1945, a report of a successful demonstration countering aspects of school harmful to children. The essential failure of schools was seen as not recognizing the developmental nature of childhood and adolescence. Teachers are skilled in making hundreds of judgments each day about "abilities, motives, feelings, attitudes, conduct and needs of the pupils" and the characteristics of the class or group and the interaction of its members; and on the basis of these judgments setting tasks, stimulating interest and learning, and choosing methods of controlling their actions. "Faulty judgments" are made where teachers have not been prepared to understand children from a developmental perspective.[115]

The results, as described by the commission, are that children struggling with developmental tasks and adjustment problems are unrecognized; those with physical problems, limited mental abilities, severe emotional maladjustments, delinquent tendencies, or who are neglected and abused are either ignored or stigmatized before being understood; the development of necessary skills, learning, or appropriate behavior is made difficult by failure to take into account a child's developmental level, progress in mastering developmental skills, and environmental and constitutional reasons for lack of experience, knowledge, interest, trust, or self-confidence; children may be left to flounder in teacher dislike or neglect and peer rejection; children's behavior is appraised in light of the environment's needs and not the child's; and control of behavior is often demeaning, humiliating, seen as unfair, and repressive of "valuable curiosity."[115]

The commission reported that, with better teacher understanding of education as "developmental rather than direct training," the same schooling processes could be used to ensure

> wholesome development for nearly all children. . . . There is no educative process for which chronological age, mental age, and score on reading test are the only important variables. Maturity level, adjustment problems, social status in the class, physical health, self-confidence, attitude toward the teacher, experience background, emotional stability and family situation are equally important factors that shape the child's motivation and determine his readiness for a particular learning task.

When all these variables are known, the needs of each child are clear. Group activities are the basis of classroom learning, but "a myriad of small and sometimes subtle variations" in handling individual children in the group can be used by the teacher.[115]

Helping teachers understand children and develop skills in handling their different needs has been the theme of other demonstrations that recognize that successful education in school is powerful "therapy." The source of assistance to teachers may be a mental health team,[32,116] with or without nonprofessional aide extenders to work directly with maladapted primary school children.[117]

The effectiveness of one program in elementary school, evaluated after 2½ years, was shown by an increase in student responsiveness to the positive developmental factors present in the school situation. The researchers had two conclusions regarding future programming: (1) In a reasonably adequate school the growth and developmental factors inherent in the school are adequate agents for the progress of most children; such strengths can be reinforced by mental health consultation to teachers on classroom management and to administrators on improving the school environment and by increased liaisons between parents and school. (2) Children with serious personality or learning problems need mental health treatment so that they also may respond to the positive atmosphere that can exist in a school, and grow.[118]

One study commented on the mental health role of the school nurse.[116] Public health nurses have developed collaborative efforts with mental health in a variety of areas,[119] including parent education,[116] and have been noted to have keen observation, easy access to children, and at times the ability to be the "only school staff able to achieve rapport with students in crises."[116] They carried out such clinical functions as interviewing parents, filled social work roles where no social worker was available, and used their strategic position with parents, school physicians, family physician, and administrators to deliver preventive services.[116]

Learning Problems.   Apparently normal children with normal intelligence who have difficulty in school may be classified as learning problems. The various types are:

1. *Organic* neurologic problems, for example, hydrocephalus, muscular dystrophy.[120]
2. *Environmental deprivation*, in which inadequate cognitive stimulation in impoverished environments produces children who have failed to develop skills in spatial relationships, time, number, classification of objects, and vocabulary, so that previous learning and schooling are not a continuous process. Lack of socialization, with hyperactivity and limited gratification delay, may also be present. Such children emerge from low socioeconomic backgrounds and situations of neglect. Structured preschool experiences, such as Head Start, can favorably affect intelligence measures.[121]
3. *Emotional problems*, including depression, fear, anxiety, and thought disorders. Neurotic reactions around various

aspects of learning have been described as due to individual emotional reactions to such family relationship problems as alcoholism, family brutality, defensive communication patterns, parental rivalry with the child, and derogation of the child's efforts.[121] These dependent, devalued children become more than normally anxious when faced with new learning situations in school. The anxiety either inhibits a child's acquisition of skills (inattention) or blocks ability to produce work (lack of cooperation). There are more boys than girls with emotional problems, possibly reflecting early school difficulties due to the slower neurologic maturation of boys, higher achievement pressure, and less (female) teacher tolerance of behavior unconformity. Successful intervention may require both psychological help and remedial education.

4. *Inadequate schooling* for a child due to poor teaching, crowded classrooms, frequent absences, or frequent changes of schools.[120]

5. *Poor communication,* which may have its origins in visual handicap,[120] hearing loss,[122] or a primary language other than English.

6. *Learning disability,* which affects 5 to 10 percent of the school-age population.[120] Difficulties are encountered in abilities to read, write, do math, comprehend and/or express language, and orient right-left. The cause is not clear. There is some association with prematurity, perinatal difficulties, encephalitis, and meningitis, and there appears to be a generalized underlying brain dysfunction. The condition appears to be related to "minimal brain dysfunction" (MBD), in which hyperactivity is present and learning problems appear in up to 90 percent of the cases.[123]

Minimal brain dysfunction is marked by short attention span, hyperactivity, fine and gross motor incoordination, perceptual cognitive disabilities in spatial or auditory discrimination and in transferring information from one sensory modality to another, poor impulse control, and inability to think ahead; a child is extroverted, resistant to social demands, and irritable and has temper tantrums. Attentional and perceptual-cognitive difficulties impede academic progress, especially in reading.[123]

Difficulties in socializing a child frequently lead to family problems because of guilt. There is an increased prevalence—about 50 to 60 percent— of "soft" neurologic signs and minor anatomic abnormalities. Children may present with hyperactive, neurotic, psychopathic, or learning disorder manifestations. There may be changes over the years depending on the response of the home and school environment. The irritable baby, constantly moving toddler, distractible and aggesssive kindergartner pleasing neither peers nor teacher, third-grader hostile when faced with increasingly difficult learning tasks becomes increasingly antisocial and is viewed as delinquent by the school. Often behavior in a group setting compared with at home or in the doctor's office is wildly distracted; thus the teacher is a prime source of diagnostic information.[123]

It is believed that MBD is a manifestation of several different etiologic conditions: brain insults, genetics, intrauterine development, fetal maldevelopment, and psychosocial experience. How the disease exerts its effect is not clear, but it is hypothesized that the central nervous system neurotransmitter nor-epinephrine is reduced, hence accounting for the often dramatic response to the drug amphetamine or the tricyclic antidepressants. Prognosis is not known. Some evidence that the condition persists into adulthood, but often with altered manifestations, needs further study. Drug therapy, family counseling, and remedial education are used in treatment. Particular vocational education and placement may be necessary for those still unable to read by adolescence.[123]

Secondary and tertiary prevention of learning problems appears possible based upon such longitudinal studies as the 12-year prospective study of reading retardation from Winnipeg, Canada. That study showed characteristics, detectable at school entry, associated with reading problems in later grades. Unevenness in specfic developmental patterns, such as auditory, visual-motor, and/or kinesthetic skills, at school entry were reflected in poor adjustment and performance in the first year. Noncongruence of mental and chronological age resulted in 23 percent of children failing to reach a satisfactory second-grade beginning level. Children referred to remedial reading class in third grade had scarcely begun to master basic skills, and by that time poor study habits and attitudes proved resistant to therapy.[124]

Reading problems were found to be closely correlated with IQ and the socioeconomic status of the child's family. Boys had rates similar to girls', a finding at variance with other clinical studies, suggesting that boys with school difficulties exhibit behavior likely to cause problems in the classroom and home and hence a speedy referral.[124] It is interesting that techniques that measure stress in school students and find it related to low socioeconomic status and school failure have described higher stress scores in girls than in boys,[125] suggesting that the difficulties experienced by girls remained unnoticed.

The Winnipeg authors suggested that many aspects of a child's future academic and social performance, such as competence, self-concept, stability, awareness, interest, and set toward further learning, have been determined largely before the child enters school. The view is supported by data showing correlations between preschool tests, sixth-grade achievement, and academic performance in the twelfth grade. The implications for schools are placement of children in programs geared to their level of competence in order to experience some early success, to remove pressures for impossible performance, and to reduce the likelihood of behavior problems and psychosomatic illness.[124]

School Phobia.   In the classic form of the school phobia a child exhibits severe anxiety and apprehension about coming to school and psychosomatic complaints. School phobia can occur at any age from kindergarten to adolescence but has two peaks: at the third and tenth grades. It affects girls more than boys, and usually there is no problem with school ability or performance. Physical complaints usually seen include morning nausea, abdominal pain and vomiting, and pains in various parts of the body. It is believed that the child fears leaving the mother because of the mother's anxiety and a "general family climate" in which the parent of the opposite sex has been rejected and the child is experiencing delayed grief reaction. Prognosis is excellent in the younger child and is aided by early detection, prompt intervention, and school and family cooperation. Successful counseling on the school premises has been reported. "Spontaneous" recovery without special therapy is no doubt due to the individual help and guidance given by teachers.[121]

Depression.   "The question of depression in children and adolescents has continued to receive little attention"[59] partly because adult-type disease entities have been looked for; yet McConville et al. described depression as the second most common symptom presented by children six to thirteen years old in an inpatient child psychiatric facility. They described three types of childhood depression: (1) affectual, more common in six-to-eight-year-olds, characterized by feelings of loneliness, emptiness, and alienation from parents and peers; (2) negative self-esteem, more common in eight-to-ten-year-olds; (3) guilt, more common in ten-to-thirteen-year-olds and usually following an acute loss or recent bereavement in which the children felt they were "wicked" and should make amends through suicide attempts.[126]

Symptoms that are relatively easy to detect in a school health program include headaches and somatic complaints, hypochondriacal complaints, loss of appetite, sleeping disorders, fatigue, fears of death, feelings of inferiority, boredom, restlessness, isolation, emptiness, and difficulty in concentration. No information is available on the effects of childhood or adolescent depression on future psychic function.[59]

Delinquency.   Delinquent children are describing as having severely inadequate homes with alcoholism, irresponsible and ignorant parents, rejection, physical and sexual abuse, and intolerable pressure to perform. In most cases schools recognize the child's problems but are unable to mobilize appropriate resources. James claimed that, in at least 80 percent of all cases taken to court, a school problem is an important factor and is noted again and again by teachers in the child's record.[127]

The causes of delinquency and even its definition are not decided. English work showed that the particular generation of children born between 1935 and 1942 and thus experiencing the dislocations of the Second World War were more delinquent in their teens than any other cohort.[128] Matters of social and political inequality, especially lack of economic and educational opportunities, rather than individual pathology and personal failure, are sought as causes.[129] The lack of understanding of causes has been filled by speculation and attempts at situational and systems approaches. Another view is that all children engage in deviance but they become "deviants" only "through contingencies, complaints, and decisions of human beings with some authority. The things which have been called delinquency are with small exception normal problems of socialization."[130] The problem arises as some but by no means all so-called deliquents are diverted into the juvenile justice system, with all the negative consequences of the label and the experience.[131]

The school may play two different roles in the current system. In the first, concern in schools for order, together with a low tolerance for male misbehavior, a tendency to see student behavior in terms of morality, and labeling of the deviant, provide a route from school into the juvenile justice system. "Conceptions of student problems held by diagnostic and remedial specialists in the schools tend to be subordinated to the strategic and administrative needs of the school as a whole, centered in the authority problems of the teacher-student relationship and the embattled position of schools in the community." In the second, systems have been established to divert deviants from the juvenile justice system to specialized classes and schools where there is evidence of lessened truancy, vandalism, and difficulties with teachers. Voluntary attendance, reduced expectations, individual instruction, and removal from competition change students' environment and set the stage for reduction of problems.[131]

The possibility of early detection exists not only in school records but also in medical histories. In the age-groups zero to four and fourteen to sixteen, delinquent children use hospital services for injuries significantly more than nondelinquents. Both age-groups are characterized developmentally by increased motor capacities and an imbalance between inner behavioral controls and heightened impulses. In both age-groups lack of parental control and structure results in more frequent injuries.[132] Early intervention might reduce the intrafamilial disturbance and prevent delinquent behavior.

Delinquent Gangs.   Theories offered for this behavior, usually by males, include that of "social disability" derived from an early life of harsh rearing, lack of cognitive stimulation, limited language use, and poor social skills. With these handicaps and generally lower intelligence, the boys are less rewarded by their schoolwork than are their brighter peers and are less able to get along with teachers and classmates. "In an effort to meet the universal need for relationships with other people, they drift into gang membership."[133]

Gang membership is a phase of life. The problem is that it offers few constructive tasks and inhibits the individual in exploration and achievement relevant to future life. In addition, delinquent activities and trouble with the law are more frequent the fewer are such other activity opportunities as "recreational centers, counseling agencies, churches, schools, chances to work." Possibly the most powerful preventive measure—at least for the older gang member—is a job immediately upon leaving school.[133]

Runaways.   Runaways, estimated at 600,000 to 1 million per year, represent a recently revealed underside of life in which the end result may be male and female prostitution, drugs, disease, rape, pregnancy, jail, and even murder. Many runaways, however, do move in with relatives or friends, find work and become self-supporting, or return to their families and attempt to solve problems.[134]

There is no doubt that some runaways have disturbed and rejecting families who do not want them back, but it is also true that work with those contemplating running away can prevent the trauma, possible tragedy, and interrupted education of that move while acting to reduce the family problem that led to the child's plan. There are reports from special police officers in schools,[134] child welfare agencies, and school nurses of successful intervention efforts based on "tips" from students or teachers or direct appeals from students to a listening adult, usually at school: "If something doesn't happen at home, I'm going to run away."[135]

Nutrition

Since the 1960's renewed attention has been paid in the United States to the effects on intellect and school achievement of poverty and poor health. In regard to the latter, nutrition has been seen to be a ubiquitous factor affecting growth, development, motivation, and resistance to disease. Unfortunately, as noted by Birch, "clarity of thought and concept has not kept pace with zeal" either to claim or disclaim the connection between nutrition and learning.[136] Given all the facts it can be concluded that:

1. Inadequate nutrition adversely affects growth and mental development.
2. The impact of inadequate nutrition depends to a large extent on its severity, timing, and duration.
3. Some degree of malnutrition is relatively widespread among poor children.[136]

Enormous gaps in knowledge remain on the quality or types of malnutrition; their severity, incidence, and duration; and the true prevalence of the various malnutritions. "The absence of such knowledge must not be taken to reflect the absence of the problem but rather the lack of attention which has been devoted to it."[136] Any analysis of the connection between poor nutrition and poor education brings into view a web of circumstances involving low income, poor housing, poor health, unemployment, and welfare status which constitute the physical, psychologic, social, economic, cultural, and political environments with which children interact in their growth and development.[136] A "web of causation" (Figure 3–7) has been constructed to show some of the relationships among these environmental factors, malnutrition, and poor school performance.[9]

Malnutrition and subnutrition are reflected in anthropometric measures.[136,137,138] The basic recommended measures are height and weight, triceps skin fold, and arm circumference, from which muscle mass can be calculated.[136] Interestingly, schools have performed height and weight measure for decades, often for health education reasons staff have forgotten, and therefore unfortunately at low levels of quality and without use of the best measurement norms. School data collected over the years cannot be used to establish the nutrition level of school-age population. An incredible waste!

The relationship between antecedent malnutrition (and thus depressed growth) and mental development has been demonstrated in population studies and in the follow-up of children hospitalized for a severe episode of malnutrition.[138] Animal studies have shown that

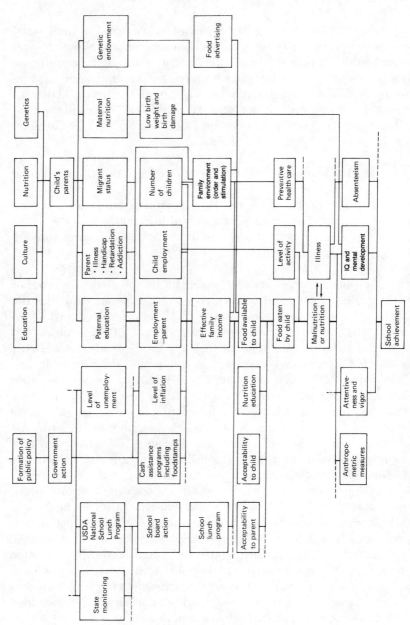

Figure 3–7.   Web of Causation: Malnutrition and Its Association with School Achievement, Adapted

severe and modest degrees of nutritional deprivation, experienced at the time that the nervous system is growing most rapidly, result in reduced brain size and myelination. These deficits are *not* made up later, when good diets are introduced. The human brain goes through its most rapid growth from midgestation to the age of one year, when it has achieved 70 percent of adult size; growth continues more slowly until body growth is completed in the late teen years.[136]

A relationship has been established between IQ and head circumference (an indirect measure of brain size).[139,140] Children whose head circumference is proportionally small have been shown to have significantly lower academic achievement scores.[139] Some recent work has found all anthropometric measures, particularly body weight, correlated with school achievement scores.[141]

The relationship between malnutrition and other possible etiologic factors in a child's environment is as follows:

1. The mother's genetic endowment and antecedent nutritional history when a child (a) affects intrauterine growth of the fetus, leading to greater prematurity (low birth weight), and (b) results in decreased maternal height and pelvic size, which with prematurity places the child at increased risk for brain damage at delivery. Lower birth weight is associated with lower IQ. Low birth weight affects 7 to 19 percent of births in the United States.

2. The proportion of children receiving poor diets rises as family income and education falls.[142] In 1965, 18 percent of families with incomes below $6,000 had poor diets containing less than two-thirds of the recommended allowance of one or more essential nutrients. Poverty has been associated with deficiencies in calories, lack of iron, and nutritional anemia;[142] vitamin C, calcium, and riboflavin deficiencies; deficiencies in all nutrients; lack of breakfast; and "irregular eating habits." In the latter group were "teenagers who appeared to be fending for themselves." Welfare status has been linked to the increased likelihood of poor diets.[136]

3. The link to illness is two-way. Nutritional inadequacy increases the risk of infection, interferes with immune mechanisms, and causes illness, which further impairs nutritional levels and also causes absenteeism from school. Illness is closely linked to the socioeconomic status of families and to family disorganization, both of which reduce use of preventive health services.

4. Cultural factors related to: 1. foods indigenous to a certain country or rural setting but less available as members of the

cultural group migrate to urban or other foreign settings may be seen in the high levels of vitamin A deficiency in children of Hispanic origin,[6] and to 2. eating, as seen in the irregular habits of teenagers.

5. Federal food programs have been reported (1968–1970) as having a negligible impact on the nutrient intake of young children, except for the school lunch program, which "made a significant contribution to the daily food intake of participating children."[142]

6. An adequate state of nutrition is "essential for good attention and appropriate and sensitive responses to the environment." Subnourished children also tire more easily from both physical and mental effort.[136]

7. Factors affecting family income are associated with nutritional changes. Body weight is greater with smaller family size and with maternal employment.[143] Karp et al. described the association between increases in food costs in the inflation of 1972–1975 and decreases in age norms for height, weight, and hemoglobin for children.[144]

8. It appears that some types of malnutrition are related to psychosocial and environmental stresses. Children hospitalized for undernutrition in the first year of life were more commonly found to be from families with "paternal separation; alcohol-related problems; inadequate finances; a larger family; and the stress of one or two additional children under two years of age."[138] (The state of obesity in which combinations of lower social class, early rapid weight gain, and low activity levels resulted in a prevalence of 40 percent obesity in adolescence has been conceptualized in terms of disordered interaction between a child with an energy expenditure deficit and an environment with food excess—and possibly underlying family pathology.)[145] Reduced somatic growth has been found associated with delayed entry into elementary school.[146]

9. School health services can be important in screening children for nutritional deficiencies and exploring causes with the family. Such work has revealed children in families with no food at all, with parents who are so ill, disoriented, retarded, or addicted that they were completely unable to cope with the survival crisis at hand.[146]

The school lunch program has already been noted to make a difference in the adequacy of the diet of needy children. The National School Lunch Act was passed in 1946 as a measure to "safeguard the health and well being of the Nation's children and to encourage the domestic consumption of . . . food." The Child Nutrition Act of 1966 expanded the intent of Congress to ensure children received food in order "to develop and learn." The 1972 amendment to the National School Lunch Act emphasized again that all schools participating in the lunch program must serve free or reduced-price lunches to all children determined by local school authorities to be needy.[147]

Implementation of the program has been severely criticized over the years. An evaluation of the program in the state of Pennsylvania was conducted by the Commonwealth's Office of the Budget in 1971/72. This study found that:

> Nineteen percent of public schools were without a lunch program.
>
> Fifty-five and one-half percent of all needy public school children were not receiving free or reduced-price lunch and two-thirds of these were attending schools with a lunch program.
>
> Most schools without lunch programs were concentrated in large urban areas.
>
> Twenty-one percent of public elementary schools and 8 percent of public secondary schools had no program, but 21 percent of high schools with needy students had no program.[147]

School boards are responsible for entering the program but in 22 percent of cases in Pennsylvania seemed to have delegated the authority to school administrators. Schools violated various requirements of the law: only 47 percent announced the program to the public as required; 13 percent did not send applications home; 42 percent investigated the family's application; about 25 percent did not protect the anonymity of the children receiving free and reduced-price lunch; 22 percent did not follow up to find needy, nonparticipating children. Regulations for the programs are issued by the U.S. Department of Agriculture; the state department of education may withhold reimbursement to force compliance; otherwise the school districts control their own programs.[147]

The school administrator's understanding of the importance of the program and willingness to find kitchen and dining room space in buildings designed without either are key issues. Poor scheduling so that children have no time to eat, noisy and dirty surroundings, lack of food choice, unsatisfactory menu planning, and poor and unattractive food preparation are all barriers to children's participation. The food program can be a potent lesson in health education, contributing to current and future nutrition, if the following occur:

School feeding is considered an integral part of the school program and not an irrelevant side activity.

The program runs at a price parents can afford.

Simple foods suited to the ethnic and cultural background of the children are served.

Lunch supplies one-third of recommended dietary allowance of nutrients and is attractive in color, flavor, and appearance.

New foods are introduced to enlarge children's food experiences.

The psychological value of hot food, at least in the winter, is considered.

Teachers and food service personnel collaborate in providing knowledge about nutrition based on the foods eaten in the program.[148]

Dental Health

Dental diseases are the most prevalent chronic conditions of children in the United States.[149] They account for much pain and disruption of time and attention in school. They are, without care, progressively destructive of teeth, gums, and bony supporting structures and of their physiologic functions of speech, mastication, and deglutition. In addition, the teeth and oral structures have profound psychological implications in their contributions to "facial harmony [which] is high among human values in our culture,"[150] to participation in socially important eating occasions, and to occupational opportunities. The amount of school time lost for dental causes—disease, prevention, and treatment—is not known. A figure of 4½ workdays lost per employee per year has been given for adults.[151]

The major dental conditions that affect children are:

1. *Dental caries,* a disease of early life affecting 40 percent of two-year-olds,[152] 80 percent of six-year-olds, and 98 percent of adults,[150] is caused by complex interaction of genetics, fluoride, diet, socioeconomic status, mouth hygiene. The condition can be halted by dental care as teeth that would normally decay and be lost are filled.

2. *Malocclusion* may occur as a gross birth deformity associated with such conditions as cleft palate; and a condition detected in about 25 percent of thirteen-to-fourteen-year-olds[153] as the second dentition, virtually complete, reveals its malformed "foundation" caused by congenital malformations of teeth and face or deformities acquired from premature loss of deciduous teeth, loss of the six-year-old molars, dental

disease and injury, and faulty dental repairs.[150] In 8 percent of cases the condition is more than a cosmetic problem and is handicapping of speech and other oral functions.

3. *Periodontal disease,* inflammation and degeneration of tissues surrounding the teeth, has its beginnings in childhood and the teen years and constitutes the major reason for loss of teeth in adults in their thirties and forties.[150] Some gum disease is present in 45 percent of six-year-olds. Actual gingivitis is found in 10 percent of fifteen-year-olds.[154]

4. *Trauma,* or injuries to teeth, occurred in school accidents ranging from 4.7 percent of accidents in elementary school to 1.5 percent of accidents in high school.[72] Statistics from high school football show the importance of protective devices:

2.3 injuries per 100 players with no protection
1.8 injuries per 100 players with face guards
0.4 injuries per 100 players with face guards and tooth protectors[155]

Dental diseases have a high incidence in the general population, but their life histories and the resultant severity and prevalence of the diseases are affected by use of dental preventive and restorative services. Use of dental services by children of all income and racial groups has increased, but the gap in use of dental services between the poor and nonpoor has not diminished, partly due to the limited coverage of dental care under Medicaid. These differences can be seen in the fact that nonpoor children make one visit per person per year more than poor children[156] and in the effects on pathology, such as among children twelve to seventeen years old in 1966–1970 as shown in Table 3–22. "Poverty—or even a middle level income—would still appear to be a serious barrier to dental care."[157]

Table 3–22. Percentage of Children, 12–17 years of Age, with Dental Pathology, by Family Income, 1966–1970

Family income range	Decayed & missing teeth	Filled teeth	Total DMF (decayed, missing, filled)
Under $3,000	3.9	1.6	5.5
$5,000–6,999	3.0	3.5	6.5
Over $15,000	1.0	5.4	6.4

Source: National Center for Health Statistics.[158]

Children with chronic and handicapping conditions remain a dentally underserved group, with a variety of dental needs caused by or related to their underlying conditions: the basic disease condition may cause abnormalities or maldevelopment of teeth; therapy for the condition (e.g., sugars used in phenylketonuria and cystic fibrosis as calorie sources or sugary syrups used as bases for medication) may stimulate caries, the condition may inhibit dental treatment (e.g., hemophilia inhibits extractions, and cardiac conditions inhibit administration of anesthesia); side effects of treatment may produce dental disease (e.g., Dilantin produces a gum hyperplasia); frequent candy snacks during hospitalization and candy given as a reward in school causes caries; dental treatment providers often resist caring for the handicapped, especially those with mental retardation, cerebral palsy, or epilepsy; families of the handicapped lack financial resources needed for dental services.

Schools have played a considerable role in delivery of dental services to children from the earliest days of school health. All the following services are currently provided by some school or have been successfully demonstrated by some school in the past:

> For dental caries: fluoridation of school water supplies, administration of fluoride tablets and/or topical fluoride application to children, instruction in brushing and flossing, less sugar in school diet, nutrition education, dental hygienist cleaning and scaling, screening and/or examination, referral for treatment, provision for treatment on school premises with high levels of restoration and diminished loss of school time
>
> For malocclusion: screening and referral, provision of special funds for orthodontic treatment of the most severely handicapped from poorer families
>
> For periodontal disease: brushing and flossing instruction, dental hygienist cleaning and scaling, screening and referral for treatment
>
> For trauma: manufacture of mouth guards, safety education, first aid instruction and provision

Adolescent Health

Adolescence has been defined as "the stage in life that starts with puberty and ends when the individual's independence from his parents has attained a reasonable degree of psychological congruence." This definition has been translated in a recent authoritative work on adolescent health into the age-group ten-to-nineteen, in which individuals may "unequivocally be labeled adolescents."[159]

"Adolescents have achieved an identity as a population group showing certain common characteristics that transcend the confines of geography, economics, education, culture, and race."[159] Health problems arise partly from the developmental process involved in adolescence, partly from the developmental disjunctions arising from the prolongation of dependent behavior beyond puberty, and partly from the lack of institutional arrangements, including health services, to meet the new needs of this population group. Each of these three factors will be discussed briefly before specific health problems are reviewed.

Developmental Process.   The World Health Organization characterized adolescence as "a series of biochemical, anatomical, and mental changes that are not found in members of other age groups. It is these rapid, extensive changes that differentiate adolescents from children and from adults and that must be taken into account when adolescents and their health problems are being given attention."[159]

The major developmental tasks of adolescence include the following:

Completing physical growth and attaining full physiological maturity

Resolving conflicts about dependence, independence, and interdependence

Developing personal systems of values and weighing the values of peers and parents

Making a vocational choice—a supreme challenge for many adolescents, given uneven distribution of options and of good education and insufficient development of skills and competence

Developing conceptual thought at an abstract level

Continuing moral development

Developmental Disjunctions.   Many of the difficulties of adolescence can be better understood in terms of developmental disjunctions, best illustrated in the matter of reproduction where:

Biological ability to reproduce (age twelve)

precedes

attainment of physical maturity in females (age seventeen and one-half) necessary to ensure optimal nutrition and weight of the infant

and also precedes

attainment of optimal cognitive function (age fifteen), with its
ability to fully comprehend the concepts of risk and the future

and

completion of the psychosocial task of establishing a sense of
identity (age twelve to eighteen) as a necessary foundation for
the subsequent stage of committment and fidelity to other
persons and to work.

the above stages precede

the cultural norms for first childbearing (about eighteen to
twenty-one)

and all precede

the social and economic ability of young people (twenty-one to
twenty-five) to provide the supplies necessary for optimal development of a family and children.

Lack of Institutions and Health Services.   As adolescence—a prolonged period of dependence—has emerged as a separate phase in the
life cycle, the problem of where this transition[160] between childhood
and adulthood will occur has been raised. The family no longer prepares the child, as formerly, for the simpler tasks of farm and house.
School provides the setting for acquisition of the range of skills adolescents package together to form the basis of their future lives as welders,
hairdressers, accountants, astronauts, or lawyers. The school and peer
group are the major socializing influences. Cross-generational relationships are limited.

Some observers see the social setting for the raising of adolescents
as ambiguous and without structure: "Adolescents live, survive or exist
in an ambiguous, poorly defined social and cultural milieu. In response
to the ambiguity, they turn to the peer group for order, status and
prestige. Acceptance by the peer group becomes extremely important
for their social health."[159] Others see the current situation as incomplete:

> The way of life we have institutionalized for our young consists
> almost entirely of social interaction with others of the same age and
> formal relationships with authority figures. . . . The objectives to
> which environments for youth should be addressed consist of two
> broad classes. One . . . concerns the acquisition of skills. . . . Schools
> have traditionally focused upon this class of objectives . . . a second
> class of objectives . . . concerns the opportunity for responsibilities
> affecting other persons. Only with the experience of such respon-
> sibilities can youth move toward . . . social maturity.[160]

There are no institutional arrangements to provide the opportunities necessary to accomplish development of social maturity.

Health services share society's lag in providing for adolescent needs. The problem has three parts: (1) lack of institutions providing services to adolescents, (2) lack of content relevant to the needs of adolescents, and (3) impediments to access by adolescents. Adolescents, as neither children nor adults, are not welcomed by pediatricians or internists. Hospitals and children-and-youth programs often cut off pediatric services at age thirteen, or at fifteen or sixteen. Adolescents may see their family physician as being a parental ally and therefore not respecting the confidentiality of the adolescent patient. Adolescent specialists and adolescent clinics are still small in number.

Where pediatricians serve adolescents it is often for organic complaints and rarely for sexual and behavioral problems.[161] Most pediatricians do not include screening for gonorrhea in the routine evaluation of their patients.[162] Consequently only 8 percent of 7,479 pediatricians diagnosed or treated any V.D. in 1968.[163]

The lack of services for sexually active and pregnant teens begins with the fact that only 30 percent of high schools provide family life or sex education courses, and of these only 40 percent provide information on birth control. (Yet the general community approves such courses at the 80 percent level.) Lack of prenatal care in the first trimester affects 70 percent of pregnant girls under age fifteen and about 23 percent of those older. There are few special programs for the pregnant teenager; most assist with emergency aid in the prenatal period. A study of 128 "comprehensive" centers in 1972 showed that 40 percent offered no prenatal health services; 50 percent offered no delivery services and 66 percent, no pediatric care for the baby; an astounding 75 percent offered no contraceptive services. Once the baby arrives, the teenage mother finds that 80 percent of day care centers will not care for children under two.[164]

About half of the 3.7 million fifteen-to-nineteen-year-old girls who are sexually active, and thus at risk of unintended pregnancy, are not receiving birth control services from a clinic or private physician. From the time of the Supreme Court decision in 1973 the teen abortion rate has risen by 60 percent. Yet teenage access to abortion varies because of lack of local services and transportation costs so that about 125,000 unwanted children are born to teenagers annually.[164]

School programs for prevention of youth alcohol and drug abuse have not advanced to the stage of some businesses, which have special programs to detect alcoholism early so that treatment can be instituted before physical, economic, occupational, and social damage becomes apparent. Treatment and rehabilitation is limited in many communities to drug abuse. There are few if any diagnostic, treatment, and rehabilitation services for the young person abusing alcohol or cigarettes.

Teenagers lack health insurance with which to purchase health services. Coverage under a parent's policy usually ends with attainment of majority or leaving school, and coverage under group policies usually comes only with regular employment. Only 70 percent of those aged seventeen to twenty-four have hospital insurance.[165] Less than 25 percent of girls seventeen years old and younger who give birth have health insurance. Only 20 percent are covered for hospital or doctor bills and fewer for prenatal care. Twenty-two states do not consider low-income pregnant women eligible for public assistance until the baby's birth; thus medical assistance is not available for prenatal care.[164]

The age at which young adults may consent to medical treatment varies from state to state. Young people often do not receive medical care because they are considered too young to give their own consent for medical evaluation and treatment. In these cases parents may not be available to give consent or the teenager may not wish them to know about problems in socially sensitive areas.[159]

Health Problems.   Observers of the field of adolescent health care agree that additional services are required directed toward a broad range of concerns in physical health, social-emotional needs, and health information.[163] Studies of teenagers provided with comprehensive health services reveal some of the unmet needs and leave "no grounds for complacency" about the deficiences in the current piecemeal arrangements.[159] Two hundred sixty-nine Neighborhood Youth Corps adolescents examined by medical history questionnaire, brief physical examination, and screening tests in 1966–1967 showed treatment was needed immediately for uncorrected vision defects (17–34 percent), dental pathology (50 percent), emotional problems (34 percent), and anemia (13 percent).[166]

Six hundred and eighteen children aged fourteen to sixteen were examined in 1966, as part of a summer work program, by a brief medical questionnaire, physical examination, and screening tests. Forty-seven and one-half-percent of the children had physical abnormalities: 99 had major problems and 274 minor. Inadequate treatment had been received for 52 percent of the major problems and 34 percent of the minor; that means that almost one adolescent in four had an untreated health problem. Extensive dental treatment was required by 29 percent.[167] Two hundred fifty-five "healthy" female adolescents aged eleven to seventeen attending a family-planning clinic were examined by medical and psychosocial history, physical and gynecologic examination, and certain tests. Sixty-three percent revealed undiagnosed medical conditions requiring treatment, and 53 percent had psychosocial problems including one alcoholic and three drug addicts.[168]

Some writers have classified the health problems of adolescence as shown in Table 3–23. Adolescents cite drug and alcohol abuse, communication with adults and peers, school difficulties, health worries, nervousness, sex, work, adaptation, and religion as their major problems.[159]

A number of adolescent health problems have been discussed in previous sections. A few of importance will be briefly reviewed here.

Drug and Alcohol Abuse.   The Gallup Youth Survey of May 23, 1977, reported that teenagers across the country considered drug and alcohol use and abuse the first and third largest problems, respectively, facing them. However, patterns of adolescent use appear to be changing: toward a lessening of drug use,[170] lower use of cigarettes between 1974 and 1977,[46] and no indication that levels of alcohol usage have increased over the 5 years from 1972 to 1977.[46] In contrast, the use of marijuana within 1 month before survey has increased from 10 percent of sixteen-to-seventeen-year-olds in 1971 to 29 percent in 1977.[46]

Results of national surveys on adolescent drug and alcohol abuse

Table 3–23.

Primary problems of adolescence	Problems made worse by adolescence	Problems with origin in adolescence
School/learning problems	Mental retardation	Hypertension—labile
Anorexia nervosa	Chronic disease	Hypercholesterolemia
Scoliosis	Handicaps	Duodenal ulcer
Slipped epiphysis	Dying	Irritable colon syndrome
Sports injuries	Automotive injuries	Migraine
Body image	Suicide	Obesity
Mononucleosis	Menstrual dysfunction	Alcoholism
Hepatitis	Pregnancy	Marital conflicts
Primary amenorrhea	Abortion	
Sexual dysfunction	Gynecomastia	
Venereal disease	Tuberculosis	
Drug abuse	Diabetes	
Delinquency	Inflammatory bowel disease	
Acne	Dental caries	
Goiter		

Source: Cohen et al.[169]

Table 3–24.   Adolescent Drug and Alcohol Use, National Survey, 1977

		12–17 Year-Olds, %	High school students, %
Ever tried:	Alcohol	50	90
	Cigarettes	50	76
	Marijuana	25	56
Used within	Alcohol	31	71
30 days:	Cigarettes	22	38
	Marijuana	16	35
Used daily:	Alcohol		6
	Cigarettes		29
	Marijuana		9

Sources: 12–17-year-olds, Abelson, Fishburne, and Cisin;[171] high school students, Johnston, Bachman, and O'Malley.[172]

in 1977 appear in Table 3–24. The pattern showed high levels of experimentation and lower levels of regular use; both increased with age. It was also noted that about 18 percent of the high school class had tried tranquilizers and 17 percent stimulants, whereas 36 percent had tried hallucinogens, inhalants, opiates, or cocaine.[172]

Alcohol abuse is recognized among school students, but the actual size of the phenomenon is not determined. Some observers believe that alcohol abuse is increasing among young people.[173] Morris E. Chafetz, former director of the National Institute on Alcohol Abuse and Alcoholism, reported full-blown alcoholism in children as young as nine to twelve years of age and the establishment of Alcoholics Anonymous groups specifically for teenagers since 1970.[174] Others emphasized alcohol abuse by high school students: drinking before school, drinking on school premises, and drinking in order to get drunk. They also noted that emergence of the fully fledged alcoholic may be a rapid process in adolescents, a matter of months compared with years in adults.[175]

The causes of alcohol or drug abuse are not known. Studies of young, middle-class alcohol abusers referred by the courts revealed evidence of "general life problems" before the beginning of drinking; 40 percent had been suspended or expelled from school, and 20 percent had failed school courses; 12 percent were sociopaths.[176] Much information basic to an understanding of drugs and their effects (physical, mental, social) on health is lacking; abuse is hard to define without drug dosage/health outcome formulas; little is known of the life history of certain types of drug abuse. Partly because of these deficiencies, data on the incidence and prevalence of drug use, drug addiction, and alcoholism are lacking. Group pressure acts to encourage experimental use, but except in the case of cigarettes we do not know of its role in turning use into abuse.

Experience in Pennsylvania's school health program shows the following community patterns of drug and alcohol use:

Virtually no problems exist in communities with a culture of abstinence.

A rising alcohol problem is evident in working-class ethnic groups, but also in suburban areas, where there are reports of drinking on school premises and of alcohol ingestion associated with motor vehicle accidents.

A heroin problem persists in large cities but is subsiding.

Suburban youths experiment with many drugs. Schools report cardiac arrests associated with poly-drug abuse.

Widespread solvent "huffing" is found in some white, ethnic working-class communities in association with theft of solvents from nearby industrial sites.

An occasional acute epidemic of drug abuse has occurred in high schools, with up to 40 students in need of care for overdosage. A response is usually obtained from the police, but not from health officials, who do not see that an epidemiological investigation is required here as for an outbreak of acute food poisoning.

Community facilities to treat youth with drug problems vary. Few locales have specific programs for the youthful alcoholic.

Gonorrhea.   Gonorrhea has stabilized somewhat since it peaked (at three times its 1950 rate) in the mid-1970's, at 12.9 cases per 1,000 fifteen-nineteen-year-olds.[46] Gonorrhea is a particularly silent disease (90 percent infected are asymptomatic) in female adolescents, resulting in sterility in about 5 percent of cases.[177] Studies of sexually active youth aged twelve to sixteen in a large city showed silent gonorrhea in 1.9 percent of boys and 7.0 percent of girls.[178] Although spread of the disease is somewhat contained by the predominant adolescent pattern of a constant sexual partner,[177] (not the "promiscuous" pattern alleged), nonetheless a 1.9 percent carrier rate in adolescent boys represents an important reservoir of infection.[178] The prevalence of gonorrhea in delinquent girls has been estimated at 11 to 13 percent.[177]

Pregnancy.   Data from two national surveys show that increasing proportions of unmarried adolescent girls have had sexual intercourse and they have this experience at an earlier age: 18 percent of fifteen-year-olds and 41 percent of unmarried seventeen-year-olds reported in 1976 having had intercourse at least once. If all other factors had been kept constant, such an increase in sexual experience would have increased fertility. Birth rates, however, have declined in the fifteen-to-seventeen-year-old group from 39.2 per 1,000 in 1972 to 34.6 per 1,000 in 1976 because of greater contraceptive use and more abortions.[46] In the fifteen-to-seventeen-year-old group the abortion rate in 1976 was 21.9 per 1,000. Still, it is estimated that 70 percent of teenage conceptions and 46 percent of teenage births are unwanted.[179] A particularly pathetic group are girls below fifteen years of age —not yet beyond their own childhood—who become mothers at the rate of 2 per 1,000 per year.[46]

Pregnancy and childbirth among adolescents carry immediate, intermediate, and long-term health consequences. The immediate effects are low-birth-weight babies with high mortality and neurological and other handicaps, eventually entering special education classes. Maternal mortality in pregnancy is higher.

Subsequent fertility is high in teenage mothers, and mortality and morbidity among the second and third infants is higher than among the first.[180] The rate of attempted suicide is high among females pregnant as teenagers. Pregnancy is the reason most often cited by female dropouts for school discontinuation.[179] Loss of education and of earning capacity, with greater poverty and welfare dependency, is found in teenage mothers as a group.

Data showed that 24 percent of adolescent mothers gave inadequate stimulation to their infants; the child's developmental process of separation and individuation was retarded, compared with 11 percent of adult mothers; the adolescent mothers experienced one and one-half times more crises.[181] With fewer personal and social supports the stage was set for feelings of inadequacy and failure.

It has been shown, despite methodological problems,[182] that special programs reduce subsequent pregnancies,[183] improve the educational,[184] occupational, and economic outcomes for the teenage mother, and improve the health of the baby at birth.

The reasons for adolescent pregnancy have been less well studied than the consequences. Psychiatric studies of 40 unmarried pregnant girls aged twelve to seventeen revealed high amounts of social disruption, conflicts between the girls' desires and those of parents/guardians, unconscious parental wishes for sexual activity by the girls, and a frequent recent loss, by death or separation, of a significant other person in the girl's life.[185] Studies of school achievement showed a correlation with both above- and below-grade attainment and pregnancy suggesting that such age/achievement incongruity may reflect the presence of psychological and maturational factors.[186] A study of suicide attempts by women who had delivered an infant when seventeen years of age or less revealed patterns suggesting that the cause of the suicide attempts lay in the stress of the pregnancy and child rearing or that both the pregnancy and suicide attempt/threat were forms of disturbed adolescent behavior.[187]

ENVIRONMENT

The lip service given the health consequences of the school environment is repeatedly apparent in the literature. The Maine School Health Demonstration of 1947–1953, for example, set as the first of its seven goals "to provide and to maintain a healthful school environment,"[95] yet specified no activities whatsoever to accomplish this goal. The advances made by public health in its early history, centering on improvements in the environment, "anticipated the fundamental truth of preventive medicine, that the health of the individual is intimately and indivisibly tied up with the social as well as the physical environment."[188] Schoolchildren live in the environment of three worlds: family, school, and community. An employee of a lead battery melting operation may take lead dust home on his clothes,[189] causing lead poisoning in his children and thus adversely affecting their schoolwork.[190]

Public health stopped expansion of its environmental health operations in schools once schools had reached a certain level of basic building acceptability. Since then there has been a tendency for responsibility for environmental health and safety to be split among a variety of agencies and for no one agency to be alert to the development of new hazards in the school. To a large extent schools have been forgotten as places with environments subject to introduction of the same modern physical, chemical, and biological agents and hazards as the rest of society. The recent discovery of asbestos in ceiling tiles in schools illustrates the lack of health monitoring of the environment. Similarly, some years after the U.S. Occupational Safety and Health Administration had been formed and had established standards for workplaces, it was pointed out by an astonished workman at an adult evening class at a vocational-technical school in Pennsylvania that the school was still using asbestos around the welding cubicles, a practice long abandoned by industry. The concern about asbestos is of course related to the risk of severe long-term health consequences:

Pulmonary fibrosis
Asbestosis
Lung cancer
Mesothelioma
Gastrointestinal cancer

All the environmental factors mentioned below have known or suspected ill effects on health. Inadequate hygiene of school toilets is associated with increased risks of diarrhea in children.[191] The deleterious effects of exposure to low levels of chemicals and other hazards are just being recognized; it was known that clinical lead poisoning was toxic to the brain and central nervous system, but recent work suggests that exposure without symptoms is associated with neuropsychologic deficits that may interfere with classroom performance.[190]

What follows is a rough listing of environmental factors with potentially adverse effects on health which are found in schools, found in community environments and affecting schools, or found in home and/or community environments and affecting children who go to school. This listing serves simply as a reminder of the size and complexity of a task that has hardly been considered an issue by those who blithely mention "healthful school environment" without pausing to define it.

Conditions Under Some Surveillance

Conditions under the standards and/or surveillance of an official agency appear to be divided as follows:

> Inspection of water supplies, sewage systems, toilets, and refuse disposal and for insects and rodents; of buildings and their walls, floors, lighting, heat, and ventilation; of classroom seating, lockers, food preparation, and swimming pools is usually a matter for the department of health or for a special environmental department if there is one. Shortage of staff may limit the annual inspection to:
>
> Independent water supplies
> School cafeteria
> Swimming pool
>
> Standards for school building construction, materials used, and heat, light, ventilation, etc., are usually the responsibility of the state department of education.
>
> Fire safety is often the province of a department of labor.

Safety standards for school buses and drivers may reside with a department of transportation.

Conditions in the School and School Program

Conditions reported to exist in schools, where one or a number of examples have been cited but data on prevalence are unknown, include:

Use of hazardous and toxic materials in art classes without appropriate hygenic handling or proper venting[192,193]

Use of laser beams in physics

Use of microwave ovens in home economics

Concerns regarding hazards in chemistry laboratories including contamination by mercury[194]

Safety standards in biology laboratories

The hazards introduced by animals, for example, infected turtles, in preschool and kindergarten[195]

Safety standards and appropriate machine guards, supervision, and instruction in "shop"

Care with dust, fumes, and asbestos in vocational-technical classes

Lack of preventive programs in agricultural high schools, with dangers from heavy machinery, falls, large animal bites and kicks, and infections, stings, noxious plants[196]

Ultraviolet radiation in gym

Lack of appropriate conditioning, protective equipment, and correct age selection for sports[197]

Radiation hazards from overzealous use of chest Xrays by school physicians (urged by mobile chest Xray unit operators as the calls for their community services drop)

Peeling lead paint in centers used for preschool programs

Safety standards for stairs, hallways, gym

Conditions in and Around School Buildings and Grounds

Littering of playgrounds with glass and refuse

Safety standards and maintenance of playground equipment

Lack of safety fences around school playgrounds with traffic hazards to running children

Lack of supervision of playground activity

School bus safety standards

Lack of seat belts in school buses

Use of pesticides and rodenticides in and around schools[198]

Drug pushing in and around schools and school grounds

The problem of violence and vandalism in schools and on school property (which in New York City in 1973 was almost 10,000 reported crimes, including 3 murders, and 26 rapes)[199] which is underreported and apparently much due to outsiders gaining entry to school buildings and property; how much the physical safety of children and teachers is affected and how this situation affects the psychologic well-being and learning ability of students is not known.

Conditions in the Community Environment

Schools are part of the general community and may find their environment influenced by neighbors:

Dump sites for toxic wastes (e.g., Love Canal) asbestos, P.C.B.

Nuclear plants

Steel mills

Chemical works whose emissions cause eye and skin irritation

Lead-smelting operations[200] or lead paint manufacturers

Smelters using cadmium[201]

Burners of high-arsenic coal[202]

Highways with high lead levels

Farms using toxic pesticides

General air pollution with varying amounts of carbon monoxide, oxides of nitrogen, and sulphur dioxide, which affect lung and cardiac function[203] and may necessitate reduction in the strenuousness of school physical education and athletic programs—a fact not appreciated by many school personnel[204]

Noise pollution, with its debilitating effects on concentration and learning

The existence of neighborhood gangs, a problem to schools when gang members have to cross into the territory of another gang in order to get to school, and when animosities provoked as rival gang members meet in class and throughout the building are played out in violent behavior either in the school or after school in the neighborhood

Conditions in Community and Home Environment with Specific Impact on Children

Schools have traditionally recognized certain hazards in the general nonschool environment with specific impact on children and have established programs to assist students to conduct themselves with greater safety, going as far as providing instruction in the appropriate use of certain products: driver education, education in safe bicycle use, pedestrian safety, consumer education as part of home economics. The pattern is somewhat spotty, and little effort has been directed to:

Use of seat belts in cars, which is less than 89 percent for those over ten years of age and below 93 percent for those under ten[205]

Skateboard safety

Home fire prevention

Home poisoning prevention

Selection of safe summer camp[206]

Safe use of drugs and medications

Overexposure to the sun

Ear protection with rifle use

Ear damage from overexposure to loud rock music

Appropriate medication of children; this consists of two problems: (1) overmedication of children by professionals and parents so that on any given day 35 percent of all children receive medications, half of which are prescribed, and (2) lack of any organized method to study drug reactions in children, as exists for adults, even though there is evidence that children sustain more adverse reactions than adults[207]

Care in the use of dinnerware or food containers coated with lead and/or cadmium-containing glazes

Selection of such consumer items as clothing and toys

Exploding of glass bottles containing carbonated beverages

Fencing of swimming pools to prevent drowning

Teaching swimming and water safety to all children as part of the curriculum objective

It is interesting that where adult health is involved, for example, cigarette smoking, children have been used to carry the message to the adult generation. There has been little of the same zeal for conditions, such as traffic accidents, so painfully felt by the children themselves.

Specific Vulnerability

Schools contain groups of individuals with particular sensitivity to environmental conditions. With new lives now beginning when parents are at school and with more fetuses going to school—as to work—there is an even greater incentive to ensure the health and safety of the environment. Generally it is not appropriate to think of excluding the mother and fetus from a given environment because of a potential hazard, but it is necessary to recognize that if a fetus is or can be damaged so also can children and adults in the same environment. It has been recently recognized that not only does exposure of the mother to Xrays, such viruses as rubella and Coxsaxie, alcohol and smoking, vibration, noise, and such drugs as amphetamine and diethylstilbestrol (D.E.S.) have deleterious effects upon the offspring, but so also does exposure of the father. Wives of men exposed to anesthetic gases have increased rates of abortion and congenital anomalies, and work on male animals has shown associations between heroin, alcohol, lead, and caffeine and increased perinatel mortality.

Schools also hold particular groups of students who will be abnormally susceptible to certain environments whether in their current school lives or in the future, and who need to be so advised. A large group is that with sickle cell trait (not the disease), who are susceptible to sickle cell–type crises in atmospheres of reduced oxygen tension such as found at high altitudes (even 4,000 feet), in certain jobs (e.g., test pilot), or with particularly heavy physical activity levels. Others susceptible include asthmatics, in regard to air pollution; anemic children, who are more sensitive to lead poisoning; some epileptics, who are particularly disturbed by flashing lights.

New Environmental Concerns

The environment changes as new substances and technologies introduce new health hazards, and the ability to control adverse environmental factors is altered by new knowledge and methods. Some of the new environmental concerns of importance to schools are as follows:

Planning internal environments to reduce energy needs but maintain the body comfort required for optimal learning.

Disaster planning[208] which recognizes that schools have been and may be the subject of, or caught in, a great variety of disastrous events (nuclear radiation leaks, floods, fires, mine disasters, toxic chemical spills or escapes, civil disturbances, aircraft and bus crashes, earthquakes, tornadoes). In these situations, not only the physical needs must be considered but also the psychological vulnerability of children when separated from parents[209] and the value of crises intervention in preventing mental illness sequelae.[210]

Increased use of human engineering to ensure a scientific approach to design of facilities, equipment, seating, desks, machines and their controls, safety operation, etc.

Greater attention to the psychosocial impacts of the environment, especially buildings, upon the humans who work and live in them. Space, crowding, color, textual variety; how many people, the number and quality of the social roles they can play, and the relationships they can form are but a few of the issues. Some children learn well in structured settings but become lost and confused in larger, more open learning spaces.[124]

Students in small schools, compared with those in larger schools, perform in more than twice as many responsible positions in the settings and report they are more likely to be challenged, to be involved, to feel valued, to gain moral and cultural values.[211] Overcrowded schools with double scheduling reduce the services, such as lunch, private learning, constructive social activities, and extracurricular explorations, the school can provide children. Busing alters the experience of the transitional environment between home to school. An English study found poorer school adjustment in bused young elementary school students compared with those who walked to school;[212] it has been suggested that busing interferes with mental contructs of the environment by which students connect home and school in space including the child's ability to mentally reverse the route travelled to school.[213]

The School's Environmental Role

There appear to be ample reasons for the school to recognize itself and to be recognized by the community as an integral part of children's ecology. There are complex interrelationships between children and the school environment; between children and the school and neighborhood environments; between children, and the school, home, and community enviroments.

The school's population is more susceptible to environmental effects than the older population and often susceptible in different ways. In this regard Finberg noted that the chemicals of this technological age and their by-products not only are rapidly increasing in number and complexity but also "have special implications for infants and children because maturation and growth processes are often qualitatively or quantitatively different from mature systems and because the infant and child have different environments from adults. In turn the effects may be immediate or delayed" until later stages in the life cycle.[214]

Other components of the environment besides chemicals may be similarly regarded: their number and nature and the complexity of their relationships in the human ecology are being increasingly understood and appreciated; they have special implications for children both because of the immaturity of the organism and because of the growth and development taking place; children's environment is a special subset in the whole human environment.

School is a constant feature in children's environment, providing the medium for exposure to certain environmental elements, on the one hand, and a mechanism or tool to assist in mitigation of many deleterious influences in the total environment, on the other. The school could carry out its mitigating role by:

1. Recognizing, through specially trained staff, the elements in its environment and in the total environment of its students that have the potential for deleterious effects on health and on optimal growth and development; and instituting actions, where possible, to eliminate or reduce the hazard(s).

2. Developing school programs to reduce current hazards while teaching students skills in dealing with the environmental hazards of their future lives. Thus environmental influences that are part of the school program, such as the use of toxic materials in art class or the possibility of playground accidents, could be approached as problems in occupational health—for staff and students—so that students, in learning the safe use of potential hazards, enter their adult world of work better able to act intelligently in the face of dangers encountered. Environmental factors that impinge on the school from neighborhood influences could become exercises in environmental hygiene and the use of community development techniques. Baumgartner, in 1946, described a joint school–community–health department effort to control rats in a certain waterfront neighborhood in Boston in which the greatest benefit may well have been the sense of power the program imparted to students in exerting a positive influence on their environment.[215]

3. Participating in regional, state, or national efforts to recognize environmental effects on child health, the school could use the particular abilities it possesses to observe health

and function in individuals it is in contact with for 13 years, with appropriately designed methodologies, to enhance knowledge of the effects of the biophysical and psychosocial environments. Methods could include surveillance of frequency of certain conditions, (e.g., those found on school entry), maintenance of registries of rarer conditions, use of an "alert practitioner reporting system"[21] to spot conditions and possible environmental influences (e.g., the occurrence of abuse of the children by parents who are workers in certain chemical plants is an alert for the possibility of short-term central nervous system toxicity), and record linkage. This latter has been demonstrated as an important tool in epidemiology in England and Canada: "Events during pregnancy can be linked with the health of the child at various ages, through the use of data on the obstetric charts; birth and death certificates; and hospital, school, and employment records. In this way it is possible to study etiology of disease not only in individuals, but also in families."[216]

4. Participating with others in efforts to prevent or reduce certain general environmental influences deleterious to children. For example, television has been implicated in the etiology of such problems as tendency to violence, consumption of excessive amounts of sugar, dental caries, sedentary life, and tendencies to use medication as a solution for life's difficulties and minor problems. Schools and educational associations can be and have been involved with other organizations in actions to reduce television's negative influences. Similarly, it would appear possible for local coalitions of agencies, led by schools, to develop means to provide systems of support for families in their task of raising children so that "intolerable losses in human potential"[217] to society may be prevented.

RELATIONSHIPS WITH MEDICAL CARE

Medical Care Practitioner

School health programs developed, under strong pressure from organized medicine, as adjuncts to children's sources of medical care. The fact that many children had no such care, either because it was not available in "medically underserved" rural and ghetto areas or because the child's family lacked the financial, transportation, or other resources needed to gain access, was simply ignored. It is not surprising, then, that school health programs have had problems with and have performed poorly in improving the health of children who lacked medical care services.

The problem has eased little over time. In 1955 the Maine School Health Demonstration wrote that "school health programs commonly are planned on the comfortable premise of availability of adequate and competent professional personnel—physicians, dentists, nurses and auxiliary services—to staff the preventive and therapeutic measures to be employed. Community health problems are commonly assumed to be chiefly those of organization and administration."[95] Experiences in a hosptial-based health program for school students in Harlem led the authors to observe that "traditional school health programs were designed for the children of parents who have the motivation, time and financial resources to ensure adequate health supervision."[218]

What is the role of medical care in the total amalgum of health care services received by children? And what are the implications for children and for school health services when medical care is not available?

Medicine began as and continues to be a profession concerned with care of human distress as exhibited by symptoms. The symptoms may emanate from conditions roughly classified as follows:

Fatal, irreversible diseases

Chronic diseases and handicaps that interfere with ability to function

Chronic disease with debilitating symptoms

Diseases that, with treatment, may be aborted

Short-lived diseases that may be self-limiting

Stresses (environmental, psychological) acting upon the human organism

The traditional role of medicine in the care of such a constant stream of human pain and misery has been beautifully stated: "to cure sometimes, to relieve often, to comfort always."[219] Although this formulation of function still holds, it does so with modifications and extensions required by the growth in complexity of knowledge, technology, disease patterns, and population expectations since the days when a single physician practicing in an office (or sometimes in the patient's home, rarely in a hospital) could provide all that medicine had to offer. From the 1920's, when the American Medical Association laid down the principle that children needed only the care of their family physician to today, there have been a succession of revolutions: the disease pattern has shifted from acute to chronic, knowledge and technology have expanded medicine into specialties and subspecialties and shifted the locus of care to hospitals and other specialized facilities, the working population has moved from one heavily dependent on physical performance to one dominated by the need to function well in intellectual and other psychological and emotional dimensions, and environmental stresses on workers and on the population generally are different from those that afflicted their rural forebears. The population is willing to bring its new symptoms, such as learning problems, and its old symptoms with new causes, such as abdominal pain from school phobia (and not from intestinal tuberculosis), to medicine for cure, relief, and/or comfort.

At the same time that medicine has become specialized, a plethora of other professionals and occupations have grown in the health field and practice in a great variety of settings, for example, clinics, voluntary agencies, departments of health, and special schools. Schools, school districts, and regional educational authorities have seen in recent years a remarkable growth of health personnel: pediatricians, neurologists, psychiatrists, orthopedic surgeons, clinical and educational psychologists, speech therapists, audiologists, optometrists, physical therapists, occupational therapists, remedial educators, social workers, counselors, adapted physical educators, nurses, nurse practitioners, dentists, dental hygienists. The fact that educational institutions have become sites for the delivery of health services has escaped the attention of most health planners and is ignored by most departments of health, but underscores the complexity of the health care system, now well beyond its beginnings in the general practitioner.

As the system has grown in the number and complexity of services, the administrative complexities necessary to ensure their delivery have kept pace. In particular, health insurance and other third-party-payment mechanisms have become the admission ticket for the patient and bread and butter for the practitioner. Consider the care of some conditions of children commonly seen in school health services: (1) Failure on visual acuity test is followed by referral to an eye specialist, either an opthalmologist or an optometrist; use of financial resources, either medical assistance, a vision care insurance plan, or cash; and a second referral to an optician followed by checking by the school or specialist that vision has been appropriately corrected. (2) Failure on hearing screening is followed by repeated failure on threshold testing by the school nurse; checking by a physician (school or private) or nurse practitioner to exclude acute conditions amenable to treatment; referral to free diagnostic services of the speech and hearing clinic of the state crippled children's program, where examinations by the audiologist and otologist are performed, and available third-party-resources collected before the crippled children's service is billed; further care possibly involving hospitalization, surgery, anesthesiologist, different and often multiple third-party-payment methods, hearing aid, with licensed hearing aid dealer paid by crippled children's program, and speech therapist (school) and special education techniques (school).

The general physician has little to add in terms of direct care to the above web of loosely interconnected services, but could play a significant role in guiding patients through the network, helping them to use it appropriately, and acting as their advocate when the system breaks down or is nonresponsive. Such functions have been described as part of the scope and content of "primary health care": "the referral of the patient, when necessary, to appropriate resources, specialists, and other, and the guidance of the patient through various levels of health care," plus a willingness to "integrate and coordinate" the patient's care and "take responsibility and be accountable for the preservation of the continuity of care in long-term follow up."[220]

The unfortunate fact is that medical school ill prepares physicians to understand, utilize, and coordinate the resources of the total health care system. This leaves the family physician, because of specialization, no longer the best agent to care for certain conditions yet in avoiding the unfamiliar role of case manager he or she does not receive information about the patient's encounter with other professionals, and gaps of considerable magnitude, with bearing upon care, remain when the patient next presents to that physician with a set of symptoms. Although physicians complain of their exclusion from care and knowledge of care and dream of providing comprehensive, continuous, coordinated care, the facts are that to fill "this new co-ordinating role . . . implies that additional time must be spent. This time must be taken from something else—presumably from rendering traditional care. The loss of this time in turn must mean fewer services will be performed per provider. If individual income is maintained, decrease in the number of services per physician implies a higher cost per service."[221]

The medical care of children with a chronic disease or handicap presents the physician many problems requiring a case management role simply to coordinate the diverse pieces of specialized medical management. To go further and consider rehabilitation of these children requires from the physician an orientation that extends beyond the treatment of organic disease and physical conditions to concern for optimal function. Such work requires the physician to rub shoulders with others—often in a foreign multidisciplinary team setting—who represent even more diverse professions and agencies among whom case management functions are to be performed.

It has been pointed out that physicians who traditionally deal with symptoms now have a greater variety of symptoms and causes of symptoms brought to their care. Besides injuries and illnesses of an emergency, acute, or chronic nature, physicians deal with "psychosocial problems and psychosomatic responses . . . learning and retention difficulties, memory defects, and perceptual problems."[220] MacCarthy said, "the child with symptoms and no disease takes up a large part of our work," but pointed out that physicians have poor "symptom tolerance" and also little experience in direct communication with children; yet the child with certain symptoms or undergoing medical or surgical procedures or who is terminally ill "has problems which have to do with the inner meaning of these things for him and the stress he may be experiencing."[222] The patient looks for someone who combines "skill with compassion" in handling a variety of problems; however, "the payment system for medical care is weighted in favor of more complex procedures,"[221] so the physician is underrewarded for dealing with symptoms that have no disease.

The emphasis of the medical profession and its sources of payment upon complex procedures has also meant little money and effort for preventive care. Some preventive services are provided to individuals when they attend for symptom care: advising women on breast self-examination, performing Pap tests, measuring blood pressure, or giving immunizations to children. A few groups have been identified as needing routine preventive care in the absence of any symptomatic disease. These include pregnant women, infants and young children, and school-age children. The provision of special preventive care for these vulnerable groups began in public health departments. Care remains in public hands for schoolchildren. Care of the other two groups has been split along socioeconomic lines. Private medical practice provides preventive services to middle- and upper-income pregnant women and infants; public health services or public clinic services serve the low-income group. For infants and young children, a schedule of regular visits is recommended by pediatric authorities in which physical examinations, growth measurements, developmental tests, tuberculosis and anemia screening, immunizations, and advice on feeding and weaning are provided. After immunizations are completed at the end of the first year of life, most children drop out of routine care and are seen by their physicians only when symptoms (usually due to upper respiratory infection or earache) develop. Low-income children withdraw from clinic preventive care after infancy and receive their episodic acute care from emergency rooms, hospital clinics, or general practitioners as considered appropriate to the needs of the child and accessibility by parents.

The reason for much parent withdrawal from preventive programs for children is that the content is geared to performance of the physical aspects of child supervision and little effort is made to assist mothers to gain skill and confidence in child rearing, to answer their questions, to advise on problems, and to give anticipatory guidance and health education. Pediatric nurse practitioners were found to conduct well-child visits differently from pediatricians. Their child health supervision was just as complete but "the nurses discussed developmental and child behavior topics in significantly ($p < .05$) greater depth, they asked more open-ended questions, made more specific recommendations, provided more maternal support, and the parents spoke a greater proportion of the time."[223]

The difficulties experienced by the usual practitioners of medical care in providing preventive services to children, in acting as case managers for care in a complex medical care system, and in working within a rehabilitation model to increase the function of the multihandicapped and chronically ill leave many tasks undone for schoolchildren—if they rely only on their private physician.

Insurance Coverage

The National Center for Health Statistics studied health care coverage in 1976. Persons aged six to eighteen had no coverage (12%), Medicaid only (9%), or private hospital insurance (75%).[224] Medicaid coverage increases with decreases in family income, but the largest percentage of families without any coverage are in the lowest income levels (see Table 3–25). Those with no health care coverage make less use of physicians and hosptials.

Table 3–25.

Family income	Medicaid, %	No coverage, %
Under $3,000	24	22
$5,000–$6,990	12	21
$10,000–14,999	2	8

Follow-up

Follow-up of health problems detected by the school and referred for diagnostic and/or treatment services has presented a problem since the first days of school health. The Maine School Health Demonstration of 1947–1953 commented: "There were too many refusals for the needed care that was advised. And this was despite the earnest support of professional and volunteer workers."[95] A number of factors were considered: the difficulty in getting to special services in an isolated community, economic depression, family movement, and limited medical social work services.

Few studies have been conducted to identify factors influencing the outcome of referrals from a school health service program. In the Los Angeles City School System, 458 fourth-grade students were identified by school personnel as needing medical or dental care; parents received at least one notification of the defect and of the need for care. In respect to actual parental follow-up, it was found that the notifications, number of persons making notifications, and number of contact techniques employed were three times as potent as social rank and eight times as potent as the parents' rating of the urgency of the condition.[225]

The survey methods used in the above study were designed by Gabrielson, who used them to study follow-up of referrals from school medical examinations of low-income fourth-grade students in New Haven. Parent action to follow school recommendations was associated with:

Parent perception of the seriousness of the condition

Parent belief in the effectiveness of medical care

Availability and accessability of care to children as noted in such factors as available health insurance and literacy of parents

A similar Canadian study showed a positive relationship between seeking professional care and:

Health insurance

Prior health care of children

Parental belief that the health problems would interfere with schoolwork[226]

Family health insurance coverage was found to be associated with a greater likelihood of receipt of care for school-detected defects. The benefit is extended to items covered by insurance (medical problems) but not to such uninsured problems as dental and visual defects.[227] Children in the lower social classes, when covered by insurance, received more follow-up care,[227] a phenomenon noted by others,[228] and apparently due to the removal of fiscal barriers to care by insurance and the greater health needs of children in lower socioeconomic groups.

Recommendations to parents made by a multidisciplinary medical clinic evaluating children with school-related problems were implemented in 90 percent of instances where the recommendation was pertinent to the child's learning problem and in 45 percent of cases where no such relationship existed.[229] Gabrielson emphasized that the existence of other family problems reduced the proportion of children receiving professional care.[226] Family problems are more likely in larger families, in the presence of family disorganization, and where the family has few financial resources.[228]

In the presence of strained family resources, inadequate health insurance, and lesser knowledge of health conditions and their consequences, special follow-up services using nurses,[230] or nurses and paraprofessionals,[218] have been shown to be effective in increasing the follow-up rate. As noted of the Harlem experience, "some families may require assistance from health providers simply to locate and negotiate the complexities of the health facilities recommended for their children."[218]

A completely different follow-up problem is presented after medical care has been obtained, that is, implementation of recommendations by the school. The only study found on this subject was that of the multidisciplinary medical team referenced above.[229] Recommendations to the school for care of children with school-related problems were followed:

Multidisciplinary team conference followed by letter to school, 57 percent

Multidisciplinary team conference plus letter, with follow-up by team in schools, 83 percent

Multidisciplinary team conference attended by school personnel, 85 percent

Multidisciplinary team conference attended by school personnel, with team follow-up in schools, 92 percent

Chapter 4

RATIONALE FOR SCHOOL HEALTH SERVICES

Health of mind and body is so fundamental to the good life that if we believe men have any personal rights at all as human beings, then they have an absolute moral right to such measure of good health as society and society alone is able to give them.

—Aristotle*

Society sends children to school for many years to learn what is needed in order to accomplish the developmental tasks of childhood and to be prepared for future roles as workers, parents, and citizens. Three areas of health concern arise out of the fact that children go to school:

1. Students, like all workers, need to be protected from the physical, mental, and social health hazards of their workplace. The state has a general duty to protect the health of its citizens and a specific duty to protect from hazards those

*Quotation attributed to Aristotle, without title of work, appeared in Department of Health, Commonwealth of Pennsylvania, "Policy Planning for Public Health," Report No. I, Policy Planning Council to the Deputy Secretary for Public Health Programs, January, 1976.

who have been placed in certain settings by the state. A school health program is an expression of both responsibilities.

2. Students need to be in their highest attainable state of health in order to function optimally at their work of education. This rationale for a school health program is so basic that it occasions no argument. As Brockington wrote: "The relationship of health and education is close. Education is fundamental to health and health to education. Unhealthy children cannot be properly educated; uneducated children cannot be healthy; the normal happy state of mind in childhood cannot be achieved when a child knows himself to be behind his fellows."[1]

3. Students need to be given the knowledge and skills necessary to protect their own health during their school years and to protect, in addition, the health of their families and community during their adulthood. Knowledge of the health hazards specific to each developmental level of human life as affected by the family, school or occupation, and community environments needs to be matched by skills in individual and group actions aimed at hazard removal, avoidance, or neutralization and self-protection. Similar mixes of knowledge and skills are required to personally care for the sick and injured in one's family and for those requiring emergency attention in one's immediate vicinity, to obtain health services for oneself and others entrusted to one's care, and to contribute to community decisions affecting health.

The essence of this rationale has found expression in the objectives of school education. In 1973 Pennsylvania's 10 goals for quality education included:

Acquisition of good health habits and understanding of the conditions necessary for maintenance of physical and emotional well-being

Understanding of self

Development of a positive attitude toward the learning process

Acquisition of habits and attitudes associated with responsible citizenship

Appreciation of human achievement in the natural and social sciences

Preparation for a world of rapid change and continuing education[2]

The World Health Organization appeared to agree with these goals when it placed special responsibility on education for the future healthy functioning of society:

A society that regularly monitors patterns of physical, mental, and social development, and takes steps to prevent deterioration and encourage progress, is more likely to promote human development than one that reacts only when changes become too obvious and too radical to be ignored. Formal education services bear a special responsibility for the forecasting, recognition, and understanding of changes, for the identification of means to cope with them, and for the teaching of the relevant ideas and techniques.[3]

4.   A fourth rationale for certain activities in the school health program may be discerned in a review of the history and current practices of the field. The community expects that schools will conduct certain health services for the primary benefit of the community: (a) Protect the community from diseases that arise in and/or are spread from the schools, such as communicable diseases. (b) Cooperate with the community in carrying out certain services to improve the health of the community, by capitalizing on the captive nature of the total population of the community's school-age children; an outstanding example is rubella immunization of young school-age children, which confers little direct benefit on them but decreases the community's pool of cases and the chances of the community's pregnant women becoming infected; the next generation is thus protected from the rubella-induced deformities of blindness, deafness, cardiac abnormalities, and mental retardation.

School health has the same concern for students as the field of occupational health has for workers: protection from the hazards of the work place, attainment of optimal health for the job to be done, preparation for healthy function in the next developmental stage of life (retirement for workers and adulthood for students), and capitalization on the captive nature of the group. School health and occupational health, in their concern for population groups, are specialty fields within the general field of public health. The essence of public health is that the health of a population group is advanced, a fact determined only by the use of population health measures or statistics. Such measures may be used to gauge the effect of school health services in improving the health of students in those areas, discussed above, considered by society to be basic to the process of schooling.

1. The effectiveness of any reduction in health hazards caused in total or in part by the school may be measured by reduction of the conditions caused by those hazards; for example, decreased school accidental death and injury rates, sports injuries, and dental trauma; reduced incidence of communicable diseases; decreased prevalence of intrapsychic stress and behavior problems arising from learning disabilities; and reductions in nutritional deficiency, dental caries, pregnancy, suicide, drug abuse, and delinquent gang activity.

2. Health services designed to improve the health status of students, in order to enhance their education, may be evaluated by recording reduction in the number of health conditions, both acute and chronic, per child over time and/or by data on reductions in disability days and school days lost due to illness.

Intervention in the life history of diseases and conditions essentially occurs at two levels: the case level, where secondary and tertiary prevention is possible, and the population level, where primary prevention of the actual occurrence of the disease is the aim. Case intervention may be evaluated by measuring, in the case of dental services for example, reduction in decayed and missing teeth, increase in number of filled teeth, and reduction in adolescent malocclusion; in the case of nutritional services, reduction in anemia; in the case of identification of teenage depression, reduction in suicide attempts; in the case of services to the handicapped, increased physical, educational, and social function; in the case of services to pregnant students, increased return to school and improved parenting skills.

Examples of primary preventive intervention are safety education and environmental manipulation resulting in reduced injury rates and fewer school days lost to injury; sex education and counseling services resulting in reduced pregnancy rates and female dropout rates; dental fluoride tablets reducing dental caries; swimming education resulting in lowered drowning rates; family crisis counseling reducing the incidence of emotional disturbances and learning problems in children.

3. The effectiveness of health education services designed to provide knowledge and skills necessary for students to protect their own health as students and that of themselves and their families, work places, and communities as adults may be assessed by: (a) improvements in health status items that were the targets of specific knowledge (rates for unwanted pregnancies, periodontal disease, obesity, immoderate alcohol consumption, maldevelopment, and emotional disturbance of children); (b) effective health-seeking behavior by graduates in their roles as parents, consumers, workers, community members; (c) appropriate processing of new health knowledge; (d) use of skills in decision making in health matters.

4. Effectiveness in meeting certain of the community's health needs may be measured only if the needs of the community are specified and the rationale for the school's involvement clearly stated, including the advantages and disadvantages of school involvement compared with other available courses of action. Measurement of community health needs and development of rationales for action require a community-planning process and a health services decision-making structure (with the school as a participating member) that clearly do not now exist. Agencies with an ability to affect a community's health services for children include, but are not limited to:

Public health services
   Federal—central and regional
   State—central and regional
   Local
Health systems agencies
Mental health/mental retardation services
Welfare departments
Insurance companies
Unions
Health maintenance organizations
Voluntary agencies
Hospitals
Medical schools
Private practitioners
Group practices
Private and public clinics
Child guidance clinics
Family service agencies
Advocacy organizations

That these agencies rarely alert each other and schools to the health needs of children as they see them and rarely work together on commonly perceived problems are measures of the total lack of community structures for planning and delivery of health services to children. In the absence of a rational community process, schools are sometimes commanded to perform certain services (e.g., immunization requirements for school attendance) by those who have or appear to have governmental power, or pressure is brought to bear on them by voluntary agencies or professional organizations to provide certain activities of dubious value (e.g., training in cardiopulmonary resuscitation—CPR, scoliosis screening, visual perception training).

The basic reasons for the existence of school health services, discussed above, express the obligations of the school and society to protect the health of children in areas beyond the capacity and responsibility of parents. Those who express the view that a child's "good health is basically his parents' responsibility"[4] are excusing those responsible for conditions inimicable to child health, such as air pollution, unsafe toys, lead paint, uncontrolled traffic flow in residential areas, unsafe school buses, and lack of insurance for preventive medical care, and are placing the burden on the victims—children and their families.

Parents reign supreme in determining the home life of their child and the quantity and type of personal health care services received by the child. Thus parents may not provide a toothbrush, seat belts, adequate nutrition, or a stimulating environment for a child's development. They may not seek immunizations or preventive health examinations and may not seek care for the child's strabismus, deafness, or congenital heart disease.

School health programs cannot force the issue unless the health of others is endangered, in which case schools must be empowered by society to act against the wishes of parents, as with immunization laws and laws requiring exclusion from school for certain contagious conditions. Except for those rare circumstances, school health, as a branch of public health, subscribes to the belief that parents desire the best for their children and parental behavior not in accord with this objective may be due to one or a number of causes: lack of knowledge, lack of resources, lack of availability and accessibility of needed services, competing family priorities of a more basic nature, lack of transportation, language and cultural barriers, and lack of parent availability due to work, separation, illness, death, or lack of intelligence.[5,6]

School health may attempt to affect some of the causes by educating parents, arranging for special services, such as immunizations, where none formerly existed, or providing transportation, financing, or interpreter service. Such actions increase the knowledge base and options available to parents, and in essence provide them with greater freedom in their decision making regarding the home environment and health services to be received by their children.

It is reasonable to consider that only two agencies in society are expressly concerned that children attain their optimal level of health: the family and the school. Their responsibilities to ensure the health of their children are different but interdependent. From the earliest days of school nursing, schools have shown that they can assist families in provision of health care to children, by knowledge, by provision of resources, and by assistance in overcoming barriers to the use of resources. A fifth rationale for school health services in the United States could be to support and assist families in provision of health services to children. In 1971 the School District of Philadelphia expressed this as a goal of its activities:

> To develop a partnership with the families of school children in protecting the health of children and in providing opportunities for their optimum growth and development.
> a. In this society, the family and the school are the two primary institutions caring for children and preparing them for independent function as adults. The aim of both partners is the healthy growth and development of children in all areas—physical, mental and social.
> b. Families, particularly as a result of social circumstances, vary in their ability to fulfill the functions they would desire for their children's maximum healthy growth and development. Thus, the school will be expected to vary the contribution it makes to its partnership with families, depending on the capabilities of the families.[7]

Chapter 5

ANALYSIS OF CURRENT SCHOOL HEALTH SERVICES

"In the old days it was reasonable. I put the lamp out in the morning, and in the evening I lighted it again. I had the rest of the day for relaxation and the rest of the night for sleep."

"And the orders have been changed since that time?"

"The orders have not been changed," said the lamplighter. "That is the tragedy! From year to year the planet has turned more and more rapidly and the orders have not been changed!

... The planet now makes a complete turn every minute, and I no longer have a single second for repose. Once evey minute I have to light my lamp and put it out!"

... And he lighted his lamp again.

As the little prince watched him, he felt he loved this lamplighter who was so faithful to his orders.

—Antoine de Saint-Exupéry, *The Little Prince*

The analysis presented in this chapter will attempt to deal with the paradox of current school health services. On the one hand, there are rationales for the existence of school health services which have the strength of moral imperatives and have been accorded general consensus within society. Some form of school health services exists in all states in which state departments of health report themselves as having roles. The health needs of school students are pressing, multiple, varied, and complex, with profound consequences for current and future health and functioning. On the other hand, the school health services of today provide a basic core of physical examinations, screening tests, first aid, and some school nurse follow-up. These services were developed for the needs of students at the turn of the century and provide little of relevance for the health needs of today's students. It is little wonder that school health services are poorly recognized and poorly understood by the health care and education communities.

This disparity between needs and services is even more remarkable given the early history of school health, in which the enthusiasm of its practitioners, their flexibility of operation, and the rapid diffusion of new ideas were notable features. The profundity of the change that overtook the field, somewhere in the 1920's, can be best appreciated in the differences in the tone of writing on school health between the first two decades and the fourth decade of this century. Dr. S. Josephine Baker, first director of the Bureau of Child Hygiene in the New York City Department of Health, wrote with enthusiasm, in 1906, of "a plan of great importance" to obtain a complete physical examination of each school child;[1] by 1939 she wrote of the work as a "dismal failure" and was unable to analyze what was interpreted as resistance on the part of practitioners, parents, and school boards.[2]

In 1917 Lina Rogers, the first school nurse in the nation, wrote of her experiences in a glowing book full of innovative responses to the health problems of her students, including a Young Parents Club in which students responsible for the care of infant and preschool siblings could bring them to school for demonstrations of proper dressing, feeding, care, and play.[3] In 1931 Mary Ella Chayer described the school nurse's role as one cramped by the requirements of others, especially school administrators, whom nurses were advised to please in order to perform any nursing services at all.[4]

Some observers maintain that the change was due to state laws requiring school health programs and specifying a rigid set of services to be provided. Others find fault with the lack of laws. Some see the problem in the local administration of school health services by school districts, thereby avoiding the 40 percent of school health services administered by public health departments. The fact is that school health services are very much the same no matter what the country or administrative pattern.[5] The problem of school health—its inability to shake free of services designed for the past and grapple with the needs of the present—has to do, I believe, with deficiencies in the administration of public health services.

Disabilities in Public Health

It has already been noted that the administration of education is different from that of public health. In education the objectives remain the same, services are essentially similar from year to year, only the classroom content changes as new knowledge and methods are added or deleted. Public health must be prepared to change both its objectives and its methods depending upon the disease pattern of the population. Thus a health department in a rural county will, with the advent of an industrial park, find itself responsible for a larger population possibly subject to air pollution, toxic wastes, occupational hazards including radiation, increased traffic patterns, strain upon local hospitals and maternity units, relocation neuroses, and manifestations of stress and of cultural and social isolation.

Public health is not easy to understand for either the public or politicians. It is less predictable than such service delivery systems as education. It is proactive whereas clinical medicine is reactive. It is more a process than a fixed structure. In the process of searching out the etiology of disease, it is liable to implicate those who are powerful in the public or private sector as contributors to ill health through their products, pollution, or policies.

The core intellectual operation of public health is epidemiology, which in investigating phenomena of health and disease is able to indicate causes and thus open the way to preventive actions. The preventive actions that may be taken are, logically, as varied as the factors defined in the web of causation. They range from political and legislative activities on the state and national levels to mobilization of local resources so that children with spina bifida may be catheterized once a day at school, thus ensuring their full educational day in a normal school. Much public health work involves extensive working with other agencies, organizations, professions, consumers, sources of knowledge, and wielders of influence in a community organization approach involving elements of community development, social action, and social planning.[6]

The two elements of public health—the epidemiologic intelligent core and the community organization approach to preventive actions—were present in the environmental work that characterized the early days of public health. Unfortunately, the discovery, at the end of the nineteenth century, of the specific bacterial causes of many communicable diseases, followed by the promise of vaccine prevention and, later, antibiotic treatment, proved a heady mix that so riveted the attention of health departments (including the U.S. Public Health Service) and the epidemiologists within them that (1) epidemiology became oriented to communicable diseases, (2) the earlier ecological view of disease narrowed to consider one cause, the bacteria, and (3) medical actions replaced community organization and environmental manipulation as avenues for prevention.

Health departments thus lost their ability to understand the epidemiology of noncommunicable diseases and, in fact, to recognize that epidemiology expressed the heart of their mission. Most health departments described themselves as deliverers of a basic set of services, as purveyors of input, and not as guardians of a process devoted to the outcome of improved community health levels.

Health services for children and mothers found their way into early health departments via a different route. Early demonstrations of environmental and communicable disease services were the work of farsighted physicians in city health departments. Public health nurses and well-baby clinics, school nurses and the dissemination of school health services were developments of the child welfare field, which sprouted such other manifestations as child labor reform groups, settlement houses, social work activists, and consumer organizations and from 1912 was represented in the federal govenment in the U.S. Children's Bureau. Some of the finest community organization for health purposes ever recorded was accomplished by the U.S. Children's Bureau. The fruit of its labor was the establishment, in all health departments, of a maternal and child health service that, with federal funds, came to represent public health services for children. The history of maternal and child health services has been a drive to ensure that all children and mothers receive a set of basic preventive services. A concern with input!

School health, as a specialized field of public health, has found itself in or connected with departments of health, where its natural allies in maternal and child health have skills in application of knowledge and not in epidemiology. Those practicing the epidemiologic, or thinking, function of public health see what they do as pertinent only to communicable disease and to preventive efforts of a medical nature. There have been no epidemiologists to assist school health to understand the new disease patterns of children and design preventive interventions for them.

With the benefit of hindsight it is easy to note the inability of school health and public health departments of respond after the dramatic decrease in and in some cases the disappearance of the communicable diseases of childhood brought about by environmental sanitation, improved living and nutrition standards, and vaccines and accomplished by the 1930's. These diseases had lowered life expectancy, filled cemeteries with small graves, and rendered parenthood a matter of grief during the whole of human history. When the veil of this mortality and morbidity was lifted and the terrain of child health was subjected to an uninterrupted "gaze",[7] some observers saw nothing and declared the group "healthy"; only gradually have the variety and complexity of health problems of schoolchildren come into focus. Recognized now for some decades, these new realities have been unable to stimulate resonses for new school health services from departments of public health, as the health departments have abandoned the epidemiologic process as the way to understand new disease realities and design appropriate preventive responses.

In the terms used by systems analysts, school health became an "input" system, with its activities or "means" determined by law and tradition, its behavior "reactive," and the outcome of its behavior "fixed."[8] The objectives of most school health services were performance of a certain number of examinations or tests and employment of a certain number of school nurses and other staff. All data produced reflected such inputs to the system to the point of recording the number of telephone calls, number of notices sent home, and number of times school nurses spoke to other school staff. Rarely, if ever, were objectives set or stated in terms of improvements in health of the target population (outputs) even when such were plainly the effects of the services; for example, hearing screening performed by schools is usually reported in such terms as "number screened," "number referred," "number wearing hearing aids." The same program could describe its objectives as: "to identify in the school student population those with previously undetected hearing loss, to reduce hearing loss through appropriate otologic and prosthetic services, and to provide each child with an educational plan to maximize educational performance" and could provide data to show the achievement of these objectives.

Inability to describe the point of activities means that they soon appear pointless. Those who stand outside school health cannot decipher the value of its activities. Those in school health, with minds divorced from the effectiveness of what they do, begin to think of activities as having value; after time, they *feel* that what they do has importance but are unable to describe, in objective terms, why that is so.

Pennsylvania provides an excellent example of these matters.[9] State law has required, since 1911, that all school districts employ staff to perform the activities of physical examination, dental examination, and screening tests for height, weight, vision, hearing, and tuberculosis. The department of health was recognized, by law, as the determiner of the content and standards of the state school health program with power over a substantial state reimbursement for school districts for school health services rendered in accordance with the law. Within the department of health the school health programs usually fell under the jurisdiction of maternal and child health services.

The Pennsylvania program was appraised critically by the American Public Health Association in 1948,[10] the Joint State Government Commission in 1955,[11] and the Johns Hopkins School of Hygiene and Public Health in 1961.[12] Each report pointed out the irrelevancy of a program primarily geared to documentation of physical defects and the misuse of professsional staff used to perform tasks easily done by those with less training. As a result of the 1955 report the existing school health law was repealed and a new school health services law was passed in 1957. It established a program of examinations, screening tests, and school nurse services as a basic program "floor" upon which the department of health was given specific powers to build, including the power to release school districts from the activities required by law in return for alternative programs meeting department standards.

The department of health took no action after any of the above reports or the passage of the new law. Such inaction was totally in accord with observations made of the field of school health generally. In 1942 Nyswander wrote that the chief fault of school health "appears to be that practice does not match up with theory . . . observations of personnel at work fail to show that recommendations . . . have been incorporated into the work of the staff. The staff, so these critics say, continue to do the same kind of job they did twenty years ago."[13] In 1968 Rogers noted that many school health programs "have become established by tradition and regulation so that they continue without respect to their effectiveness or relevance to health improvement."[14]

Finally, new leadership in the department stimulated a systems evaluation of the program in 1970 which concluded:

> The evaluation of the School Health Services Program has succeeded in uncovering little reliable, quantifiable data that sheds light upon the outputs that School Health Services produce . . . [but] has, however, resulted in the conclusion that a clarification of the objectives . . . of the Program . . . are necessary to improve the delivery and assessment of results of school health services.[15]

One of the side effects of the inertia of departments of health in relations to school health was that the statements of the American Medical Association–National Education Association expressing the policy that schoolchildren are "healthy" and that school health services should consist of health education to maintain health and a few clinical services for the less fortunate was left unchallenged. Another effect was the lack of any consistent federal government activity devoted to school health, which may have reflected the general paucity of public health thought in regard to school health or may have been a practical response to the monolithic devotion of the field to the status quo. The lack of academic interest in school health is remarkable and not completely explicable. Occupational health, like school health with origins in public health and subject to neglect within departments of public health, was able to grow into a recognized field of health care with a sound theoretical basis, research, training programs, and specialization for nurses and physicians including, for the latter, board certification. The presence of these activities is revealed in the many books, articles, and journals devoted to the field. School health has none of these things. It is recognized, if at all, as an activity of dubious worth existing on the outer fringes of the health care field. It is not a discipline or specialty within schools of nursing or medicine or public health, or within departments of pediatrics. It is starved for theoretical discussions and research findings. The few books are attempts to make interesting the dull recital of the "activities" of the "school health program" and are intended for students of education. There is but one journal. The result has been a lack of thought, lack of leaders, and lack of skilled practitioners to challenge the pall of inaction. The dilemma of occupational health is to be admitted to the work place in order to apply its knowledge. The dilemma of school health, ensconced in the work place, is to become knowledgeable. This lack of knowledge of the heart of the subject and lack of any authoritative views challenging the status quo mean that state departments of education and welfare, regional education agencies, and local school districts—the other actors in the school health system—have not known that things could be different and have, therefore, not pressed departments of health to become proponents for change.

State departments of education provide standards and guidelines for a variety of functions, performed by regional education agencies and/or local school districts, that have health content or are health-related: the health education curriculum, special education services for the handicapped, pupil personnel services (school guidance counselors, attendance officers). They are also responsible for the process by which certain local health staff, usually nurses and dental hygienists, are required to be certified in order to perform in schools. It sometimes appears that staff of state departments of education believe that these activities encompass all state responsibility for school health and are willing to answer questionnaires and surveys to that effect without reference to the state department of health (as noted in Chapter 1).

State departments of welfare, in some matters involving medical assistance and the Early Periodic Screening Diagnosis and Treatment (EPSDT) program, have developed relationships with school districts as providers of certain reimbursable health services. It is tragic and also ironical that the latter program often eschews school health as a pointless, irrelevant service while proceeding to duplicate the mindless activity from which school health is now castigated for not extricating itself. In short, EPSDT consists of legally required input services—physical examination, dental examination, and screening tests for vision, hearing, growth, tuberculosis—for a specified population group, namely, recipients of medical assistance below the age of twenty-one. Better academic understanding of school health, plus some devotion to health outcome on the part of those legislating and administering health services, might have prevented the irrationalities of the EPSDT system.

The above exploration of all possible sources of challenge to department of public health passivity in the matter of school health turns to the most logical and potent source: the local provider of service, whether the local school district or the local health department. The latter institution can be dismissed; it was hampered by the prevalent public health view of school health, staff shortages, and the generic role of public health nurses as performers of activities in the varied settings of home, school, and clinic. These splendid nurses were rarely allowed to specialize in school health or given the opportunity to see the system from the inside. School nurses, employed by the local school district, were in a different situation: as members of the staff they had access to the total facility, staff, and students. The nurse's office was an open door through which anyone could pass who wanted to discuss a problem. More problems were revealed as the nurse's style, competence, and integrity became institutional facts. School nurses became and remain to this day repositories of verbal data and oral history, set in keen observations of individuals and environments, which are the basic skills of the nursing profession. What went wrong?

EDUCATIONAL LOCATION

The early history of nurses in schools reveals energy and ability successfully directed at the health needs of the students in particular schools or school districts.[3] All this stopped and stopped suddenly by the 1930's.[4] A number of factors appear to have been involved:

1. As school districts became the organizational base for school health services, school administrators were vested with responsibility for carrying out the activities required by law. The administrators extended their control to all health services, not only those specified by law, until, in many in-

stances, the law was interpreted as defining the totality of what is allowed and not the minimum required. This arrangement placed "a millstone of incredible deadening weight . . . around the neck of school health as any demand for change from the practitioners in the field could be choked off at its source." Health professionals carried out tasks, and persons without any health training at all made the policy and program decisions.[16]

2. Because school health has been seen as the provision of a set of services to individual students in individual schools, the school health staff has rarely been organized into a staff unit and the small size of most school districts has further isolated professionals from each other.

3. School administrators, finding themselves without any preparation in health care administration, responsible for the day-to-day management of school health services, often deal with their unenviable situation by avoiding decision making, or they retain their authority and control by invoking the law as a reason for inaction. Their understanding of health law is tenuous at best and is little strengthened by consultation with the school district's lawyer, whose expertise may be in real estate and property law. In this fashion an oral tradition of school health legal fables involving wild monsters of malpractice has been manufactured that bears as close a relationship to reality as did the medieval maps of a flat world. Every school nurse has stories to tell of plans to improve health services for children which were smothered at birth by a frightened educator in a position for which he or she was unprepared. Some examples of activities frequently forbidden to school nurses: taking of a full pediatric history from children before a physical examination, pregnancy screening tests (now sold over the counter) in order to obtain early prenatal care for teenagers, catheterization of children with spina bifida, nurse practitioner physical examination of male athletes, home visits for follow-up of difficult problems, and reporting of cases of child abuse as required by law. The health of schoolchildren is surely too important to be left to the ignorant.

4. School nurses not only were deprived of a professional decision-making role by the organizational changes occasioned by school health laws. They also have been subject to other forces in schools which have reduced their power and influence:

    a. They are health professionals in an educational setting.

    b. They are nurses in the health care field, where physicians wield authority.

    c. They are women working in two fields, health care and education, both of which are dominated by men.

5. The above circumstances made it unlikely that nurses could influence the field of school health with program innovation as they did once. Then certain changes in nursing education removed the likelihood of a struggle by educating nurses to be submissive to authority. Nursing education became firmly established in hospital schools by the first decades of this century. A prime reason was that the basic education of women was so poor that college education for large numbers was impossible. The hospitals worked the trainees as indentured servants and demanded discipline, obedience, and control of the nurses' personal lives. The fierce opposition to nursing displayed by the medical profession (many poorly trained in the diploma mills of the late nineteenth century) was deflected by teaching nurses excessive deference to physicians even to point of nurses' opening doors and standing in physicians' presence. The lack of college preparation led to the view of nursing as a nonprofession. Among the major women's professions—nursing, social work, teaching, and library science—only nursing has had to develop without a college background, without male members (the hospitals prohibited that), and without the support of related male-dominated professions.[17]

Having reviewed some of the major reasons for the inability of the school health system to respond to the health needs of students, we now summarize briefly some operating aspects of the current system.

SERVICES SUBSYSTEM

The major thrust of the service subsystem is appraisal of the health status of the individual child. This is usually accomplished by some combination of:

Medical examination by school or family physician on entry and sometimes in two subsequent grades

Dental examination by school or family dentist

Screening tests for vision, hearing, height and weight, tuberculosis, immunization status

School nurse services

The physical examination is seen by school staff to be the chief appraisal activity, despite the increasing number of reports indicating the
deficiency of the physical exam even when done well, compared with
the health history, in the number and relevancy of health problems
discovered.[18] Dental examinations performed by dentists are a grossly
inefficient use of professionals who are desperately needed to provide
restorative services; screening-type evaluations could be performed,
with appropriate education, by physicians as part of the physical exam
or by nurses or technicians.

Each year millions of schoolchildren are screened. Such routine
screening, performed smoothly for decades, may make school health
services the most experienced mass-screening agent in the nation.
There are problems: lack of standards of height and weight; dissatisfaction with visual acuity screening in an age in which learning problems are attributed, often with little justification, to "muscle imbalance"
and "visual perceptual problems"; lack of appropriate school facilities
for hearing screening; general lack of quality control in administration
of tests, for example, lack of training, of manuals, of supervision; use
of expensive professional nurses to perform repetitive, simple screening tests that by definition are designed to be performed by nonprofessionals; lack of understanding of the theory of screening,[19]
leaving school districts vulnerable to every group that comes peddling
its pet, unproven test, such as vision-testing machines,[20] sickle cell trait
screening,[21] and scoliosis screening.[22]

School nurse services have been defined by regulations. In Pennsylvania the regulations are marvelously vague.[23] They ascribe to
school nurses the "traditional" nursing role of assisting, offering assistance, assisting in interpreting, assisting in evaluating, advising, providing, working with, encouraging (and generally acting as handmaiden
or mother for) administrators, physicians, dentists, teachers, personnel, councils, community groups, families, parents. Three types of
activities can be discerned with which school nurses may "assist":

1. Administrative functions
    a. Program planning including environmental and first
        aid services, accident prevention, home nursing, com-
        municable disease control
    b. Program organization and implementation including
        scheduling, public relations and information, record
        keeping, instruction of first aid personnel
    c. Program budget preparation

    d.   Program evaluation

    e.   Program development including community organization

The described administrative functions diminish in the face of a set of mandated services provided without planning, evaluation, program development, or budget discretion; in addition, the school administrator does not easily give administrative prerogatives, such as budget preparation and certainly not budget control, to clinical, assisting types such as nurses. Thus the administrative functions are reduced in practice to scheduling, assisting, informing, and record keeping. (The school nurses call these functions "clerical," a caption that correctly identifies the frustrations felt but is incorrect in that these functions, particularly scheduling of large numbers of students to receive sets of services, are basically administrative in nature.)

2.   Consultation functions

    a.   Evaluation of course content and provision of information to school personnel for health teaching

Consultation functions, depending as they do upon the willingness of others to seek the services of the consultant, tend to wither in an educational setting where any high school curriculum guide tends to take precedence over other influences, where elementary school teachers are free to ignore the whole area of health instruction if they so choose, where nurses are not able to "sell" the value of their expertise given the dominant role of education.

3.   Problem management functions

    a.   Management of family, school, and community resources to resolve health problems of students

The health management function is left as the major area in which the school nurse has the chance to exert professional skill and judgment, but the freedom in time and space and the environmental supports needed to carry out follow-up are not provided in many instances.

Time for follow-up is restricted as nurses are forced to carry out the screening tests for vision, hearing, and height and weight; to perform the scheduling, assisting, and record keeping needed to implement the program; and in the absence of other personnel to perform first aid services. Freedom of movement is denied many nurses by school administrators who demand their continued presence in school for first aid functions; thus home visits and direct work with other agencies cannot be done. Few nurses have the telephone service, files and filing systems, clerical assistance, confidential office facilities, postage, copying, and other supports needed for problem management/follow-up functions. What emerges in practice for school nurse services can be summarized: 75 percent of time spent on screening tests, first aid, and clerical tasks and 25 percent spent on professional nursing in problem management and follow-up.

As school nurses have been gradually removed from their chief professional service, they have been forced into a service area about which there is much ambivalence and evasion. First aid and those services provided in the school's health room to children who have minor injuries and illnesses, are not specified as activities of the school nurse in the regulations of the Pennsylvania Department of Health; those regulations prescribe, as an activity for school nurses: "To plan for first aid services and instruct personnel responsible for giving first aid." There is no doubt, however, that the main and sometimes only reason school administrators want school nurses is for first aid.[24] The presence of a nurse gives them peace of mind; at the same time they begin to realize that someone with less training and needing less salary could do the job. A curious ambivalence sets in: the nurse, trapped in subprofessional duties by the administrator, is blamed by the same administrator, and sometimes by parents,[25] for not doing a professional job worthy of the salary.

The school nurse, as victim in a situation in which professional activities are totally controlled by a superior from another discipline, tends to react to the charge of not deserving the salary or of doing subprofessional-level work with an understandable vehemence, a tendency to dwell on the input rather than the outcome of the service, and a tendency to portray what the nurse does (i.e., is forced to do) as fully professional in nature. First aid is defended as "health counseling" and as an opportunity to detect unsuspected conditions of children—which is true save that there are much better ways to organize health counseling and problem detection services than by using first aid as a front.

Administrators know nothing about the various options available in provision of first aid services and believe that a warm nursing body on the premises is what is required. Nurses who have suggested alternatives have had them rejected.

PERSONNEL

The main personnel involved in the provision of school health services are school physicians, dentists, and school nurses. School health has not only been unable to keep pace with the changing health needs of the population it serves; it has also been unable to adjust its staffing pattern to the change in skills that has taken place over the years in which nurses have taken over functions formerly carried out by physicians and aides and technicians now perform tasks once done by nurses and physicians. School health is marked by the subprofessional use of all staff!

The lack of a theoretical undergirding of school health practice, the lack of specialization already alluded to, means that no specific training exists for those about to enter the practice of school health. There are no courses for school physicians or dentists, and there is often no specific school health content to the courses school nurses must take to become certified by the department of education. School health staff, for example, receive no particular training in normal growth and development although the major tasks facing their clients—school students—are developmental: emotional maturation, growth of independence, and social adaptation.[18]

School physicians are in short supply, so many school districts are unable to employ the numbers needed. Their main task is the physical examination, which is often done poorly. Many but not all school physicians are not interested in the job, being either at the beginning or the end of their practicing life; they are looking for part-time work to balance a less than full practice. Many physicians interested in the health of schoolchildren have been driven out by the mindless concentration on physical examinations. Yet without training programs "the school physician of today . . . is still relatively uneducated as far as the first part of his title is concerned."[26]

The subprofessional tasks currently assigned to school nurses not only are an expensive use of staff, but also lead to lack of time for real nursing functions and consequent staff dissatisfaction.

In many states nurses must be certified by the state department of education in order to work as school nurses;[27] for example, in Pennsylvania, nurses are required to have a bachelor's degree in nursing and 24 additional credits. The first requirement presented difficulties when most nurses were graduates of hospital diploma (3-year) programs and there were few schools offering bachelor's (4-year) programs. Later, the bachelor's programs that opened up, as the field of nursing swung from hospital to college education, refused to go through the additional process of being certified as approved programs by the department of education, claiming with justification that certification of nursing education programs was a function of the nursing accreditation agency, the National League for Nursing (NLN).

In the meantime, the Pennsylvania Department of Education had stimulated development of bachelor's programs in school nursing, usually at the campuses of the state university system. These programs were certified by the department of education as competent to grant bachelor's degrees to school nurses but could not meet the requirements of the NLN. Nurses who took such programs could work in schools, but were not recognized as graduates of nursing programs by schools of nursing when they went to take advanced training. For this reason many school nurses seeking higher education have obtained it in education or guidance counseling, where their bachelor's degree is recognized. The nursing field has been drained of some of its most able members in this way.

Nurses in school health are the most highly educated group after those in nursing education, as shown by data for Pennsylvania for 1972 (Table 5-1). School nursing has been able to attract able practitioners because its hours fit the needs of nurses who wish to work while raising young families. The certification requirements, which entail considerable time and expense, serve to box nurses into the field of school health, and the full-time status, the good wages and conditions, and the pleasures of working with children keep them in the field. School nurses tend to have comparatively little turnover. The average age of practitioners is high.

Table 5-1.

Highest degree held	Total percentage of registered nurses by field of employment				
	Nursing education	School health	Public health	Occupational health	Hospital
Less than bachelor's	16	24	56	79	80
Bachelor's: nursing	33	29	25	4	7
Bachelor': other	15	28	4	1	2
Master's: nursing*	17	1	4	0	1
Master's: other*	14	8	3	0	1
Doctorate	2	0	0	0	0
Other/Unknown	3	10	8	16	9
Total	100	100	100	100	100

*Philadelphia 1970/71: Sixteen percent of nurses with permanent school nurse certificates held master's degrees.[28]
Source: Morgan and Balog.[29]

SUPPORT PERSONNEL

There is no doubt that, if 75 percent of the current work of school nurses is below their professional ability, then it can be done by someone with less training. "Nonprofessional personnel with . . . competency and . . . training can make an effective contribution to the school health program and, at the same time, make it possible to focus professional efforts on professional tasks."[30] The Head Start program in Philadelphia employed former medical corpsmen from the armed services as pediatric technicians who performed all screening tests and some clerical, administrative, and follow-up functions under the supervision of pediatric nurse practitioners.[31] Some school districts employ part-time clerks or occasionally have volunteers to assist school nurses with clerical duties, dressing and undressing of young children for physicals, assisting the physician, doing height and weight measurements, answering the telephone, getting out letters, sorting permission forms, etc. Such suggestions are, however, likely to generate immediate emotional, negative reactions, partly because they clearly recognize the subprofessional nature of much of the current work of school nurses and partly because they are seen as presenting a threat to the job security of nurses.

HEALTH INFORMATION SUBSYSTEM

Health information subsystems to quantify health needs, and thus provide the basis for program planning and evaluation, are not found at the central nor local levels of the school health program and are not required in reactive, input systems. A considerable amount of staff time is used in data collection and compilation, but most data are related to activities performed rather than assessment of health status. Health data collected by other agencies are little used by school health services.

MANAGEMENT SUBSYSTEM

Management or decision-making subsystems in the school health system are rudimentary, as befits the input nature of the operation. State departments of health, making no professional decisions regarding school health rarely employ professionals or staff with management skills. In Pennsylvania, for over 10 years the department of health employed only one clerk to disburse the $14 million of state reimbursement to school districts and to answer questions from the field.[16] In the local school districts, as already noted, there are program administrators—unfortunately, without skills in the content of management of health services.

In most school districts, decisions regarding health services are made by superintendents, assistant superintendents, or the head of pupil services, who may be a counselor, a physical and health educator, or a psychologist. In most school districts there is no "director of health services." The role would be inappropriate for physicians, who are mostly part-time employees. Nurses, although full-time employees, would rarely be considered for the role, partly because of their sex and the generally low esteem in which nursing is held. If a school health program has a chief who is a nurse, the nurse is usually called "coordinator," sometimes "nursing supervisor," however, the nurse *almost never* has control over the budget for the school health program.

The control exerted by educational administrators over the total program is duplicated at the school level in the control exerted by the principal over the school nurse. The only reason advanced in school circles for absolute control when it is exerted by a school principal is "The principal is the captain of the ship." Schools are *not* ships! They are not even totally isolated communities surviving on tight discipline. They are part of their society and neighborhood and communicate with them daily. In such a system there is little reason for an expert in one field (education) to tell those in another area (health) how to conduct their business.[24] There is even less reason for such an arrangement to be upheld by those who know that administration theory clearly distinguishes administrative structure from professional content.[24,32]

Chapter 6

A NEW SCHOOL HEALTH SERVICES SYSTEM

The longing for certainty and repose is in every human mind. But certainty is generally illusion and repose is not the destiny of man.

—Oliver Wendell Holmes, Sr.*

The school health services system designed at the beginning of this century, effective in improving the health of students and efficient in its use of staff (as nurses took over classroom inspections performed by physicians and physicians began performing the new physical examinations), developed problems only when the health status of the school student population changed. A logical new system would be one containing services for the new health needs of students, but it, too, would be vulnerable to obsolescence once those health needs changed again. Therefore a system that could alter itself in an ongoing fashion would be preferable. Such a system would be cybernetic, with a feedback, or information, loop keeping it aware of changes in the health status of students, and it would also be dynamic in that it could change its services to meet new needs. Thus the system would choose both its

*Oliver Wendell Holmes, 1809–1894, described by Sir William Osler as "the most successful combination the world has ever seen, of physician and man of letters" from Harvey Cushing, *Life of Sir William Osler*, 1925, Vol. I, ch. 15.

ends (objectives) and its means (services and use of resources) and in so doing would exhibit the characteristics of a purposive system.

Such a school health system, responsive to the changing health system, responsive to the changing health needs of its target population, can be conceptualized as consisting of three subsystems (Figure 6–1):

> *Health information* to measure the level of health of the target population
>
> *Management* to make epidemiologic analyses of the health information collected, to make decisions regarding the ends or objectives to be achieved, and to plan and implement the means or services required to achieve those objectives
>
> *Services* to provide activities that significantly improve the health of the population

The problem of differences in the health status of the school student population is a function not only of time, as noted in the history of school health, but also of place and person. School students who are residents of different areas have health problems that also vary; for example, those in rural and urban areas differ in regard to environmental pollution, availability of health services, availability of drugs, and use of automobiles to name but a few differences. Characteristics of persons which affect health include age, sex, race, ethnicity, religion, socioeconomic status, parental occupation and education, and immigrant status. School districts, and indeed schools within school districts, vary widely in regard to the characteristics of persons and place, and thus health status, covered by their populations.

These differences in the health needs of school students at the local level provided a reason for the School Health Advisory Committee of the Pennsylvania Department of Health to recommend in 1973, after a systems analysis of the school health program of the commonwealth, that each school district, on the basis of the health needs of its

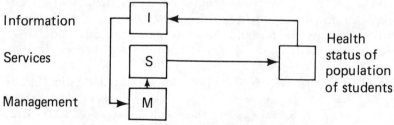

Figure 6–1. Purposive School Health System.

student population, develop and submit for state funding a plan for a school health services program to best meet those needs consistent with efficient use of available health care resources and within guidelines established by the department of health.[1] Thus would school health services "be funded in the same manner as most current health programs; flexibility to meet variations in health needs would be assured; program evaluation would be possible; a great amount of information about feasibility, efficiency and effectiveness in school health services would quickly become available in a field parched for initiative, research, and ideas."[2] In 1978 similar recommendations were made for the school health program in New York State.[3]

These recommendations recognized (1) that the only means by which variations in the health needs of students at the local level can be accounted for is by the existence of purposive school health systems at the school district level; and (2) that it is a patent impossibility for a centrally operated state institution, such as a state department of health, to understand the different needs of populations in school districts and their subdivisions, let alone plan services that reflect the variations in health care resources in those communities.

The major problem blocking implementation of a purposive school health system at the local level is the complete absence in the current system of any form of health information or management subsystem. The services subsystem, although limited in activities performed, possesses professional staff who have accumulated skills in sensing the health needs of students, in operating health services within educational settings, in recognizing the value to school health services of certain school staff and practices, and in using of health resources in the school and local community.

By 1975 the Pennsylvania Department of Health recognized that the task was to implement, at the local level, a systems change from an input/reactive model to an output/purposive model consisting of subsystems of information, management, and services, where only the services subsystem currently existed; and to do this with current resources.[2,4–6] The strategy for change revolved around the use of major assets currently in the school health system, namely, the services subsystem and the school nurses. Expanding the skills of school nurses to those of school nurse practitioners, together with releasing the nurses from the subprofessional activities of their current role, created nursing time and capacities for expanded health assessment of students and more effective follow-up of problems found. These activities increase the health of individual students (the second rationale for school health), provide more information on the health status of the population, and lead to the exercise of management functions.

The progression from school nurse practitioner education to an improved services subsystem that stimulates development of information and management subsystems has been observed in school districts of Pennsylvania where, since 1974, 233 school nurses have been educated as school nurse practitioners and 48 school districts have embarked upon the process of systems change.[7] The following chapters describe development of the subsystems of the new school health services system.

Chapter 7

SERVICES SUBSYSTEM

He who would do good to another must do it in minute particulars;
General good is the plea of the scoundrel, hypocrite, flatterer:
For art and science cannot exist but in minutely organized particulars.

—William Blake, Jerusalem

The services subsystem covers activities supported by the rationale for school health services that states that students need to be in their highest attainable state of health in order to obtain optimal benefit from their education. This objective was selected as the focus for development of a new school health services system for a number of reasons: current services, despite their inadequacies, are directed toward this objective; it is a rationale that occasions no controversy; and means were available, in nurse practitioner education programs, to immediately upgrade the scope and quality of current activities directed to this objective. It was also believed that the other rationales for school health could be more easily served after the new school health system began to operate: protection of children from the hazards of the school work place depends upon evaluation of the health status of children and a functioning information subsystem;

anticipatory guidance becomes possible with expanded health assessment; planning health education services to reach specific objectives requires an operating management subsystem, as does development of services to assist the community to reach its health goals.

The rationale selected requires that the health of each child be assessed so that those with health problems may receive case management services directed at resolution of the problems. It must be admitted that this sounds suspiciously like the old program done up with new words. Are there differences between "defects" or "conditions" and "problems"? Does "resolution" differ from "correction"? Certainly the concept of finding things wrong and getting them fixed is present in both word sets and is accepted as an aspect of owning a body, a set of teeth, or a car. The differences to be described in this services subsystem are found in the methods of assessment and in the concept of accountability built into problem resolution.

HEALTH ASSESSMENT

The foundation of assessment of the health status of individuals in this services subsystem is the health history.

Health History

The health history has always been recognized as the cornerstone of clinical practice and remains the most productive of all the assessment procedures available to modern medicine. In recent years popular magazines have informed readers that the health history is a better detector of internal illness than the physical examination or lab tests, and have explained the value of "health-appraisal questionnaires."[1] Unfortunately the medical history is more often honored in the breach than in the observance, as physicians have become enamored of laboratory tests and X rays or prefer a rapid physical examination to the time and discipline required for a good history.

A recent book on interpretation of clinical evidence noted a tendency among physicians to rely "more on laboratory tests than on clinical observation. This is unfortunate. Despite the usefulness of laboratory procedures, the bulk of the information required in diagnosis continues to come from the history and physical examination."[2]

Downplaying the value of the history by giving undue prominence to the physical examination has occurred particularly in military and school health, as noted by North: "The physical examination has become a ritual, an almost magical laying on of hands, which ... may be reassuring to the patient [but] is not very productive. In many instances physicians have abetted the public image that 'a physical' represents the sum and substance of a complete health evaluation."[3]

Some of the results of these trends are that few people appear to have had a good health history ever taken from them; some professionals confuse a health questionnaire with a health history, and some school nurses believe that a list of 10 or so questions can be classified as a health history. A basic pediatric history, however, designed to assess the overall health of a child reviews the following pertinent areas of the child's life for evidence of disease, dysfunction, hazard, or risk:

1. Prenatal and neonatal: pregnancy, labor, delivery, drugs, birth weight, resuscitation, newborn condition, hospital course, early care at home
2. Developmental: milestones, such as sitting, walking, talking, toilet training
3. Nutrition: breast or bottle feeding, weaning, food allergies, growth, appetite, current eating pattern
4. Immunizations: pertussis, diphtheria, tetanus, measles, rubella, mumps; basic and boosters
5. Past medical history: contagious diseases, other illnesses, accidents, operations, hospitalizations, medication, allergies, medical care providers, dental care providers, health insurance
6. Family health history: health of individual members of family; deaths; diseases with genetic, communicable, or serious family and/or socially disruptive characteristics
7. Family social history: family composition, age, employment and occupation, educational levels, income range, home size, plumbing and state of repair, child care arrangements, culture
8. Child's functioning:
   a. Physiologic functions, such as eating, sleeping, toilet habits, exercise and play
   b. Family functions, such as relationships with siblings, discipline, parental perceptions of child's problems and strengths
   c. Social functions, such as relationships with neighborhood children, school friends, hobbies, interests
   d. School functions and progress
9. Behavior: disturbances of physiologic function and evidence of anxiety, depression, regression, poor impulse control, hyperactivity
10. Review of body systems:
    a. Ear, nose, and throat

b. Hearing
c. Eyes
d. Vision
e. Cardiovascular
f. Respiratory
g. Gastrointestinal
h. Genitourinary
i. Neurological
j. Musculoskeletal
k. Hemopoietic
l. Endocrine
m. Allergic[4,5]

Use of some form of pediatric health history has been shown to result in detection of physical and nonphysical problems:

> In 1947 Yankauer found the New York City Astoria plan was successful in detection and care of physical defects, but a health interview with the parents of 114 sixth-grade children revealed 38 percent with "psychic and behavior problems" providing "an impression of disturbing factors in the child's home environment and emotional life."[6]
>
> Two hundred eighty-five middle-to low-income children ranging in age from three to eighteen received well-child care in a large health maintenance organization (HMO) in New Haven, Connecticut, from pediatricians who were responsive to the psychosocial data elicited by history; 38 percent of the children had "definable developmental or psychological problems requiring some action or intervention by the pediatrician."[7]
>
> In the school year 1972/73 the School District of Philadelphia assessed 1,136 entering kindergarten and first-grade students using a comprehensive pediatric history questionnaire, with parent interviews in 96 percent of cases; 31 percent of the children had behavior problems, 25 percent had developmental problems, and in 23 percent of cases the family environment was classified as constituting a health problem for the child.[8,9]

The importance of detailed and in-depth histories has been emphasized in the assessment of important conditions of childhood, for example, school failure[10] and allergy.[11] Not only does the health history find problems of a nonphysical nature, thus proving itself a valuable assessment tool for a population whose health needs are nonphysical, but it also detects problems not accessible by other methods and continues its tradition of being the most productive of assessment techniques.

In the Philadelphia study of 1,136 students, all problems identified on the history which could have been discovered by screening tests (growth, vision, hearing, T.B.), by review of immunization status, or by dental examination were removed, leaving, per examined child, 1.9 problems that could be detected only by history.[8] The Penn Manor School District reported the number of problems per child discovered by each assessment procedure as shown in Table 7–1. The Philadelphia study reviewed the records of 111 children on whom a history and physician-conducted physical examination were performed: 82 percent of the abnormalities found on the physical examination were recorded on the history. The 13 abnormalities recorded on the physical and not on the history were dental caries (4), wax in ears (3), infection of eyelids (3), warts on hand (1), posture problem (1), speech problem (1). These either are minor abnormalities hardly rating as problems or are discoverable by means other than a physician-performed physical examination.[8]

The way the health history is to be administered and the problems and errors of any method must be considered. There is an incredible paucity of studies considering the importance of the issue; if the problems found by history do not reflect reality then all information derived from such activity becomes useless and patient care, program evaluation, and research suffer. Health histories, like any form of clinical data, for example, X rays, are subject to observer error. A clinical survey of 993 coal miners made by 4 observers showed observer's bias influenced the frequency with which a positive answer was recorded to questions asked.[13] Questions requiring yes or no as an answer caused few problems. Questions eliciting more complex responses requiring observer judgment created problems of consistency.

Table 7–1.

Assessment procedure	Number of problems per student assessed	
	1974/75	*1976/77*
Health history	3.20	1.64
Neurological exam	0.59	0.76
Physical exam	0.48	0.33
Teacher observations	0.31	0.27
Screening tests (growth, vision, hearing)	0.23	0.24
Denver Developmental Screening Test	0.08	0.27
Total	4.89	3.51
Health history % of total	65%	47%

Source: Division of School Health.[12]

The more carefully defined the questions, the more consistent the replies.[14]

The Cornell Medical Index was published in 1949 as a standard health history questionnaire for adults, with 195 questions the patient answers by circling yes or no on the form.[15] The Cornell Medical Index was found inappropriate for use with adolescents. Alexiou and Wiener at Johns Hopkins University School of Hygiene and Public Health developed a similar health history questionnaire for adolescents, with 182 questions:[16] it was tested on 1,166 seventh- and tenth-grade students in a representative sample of public and private schools in Baltimore plus 3 rural and 2 upper-income private schools. A formal reliability study using a test-retest techinque gave a correlation coefficient of 90 for retests after a 2-week interval. This reliability is comparable to that of the Wechsler Intelligence Scale for Children and the Minnesota Multiphasic Personality Inventory. The test was found highly reliable for race, sex, age, and socioeconomic status. (Those with IQ below 80 or reading ability below fifth-grade level were not included.)

The validity of the questionnaire was studied by examining the relationship between students' answers and physicians' findings (examination plus screening tests of vision, hearing, color vision, height and weight, and past records.)[17] The number of yes answers by 388 students ranged from 0 to 69; the mean of 12.4. High scores on the questionnaire significantly predict health problems; however, "the statistical significance was not great enough to warrant the questionnaire's use for a mechanical diagnosis of an individual case." It was found that a clinical (subjective) interpretation of the content of the answered questionnaire produced a 94 percent "fair" to "good" agreement with hospital records of students, a finding supported by studies with the Cornell Medical Index.[18,19]

The adolescent questionnaire is one of the few health history questionnaires for which reliability and validity studies have been conducted. The findings indicate that the yes or no answers recorded by adolescents are reliable; large numbers of yes answers indicate a high probability of health problems (such a group could be scheduled first for further assessment); and questionnaires, if evaluated for clinical content, provide a more accurate understanding of the health status of the individual.

As a diagnostic tool in a clinical assessment,[17,20] the questionnaire adds to the process of obtaining a health history:

A comprehensive set of questions

Reduction of observer error through precise questions and the yes or no answers

A method for focusing the clinical interview around the meaning of the yes answers; the information obtained is listed, so that others can judge the validity of including or discarding the answer as indicating a problem; for example, if the question, "Do your gums bleed?" is answered yes, subsequent information obtained from the patient should be listed; it could be as different as:

Case 1—"1975, 5 years ago, light pink color on toothbrush once."

Case 2—"Since 2 months ago, red blood on toothbrush at least every second day. Bleeding on eating hard food such as nuts, noted about 5 times in past month."

In the first case the problem is dismissed, in the second case retained.

No health history questionnaire other than that for adolescents had been developed and tested for the schoolchild population. The Pennsylvania Department of Health adopted for elementary school enterers an untested but comprehensive health questionnaire that had been developed in 1971 by the Philadelphia School District, first for the Head Start program[21] and then with few modifications for the 1972/73 school enterer study.[8,9] The sources were the recommendations of the American Academy of Pediatrics and questionnaires used in neighborhood health centers and in the Hahnemann Department of Pediatrics. The Pennsylvania questionnaire incorporates the Behavior Questionnaire of Willoughby and Haggerty.[22]

The history questionnaire (see Appendix) is designed:

1. To be completed by a parent or guardian; therefore the questions are phrased clearly and the answers required are either yes or no or a piece of factual informaton, such as birth weight

2. To provide a comprehensive review of a child's health; therefore all areas of the pediatric history listed above are represented

3. To be used in conjunction with a health interview; therefore the questions are not exhaustive; positive answers provide indicators to be explored, and the interview process enables the skilled interviewer to hear the additional significant things being said and not said

4. To provide accountability in investigation of positive leads; therefore all answers indicating a response requiring further exploration are on the outside column of the page

5. To provide information indicating why problems were in-

cluded or rejected; therefore a blank page is provided opposite each page of the history to record the data upon which
the decision is made

6. To facilitate and respect the interview process, particularly
establishment of rapport between interviewer and parent so
that the clinical value of the history in revealing the real
issues troubling the parent and child will be enhanced;
therefore the more usual and routine health history items
and those that can be answered factually are placed first; the
history flows from pregnancy, development, past health,
family health, and review of systems to behavioral problems
and social and interpersonal functioning of the child, the last
questions are open-ended to enhance the flow of subjective
information from the parent

For the middle school students the task was more complicated.
There were no tested questionnaires as for high school, no well-tried
versions as for elementary school. In addition, the best health history
of the middle school child would appear to be one derived partly from
the parent (who knows the events of the past) and partly from the
student (who experiences the symptoms of the present). Therefore two
questionnaires were developed: one for parents, essentially the same as
the elementary questionnaire but without questions regarding symptoms; the second for students, concerning symptoms, problems, and
habits, adapted from the adolescent questionnaire but without those
questions dealing strictly with adolescent phenomena. Initial reports of
its use are good[12] and it has proven unexpectedly helpful with moderately retarded adolescents.[23]

One of the advantages of a questionnaire is that it can be sent
home, thereby giving the parent or patient greater time for completion, for discussion with other family members, and for reference to
records. In the early 1950's in San Francisco a comprehensive health
inventory was sent home to about 360 parents of children in kindergarten and first, third, and sixth grades; 89 percent of the forms were
returned completely filled out by parents within 10 days, and 93
percent were returned by the end of 3 weeks.[24]

It is also possible to offer the parent the option of taking the
questionnaire home for completion or having the health professional
ask the questions in the interview. In lower-literacy populations, such
as parents of Head Start children, 72 percent opted to complete the
questionaires at home and obviously spent considerable time and careful effort in the task.[21]

In the Philadelphia study, which began with 1,196 parents,[8,9]
some school nurses, fearful that questionnaires would not be returned,

restricted take-home to 69 percent. Careful study showed that only 1.2 percent of the records were not returned and only one form was in any way "mutilated"—with some coffee stains on it.[25] The health questionnaire was completed by the parent at home or in a nurse-parent interview at school in 95 percent of cases.[8] Given similar options in the Penn Manor School District in 1975/76, 88 percent of parents completed the questionnaire.[12]

It has been found that, following completion of the questionnaire, most parents attend the school for an interview designed to elucidate the nature of the problem behind the yes answers. In the Philadelphia school enterer study the parent attendance rate was 93 percent of 1,176 appointments made;[8] in Penn Manor it ranged from 82 percent to 92 percent in 1975/76 and included a significant number of fathers, most of whom had taken time off from work.[12] It is not known what stimulates parental participation—possibly the nature of the questionnaire or the anticipated nature of the interview—because in the same schools in previous years of the Philadelphia study, only 33 percent of parents attended for the physical examination of their kindergarten children. In Penn Manor the physical exam attendance had been only 15 percent. In the Bristol Township School District in 1976/77, 98.8 percent of parents of 1,169 ninth-grade students gave permission for their children to complete the adolescent health history questionnaire.[26]

Use of a questionnaire reduces the time necessary for health history interview. Observations during the Philadelphia study showed that histories taken by interview of the parent without prior questionnaire averaged 15 min longer than those following the questionnaire, which usually ranged from 15 to 30 min.

It appears that the health questionnaire not only secures parent information about child's health but also provides an activity around which parents and schools cooperate, thus strengthening the relationship between them.[24] School nurses report, and a survey of parents (below) supports, the idea that through the questionnaire and interview process parents see the nurse as a person interested in their child. Thus many parents take it upon themselves to keep the school nurse informed during the year of changes in the child's health.[12,21] Follow-up is made easier as the nurse and parent together decide on needed action, instead of a unilateral stream of notes and phone calls going from nurse to mother.[12]

The questionnaire provides a vehicle for health education and anticipatory guidance that, at least in the case of preschool children, has been shown to have preventive value particularly for developmental and emotional health.[27,28] Results from a health history provide information of value to teachers. In the San Francisco study 99 percent of teachers indicated that the information provided by parents, especially those sections related to emotional health, signs and symptoms of disease noted by parents, history of past illness, and health practices, was helpful.[24] A health questionnaire also provides information on the presence and use of health resources in the community.[21]

The health history questionnaire–interview format has proven successful in assessment of handicapped and retarded children receiving special education services.[23,29,30] Physical and structural problems, including family and social problems, were detected at rates beyond that discovered by any source of care previously provided to that group of children,[23] but functional problems were inferred rather than precisely indicated. Therefore a special questionnaire concerning function was developed as a supplement to the health questionnaire and has been well accepted by parents.[23,31]

Having reviewed the importance of the history in health assessment, it is now possible to consider its use as one item in an assessment schedule for students throughout their school years. Although no studies of the optimal periodicity of comprehensive health histories in assessment of ambulatory, functioning, pediatric populations are known, the advice of experts is about once every 4 to 5 years during the school years.[32] Thus school health assessment may be conceptualized as falling into two types: (1) periodic comprehensive evaluation at intervals of 4 to 5 years and (2) ongoing monitoring between comprehensive evaluations.

Comprehensive Evaluations

Comprehensive evaluations may be programmed at intervals during the 13 years of school life, such as during kindergarten and fourth and ninth grades; or, with slight variation to coincide with entering a new school and developmental phase, and thus getting to know a new school nurse and assuming increased responsibility for personal health care, see schedule shown in Table 7–2. The content of the evaluation (see Figure 7–1) is as follows:

1. Health history questionnaire and interview
2. Physical examination,
    a. On entry to school, performed by family practitioner or by school personnel
    b. At fifth grade, as indicated by history
    c. At ninth grade, not as routine assessment tool for all but (i) as a teaching device so that the student, as a future consumer of health care, knows the product called the "physical examination" (this objective may be more easily achieved in small group settings or class)

Table 7–2.

Kindergarten	Age five
	Elementary school entry
	Latency phase of industry and development of competence
	Health history from parent
Grade 5	Age 10
	Middle school entry
	Preadolescence to early adolescence
	Health history from parent and student
Grade 9	Age 14
	High school entry
	Adolescence and youth
	Health history from student

    (ii) as a means to establish rapport with some students with problems

    (iii) as indicated by the history

3. Screening tests for conditions of a hidden nature, such as problems with visual acuity, hearing, growth, color vision (once), tuberculosis, behavior, development, hypertension
4. Dental screening
5. Teacher observations of child's health and behavior

A few additional words are appropriate for some of the above items. The physical examination should cover the range of the usual pediatric physical examination, encompassing assessment of:

Measurements including pulse, respiration, blood pressure

General appearance

Skin and lymph nodes

Head and neck including eyes, ears, nose, throat, teeth, pharynx

Chest, breast, lungs, heart

Abdomen and genitalia

Extremities, spine, joints, muscles

Neurological[33]

Various aspects of the pediatric physical examination may be stressed according to information obtained on the health history; for example, a more detailed cardiovascular examination might by performed in the child with a history of rheumatic fever and breathless-

	K	1	2	3	4	5	6	7	8	9	10	11	12
emergency information	■	■	■	■	■	■	■	■	■	■	■	■	■
special health needs	■	■	■	■	■	■	■	■	■	■	■	■	■
history questionnaire parent *	■					■							
student						■				■			
history interview parent	■					■							
student						■				■			
history update parent		■	■	■			■	■	■				
student							■	■	■		■	■	■
physical examination * screening tests	■				■				■				
visual acuity	■		■		■	■	■				■		■
color vision	■												
hearing	■	■	■		■		■		■		■		
growth	■	■		■		■		■		■			
T.B.		■				■							
blood pressure	■		■		■		■		■		■		
dental screening	■		■			■				■			
teacher observations	■	■	■	■	■								
gym excuses review	■	■	■	■	■	■	■	■	■	■	■	■	■
absentee review	■	■	■	■	■	■	■	■	■	■	■	■	■
class performance review	■	■	■	■	■	■	■	■	■	■	■	■	■
temporary problem list	■	■	■	■	■	■	■	■	■	■	■	■	■
athletic questionnaire										■	■	■	■
examination							■						

* screening tests for development and behavior included

Figure 7–1.   Health Assessment Schedule

ness and a neurological examination in the child presenting with learning problems or failing in school. Experts have disagreed on the value of a neurological examination for schoolchildren. In 1976 four pediatric authorities agreed "on the importance of obtaining a detailed history and performing neurodevelopmental and psychoeducational assessments" in the evaluation of learning disorders.[34] The purpose of the neurodevelopmental assessment is to obtain evidence by "hard" or "soft" signs that some damage has occurred to the nervous system thereby increasing the *chance* that the association areas of the cerebral cortex relevant to beginning reading, but inaccessible to direct testing, may also have been damaged.[35]

The lesser importance of the physical examination and the relatively greater importance of screening tests in adolescents were shown in the work of Rogers and Reese, who demonstrated that detailed physical examinations on 985 adolescents aged fourteen to nineteen did not reveal serious disease, but did show that 45 percent had conditions that could be improved. These conditions fell into the categories of vision, hearing, dentition, nutrition, and skin and were identified by simple screening procedures (visual acuity, hearing, growth, dental screening) by simple inspection (skin) or were reported by the student on the history.[36]

Health education has been suggested by many observers over the years as the prime function of and justification for the periodic school physical examination. It is usually not made exactly clear what particular educational objective is meant to be served. Rogers and Reese suggested that the educational value of the physical examination was presumed to lie in the imparting of information by the physician to the teenager on "adolescent growth and development and its variation. In the process, the pupil is often given reassurance about the normality of his body structure and function."[36] It is obvious that other effective and certainly more efficient means, for example, health education classes combined with individual and group sessions on concerns elicited by the health history questionnaire, could be developed to meet this objective. It seems that students understand only too clearly the lack of value of a physical examination procedure lasting only a few minutes and stay away in droves—a phenomenon reversed when the health history questionnaire is introduced.[26]

All screening tests previously performed and new ones contemplated should be subject to review against standard guidelines.[37] The purpose of the test; the proven value of treatment that follows detection of the condition; the test procedure; the training and reliability of performers; the manuals; the timing; the recording of results; and the validity, reliability, sensitivity, and specificity of the test should be known. Too often tests are done when the need has passed (e.g., tuberculosis), when the value has not been proven (e.g., scoliosis), too frequently (e.g., yearly hypertension testing or color vision testing more than once), poorly (e.g., height measured against unstandardized measures and with shoes, blood pressure with incorrect cuffs, hearing without a soundproof setting), without appropriate charting (e.g., height and weight), or without appropriate standards (e.g., few schools have incorporated the national standards for height, weight, and blood pressure for children and adolescents).[38] Handicapped children must be tested so that the critical physiological functions measured by screening or screening-type procedures can be evaluated either by physical examination, special screening efforts (e.g., for growth),[39] or newly developed methods (e.g., tympanometry where hearing screening is impossible).

The Behavior Questionnaire[22] provides an interesting example of a procedure that resembles a screening test but, in the nature of the Johns Hopkins Adolescent Health Questionnaire,[16] can be extended to enhance the clinical interview. It presents the possibility that certain portions of the health history questionnaire may be replaced by questionnaires developed for specific functions or activities and tested for reliability and validity. In the health history of the infant and young child, developmental inventories of proven value can now be inserted.[40] Other questionnaires related to the home environment, as it pertains to child development, and to family routine are being developed or are currently available.

It was hypothesized that the two most important sources of information regarding the health of students were their parents and teachers. Parents know their child intimately and individually and can detect changes in the usual pattern of health and behavior; their input is obtained via the health history questionnaire and interview. Teachers know the child as an individual but from a different perspective: they see the child in relationship to others of the same age and matched against certain tests and challenges to performance.

From a clinical perspective Schoenwetter wrote, "Kindergarten teachers generally make a very good assessment of the child within several weeks of the start of school."[41] Research has shown that inventories "are reliable instruments when administered by experienced teachers. The scales [developed for the study] appear to be sensitive to psychopathological symptoms in that they distinguish known disturbed populations from control groups."[42] A recent review of the field concluded that the studies also show "that scores based on teacher checklists are a reasonably reliable and valid measure of a child's current classroom functioning . . . unfortunately, current behavior does not seem to be a very good indicator of future behavior."[43]

The situation is remarkably similar to that described for the adolescent health questionnaire.[16,17] The yes answers need to be subjected to further clinical scrutiny that will assess the importance of observations and differentiate "between those behavioral disorders that are likely to persist and those that are transient . . . [or] situational instead of internalized."[43]

A teacher's health observation form was designed to provide a structured medium for teachers to transmit their observations of children and also their concerns. The questions were derived from a variety of sources, such as neighborhood health centers, the federal Follow-Through Program, and insurance companies booklets for teachers, and were grouped into headings that reflected the nature of the teachers' observations:

Observations of child's body
Observations of child's body functions and symptoms
Observations of child's behavior
Observation of child's social adjustment

Teachers check only those observations made. They are also asked for a general opinion (one of three choices) regarding both the child's health and behavior.

The observation form was field-tested and further modified with 28 classroom teachers at all school levels in the Penn Manor School District.[44] It was found applicable only to teachers in fairly constant contact with students, such as in elementary school; special-subject teachers in junior and senior high schools did not know their students well enough to provide answers. The elementary teachers appreciated the form's content and structure and the means it provides for alerting the health staff to their concerns. Teachers complete the form, usually for a few students at a time, once a year on each student, after about 2 months into the year when the students are known to them. Following completion of the questionnaire, the nurse or other health professional interviews the teacher on the items marked, records additional data on the blank page opposite, and makes a decision regarding the existence of a significant problem.

Monitoring Procedures

The monitoring procedures that are followed between comprehensive evaluations are designed to alert the school health staff that some problem has developed or may be at risk of developing. A series of monitors that are easy to introduce or already exist in schools include

Emergency information and permission form collected at the beginning of each school year. This shows change of address, caretaker, family physician, and if not completed may indicate family distress and/or neglect. This information should be filed

(1) in the health record and (2) where all staff who may provide emergency care have ready access.

Special health needs form completed at the beginning of each school year, in conjunction with the emergency form. This short questionnaire is designed to alert the school, from first day of attendance each year, to the possible existence of serious problems that may affect performance or require certain responses from the school, such as medication; it may be used by school health staff to determine priorities for evaluation.

Updated health history questionnaire. A brief questionnaire, without interview, from parent and/or student, as for the comprehensive health questionnaire, designed to update health events of the past year, especially those occurring during school vacations.

Athletic health questionnaire and examinations. The institution of a health assessment system consisting of comprehensive evaluations and ongoing monitoring removes the need for the special athletic physical examination—which is subject to the same criticisms as the school and military physical examination. Just before each athletic season, a health questionnaire for both parent and student provides a better review of health status than the physical exam.

Screening tests according to the schedule developed for each test.

Teacher's health observation form completed once in each grade of elementary school.

Review of gym excuses.

Review of absences from school.

Review of class performance. The close relationship between school performance and higher rates of certain physical health and mental health conditions should alert staff to review the health status of those in the lowest percentiles or quartile of each class.

Temporary problem list.

The reviews of gym excuses, school absences, and class performance will be considered, together with the temporary problem list, as presenting similar types of data and problems to the health assessor. In all schools these data are present. They may not be brought to the attention of health staff. If they are, they are treated as discrete items separate from the overall health status of a child, and the events they record are not related to similar events occurring at other times to the same child. There are four steps to using these data to monitor health status:

1. The data must flow to the health room.
2. Brought to the nurse's attention are pieces of data determined as significant; for example:
   a. All gym excuses
   b. All health room visits
   c. Individual absences longer than 5 days
   d. Total absences for marking period greater than 2 standard deviations above mean
   e. Class performance in the lower percentiles
3. The nurse integrates the data into the overall pattern of the child's health status and decides if a problem is present.
4. The data are stored so that patterns over time, such as in health room visits and absences, become evident. The data pattern is reviewed each time new data are added.

The temporary problem list records use of the nurse's office or health room by the student, by date, chief complaint or condition, and notes on disposition. The record in each student's chart may be kept by a nurse or aide and replaces the health room log, which served simply to separate students' symptoms from their health records. Records of those who used the health room and their time in and out is information needed by school administrators and can be supplied by two-part cards completed by students for both health room data and corridor pass (or other administrative purpose).

That the temporary problem list may provide the first evidence of student illness or distress is strengthened by the following facts: the health room is an "open door" in the school system; frequent health room visits in high school have been associated with low academic status, poor participation in school activities, high dropout rate, and frequent absence or, in other words, life adjustment problems; the school nurse is not "psychologically threatening"; some children with emotional problems choose to present with a physical complaint in the health room as a way to discuss and get help with underlying problems.[45]

PROBLEM MANAGEMENT

The point of assessment of the health status of an individual is detection of health problems so that action (prevention, treatment, rehabilitation, reassurance) may be taken to reduce the effect of the problem on the health of the individual. This process of patient care (see Figure 7–2) has been conceptualized as problem management consisting of four steps: (1) collection of data, (2) analysis of data and formulation of problems, (3) determination of a plan of management for each problem, (4) accomplishment of management plan.[46]

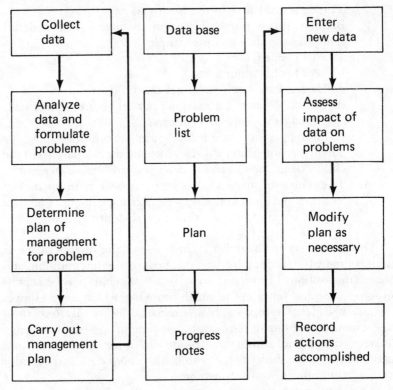

Adapted from Woolley et. al., 1974[46]

Figure 7–2.   Patient-care   Figure 7–3.   Problem-oriented Record
Process   Process

Development of the problem-oriented record by Weed[47] has given to those involved in patient care a powerful tool by which to organize the process, maintain its problem-solving logic, and ensure staff accountability in problem management.[48] The problem-oriented record (Figure 7–3) is organized around four steps that match those described in the patient-care, or problem management, process: (1) data base, (2) problem list, (3) plan, (4) progress notes.[49–51]

The problem-oriented record is particularly suited to the nature of the thinking process used by health professionals, who, when faced with a patient, take into account two knowledge sets: (1) the facts of the patient's status or condition and (2) the expected outcome, or course of illness, for that particular patient with that specific condition.[52] These two knowledge sets are integrated in the formulation of a hypothesis or assessment or diagnosis regarding the patient's condition. The hypothesis is tested through two types of actions: (1) to obtain further information on the health status of the patient (diagnostic) and (2) to alter the expected outcome of the condition (therapeutic). The results of such actions are fed back for assessment: diagnostic data alter therapeutic possibilities, and therapeutic responses constitute the ultimate test of the diagnosis; thus hypotheses are strengthened or reformulated, and plans of actions are continued or altered.

The problem-oriented record makes conscious the cybernetic problem-solving thinking process described above, through:

Collection of *data* on the health status of the individual, beginning with specified health assessment procedures or a defined data base

Analysis of the data to develop an *assessment* (or hypothesis or diagnosis) regarding the nature of the individual's health condition, as expressed in a problem list

Development of a *plan* consisting of actions:

1.   To further understand the condition—diagnostic

2.   To intervene in the course of the condition—therapeutic

3.   To explain the assessment and plan to the patient/parent and gain their agreement before proceeding—patient education

Recording, in progress notes, the diagnostic, therapeutic, and patient education actions accomplished

New data generated from the actions taken and arriving from other sources are assessed for their implications regarding the hypothesis, and the problem list and plan are altered accordingly. The plan is written in terms of diagnostic, therapeutic, and patient education actions. The cycle of: Data, Assessment, Plan is continued until the health problems of the individual are solved.

SCHOOL HEALTH RECORD

The basic structure of the student's health record designed for school health services in Pennsylvania includes both health assessment and problem management (Figures 7–4 and 7–5).

Health Assessment

The following procedures are involved in health assessment:

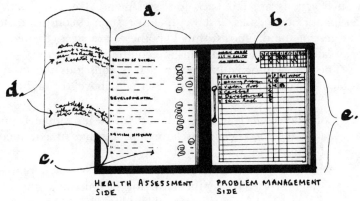

HEALTH ASSESSMENT   PROBLEM MANAGEMENT
SIDE   SIDE

Figure 7–4.

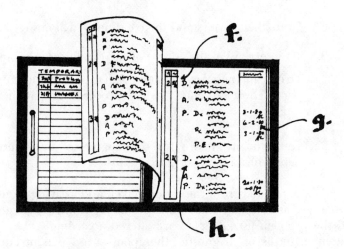

Figure 7–5.

a. Defined data base: A data base is defined as "that information to be collected from which problems are identified."[49] A defined data base is one in which the information to be obtained is specified in advance. The defined data base in school health consists of all health assessment items of the comprehensive evaluations and the annual health monitoring procedures.

b. Checklist for the items completed in the defined data base; thus the data base from which problems have been derived is easily seen.

c. Each defined item of the data base is represented by a special form, such as a questionnaire.

d. Further data concerning any positive item in the data base are recorded on blank page opposite.

The purpose of health assessment is detection of problems, which are listed on the problem list.

Problem Management

Problem management involves the following procedures:

e. Problem list: Each problem derived from the data base is listed with a number, problem description, date problem (and plan) was entered by nurse, date reviewed by physician for medical content, date problem resolved. A column for significant past problems, now inactive, is included. The purpose of problem management is resolution of problems and their removal from the problem list. The problem list provides a summary of the individual's health and an index to the record.

f. Plan: Beside the number of each problem and the date, all pertinent data (D) are listed, an assessment (A) made, and a plan (P) developed. The plan consists of diagnostic (Dx), therapeutic (Rx), and patient education (P.E.) actions.

g. Dates for planned actions are noted, and when accomplished checked.

h. Data generated by actions or from other sources are entered by problem number with data in the D,A,P format.

The student's health record provides an assessment of the student's health status, goals for its improvement, and progress made toward accomplishment. It provides a medium of communication between professionals working with the student. It provides a mechanism to audit staff performance in the process of patient management; to identify the needs of individual staff for assistance by supervision, consultation, and education; and to identify gaps in community services. The health record also provides a means for student education. In the words of physician faculty of the University of Vermont School of Medicine, who use the problem-oriented record in group practice: "Perhaps the most enlightening and emotionally rewarding aspect of our practice experience is in the way in which patients have become more active participants in their own health care. This system, because it demands explicitness and clearly defined goals, can be a truly patient centered system of health care."[53]

School Nurse Practitioner

Major problems occur when the model of health assessment and problem management is translated into schools. The model requires a health professional, which in schools would be either the physician or the nurse. In Pennsylvania nurses were selected, being more numerous,[54] working full-time, serving fixed schools, expressing interest in obtaining comprehensive histories, having had the role of collecting the short list of health questions in the old program, having a mandated role in maintaining children's health records, and exhibiting skills in follow-up. Nursing staff taking comprehensive histories would, judging by the median salaries of both professions, cost 25 percent of the physician's rate, and would also save the physician's time, enabling the physician to deal with a smaller number of children with difficult problems requiring the clinical and analytical skills of a medical consultant.

In Philadelphia the health assessment–problem management model had been developed for a team consisting of a pediatrician, pediatric nurse practitioner, and health aide.[21] In 1972/73 the model was tried by a group of 32 school nurses and 8 physicians selected for their quality, willingness to be involved, and distribution across the city. It was demonstrated that the nurses did not have the ability to conduct disciplined, in-depth interviews concerning positive items on the history;[8,9,26] they missed physical and medical abnormalities later noted on physician review of the history. Also, not surprisingly, both nurses and physicians experienced great difficulty handling the problem-oriented record.

Based on this experience, the Philadelphia nurses requested a continuing education program to expand their skills to those of a pediatric nurse practitioner. What is this nurse practitioner? The movement began in 1963, when it was reported that public health nurses saw children and parents, without physicians present, in well-child care and provided educational and supportive services.[55] In 1965, responding to the shortage of pediatricians, Henry Silver and Loretta Ford used the term *pediatric nurse practitioner* when establishing their education program at the University of Colorado.[56] The practitioner was at that time seen as a provider of physician-type services in underserved areas.

Definitions of the nurse practitioner vary. According to the American Nurses' Association a nurse practitioner is a registered nurse who has completed a course of study leading to competence in taking medical histories, assessing health and illness, and managing a regimen of care.[57] In 1970 the first *school nurse practitioner* education program was opened by Henry Silver at the University of Colorado.[58] Many school nurses have received comparable preparation in courses for pediatric nurse practitioners. In 1974 the American Nurses' Association and the American School Health Association issued recommendations on the role, function, and education of the school nurse practitioner. The function was seen to be directed toward "comprehensive assessment and remedial action" in order to identify a broad range of health problems and conditions including "learning disorders, psycho-educational problems, perceptive-cognitive difficulties, and behavior problems, as well as those causing physical disease."[59]

Course content includes:

Systematic collection of physical, developmental, social, nutritional, dental, and general health information

Interviewing skills

Pediatric physical and neurological examination using techniques of inspection, palpation, percussion, and ausculation; making use of such instruments as otoscope, stethoscope, reflex hammer; and distinguishing normal from abnormal

Knowledge of normal physical, perceptual, cognitive, mental, and psychosocial growth and development of children

Knowledge of family dynamics, interactions, critical periods, sociocultural patterns, and their effects on health

Assessment and management in such specific problem areas as childhood illnesses, learning disabilities, mental health, developmental delays, handicapped, and chronically ill

Development of standing orders and protocols, and physician supervision in the practitioner's use of prescription drugs, as provided by state law; nurse management by use of nonprescription medications and protocols; school staff *in loco parentis* handling of dispensed student medication

Counseling of parents and children, including anticipatory guidance regarding growth and development and other experiences; psychotherapeutic behavior modification techniques; health education

Recognition of community resources and child health delivery systems, and use of referral process

Examination of the school nurse practitioner role and its impact on the school and school health system.[59,60,61]

It is obvious that the nurse practitioner's role is different from that of the physician's assistant, who performs many assessment and treatment procedures for the physician but not the actual processes of diagnosis and formulation of a treatment plan.

The "expanded" role of the nurse, as expressed in the functions of the nurse practitioner, was considered compatible with existing nurse practice laws by the U.S. Department of Health, Education, and Welfare in 1971.[62] Some confusion still prevailed primarily because nurse practice laws, although making it illegal for any unlicensed person to practice nursing, also forbade nurses to perform "any acts of diagnosis or prescription of therapeutic or corrective measures".[57] This proscription, formalized by the American Nurses' Association only in 1955,[63] "created an ambiguity as to where the practice of medicine left off and the practice of nursing began".[57] The problem has been dealt with by semantics: "nursing assessment" instead of "diagnosis" and "nursing intervention" instead of "treatment"; by amending nurse practice laws to include the expanded role; by using guidelines or standardized protocols drawn up by state boards of nursing and medicine; and by certifying registered nurses who have completed an approved postgraduate program and who work under the supervision[64] of a licensed physician for acts beyond the scope of professional nursing, such as prescription of drugs.[57,63]

In 1979 it was estimated that there were between 3,000 and 3,300 pediatric nurse practitioners in the United States who had completed training in formal programs.[65] Training programs vary greatly. In 1971–1973 there were 56 programs of which 7 percent offered a master's program in nursing and 93 percent provided a certificate as evidence of completion of the educational program. In 1977 and 1979 there were 190 and 202 programs, respectively with 37 percent at the master's level and 63 percent certificate program.[65,66] Not surprisingly, formal programs, not including those informal courses in physical examination skills provided by physicians to nurses, were found in 1973 to vary widely, with duration ranging from 7 weeks to 9 months, didactic components of 48 to 720 hours, and clinical components of 90 to 720 hours.[67]

In 1971 the American Nurses' Association and the American Academy of Pediatrics, in a joint statement, issued "guidelines on short-term continuing education programs" for pediatric nurse practitioners. These include nursing and medical codirectors of the program, a course content similar to the one outlined above, and a program length of at least 4 months. "The program should include a combination of classroom work, clinical practice and work experience composed of approximately four hours of class and eight to twelve hours of supervised clinical practice each week, with the remainder devoted to on-the-job experience."[68] By 1977 the mean length for certificate programs was 5.4 months and for master's programs 15.8 months.[56]

Only one study was found comparing the clinical performance of nurse practitioners formally prepared in a master's program against those having a certificate. There was no difference. There are of course other skills imparted by the master's program which are not the objective of the continuing education programs.[69]

Despite the differences within the nursing education arena, the most important result is that randomized controlled trials "have consistently shown comparable safety and efficacy of nurse practitioners and medical practitioners in several settings, for different age groups and with various outcomes."[70,71] It has also been concluded that "substantial evidence has validated the original concept that these health care professionals can provide primary care for pediatric patients."[65] In a review of studies conducted to 1974, the Yale University School of Medicine concluded that nurse practitioners compared favorably with physicians as judged by standards developed within the practice setting.[73] The most critical issue—the ability of nurse practitioners to perform accurate, comprehensive physical examinations—has been decided in the affirmative. Nurse practitioners perform as well as physicians in discriminating normal from abnormal findings.[73,74]

The quality of primary care provided by nurse practitioners in neonatal intensive care units were found "comparable and often superior" to that provided by pediatric interns.[75] The nurse practitioner has been shown to be an economical addition to private medical practice[76] by saving expensive physician time and reducing average visit costs by 20 percent.[77] Patient satisfaction with nurse practitioners has been shown to be "significantly higher than patient satisfaction with physicians,"[78] and as the result of a random trial, it has been suggested that patients are more likely to shift their preferences for services from physicians to nurse practitioners when the nurse practitioner has integrated the medical and nursing care processes of the new role.[79]

Recent studies are showing qualitative differences in the practice of nurse practitioners compared with physicians. Practitioners have been reported as more likely to obtain a detailed growth and development history, perform more thorough physical examination and screening tests, identify more signs and symptoms in patients, record more problems per patient, provide less drug therapy, provide more nondrug therapies, and give more anticipatory guidance to mothers.[80,81]

A British study showed that the accuracy of physicians' diagnoses was improved 20 to 30 percent when a nonphysician practitioner took a detailed health history in a highly structured situation.[82] In an evaluation of history taking and disposition in telephone management

Table 7–3.

| | Precentage of total possible score | |
	History taking	Disposition
Nurse practitioners	79.6	71.1
Pediatric house officers	69.1	60.1
Pediatricians	52.6	58.9

Sources: Perrin and Goodman.[83]

of five common pediatric problems, the results shown in Table 7–3 were obtained. Similarly, nurse practitioners had significantly higher scores for interviewing skills.[83] These results are not surprising to many pediatricians. One wrote: "I ran a well-child clinic last summer in a rural area of our state; a pediatric nurse practitioner worked alongside. It was evident that she did a *better* job than I in this type of work. She was more thorough both in her physical exams, and in eliciting problem areas that required counseling."[84]

There have been few studies evaluating the pediatric nurse practitioner in a school setting or the school nurse practitioner. Two studies have compared nurse practitioners and school nurses in the care of children presenting in the health room in elementary schools. Lewis et al. could detect little quantitative and only the possibility of some qualitative differences.[85] In a larger, more carefully documented study Hilmar and McAtee obtained results that suggested that the nurse practitioners provided more direct management of problems and were more focused and specific in their recommendations: parents reported less uncertainty about what to do when a child was sent home by the nurse practitioner; they reported that their children received more care; they recalled the advice given and agreed with it. Referral to physicians was reduced and, most important from the point of view of education, school nurse practitioners "excluded far fewer [about one-half as many] pupils from school than school nurses although the number of pupil visits and the school enrollments were approximately equal."[86]

Silver et al. reported that a major difference between school nurses and school nurse practitioners is that school nurses see children in "brief and essentially superficial" encounters whereas school nurse practitioners spend more time in "thorough, extensive assessments and in-depth appraisals of health problems."[60] Lewis et al. reported that, although little change in student care could be seen, the nurse practitioner's new role evoked a marked response from the school system as evidenced by enthusiasm for the new role on the part of teachers and principals.[85]

ROLE CHANGES IN SCHOOL HEALTH

The change in the role of the school nurse to that of school nurse practitioner creates change in the roles of others. These changes are illustrated in Figure 7–6.

The nonprofessional and subprofessional activities of school nurses, which may consume up to 75 percent of their time, are assumed by a trained, nonprofessional aide-technician supervised by the school nurse practitioner. Trained as nurse practitioner and with the additional time made available by the aide-technician, the school nurse assumes all former functions of the school physician; strengthens the school nurse's traditional, professional functions of follow-up, counseling, and individual health education; and adds new services: (1) to expand health assessment by health history, physical examination, and developmental assessment; (2) to improve problem management with use of the problem-oriented record and broadened anticipatory guidance; and (3) to provide more expert handling of acute intercurrent illness and injury, beyond the capacity of the aide-technician, through expanded assessment techniques, pediatric knowledge, and management skills. School physicians, no longer needed for mindless screening physical examinations, immunizations, and, in some places, skin tests for T.B., are required for lesser hours but in the professionally demanding role of consultant in medical-pediatric matters to the school nurse practitioner.

The physician who provides pediatric consultation to the school nurse practitioner may be a pediatrician or a physician from another field, such as family medicine or general practice, who has interest in and knowledge of the more severe health problems of school students. A high degree of structure makes optimal use of the expensive skills of the school's consulting physician in pediatric matters. The consultant should be engaged:

Old Role	Physician			School Nurse	
Functions	Pediatric consultation	Physical exam Immunizations Tine tests for T.B.	Medical history interview Problem-oriented medical record Problem management Anticipatory guidance Acute care diagnosis and treatment Aide supervision	Follow-up Counseling Health education	Screening tests Health room: first aid, acute care, referral Clerical Assist at physical exam
New Role	Pediatrician	School Nurse Practitioner			Aide-Technician

From Lynch.[87]

Figure 7–6.   Role Changes.

1. To be available for phone consultation with school nurse practitioners during school hours. The nature of most school problems and the daily presence of students in school mean that such consultation is rarely needed or used.
2. To attend for regular case conferences with school nurse practitioners at at rate of about 2 hours every 2 weeks per practitioner. There is some evidence from the literature that nurse practitioners advance faster in their new role when relating to one physician.[80] In the experience gained in Pennsylvania it also seems that the nurses progress faster, and the teaching of the consultant is more effective and efficient, in a group of about four school nurse practitioners meeting for about 2 hours every week with the consultant. In such a group setting the nursing aspects of problem management, in addition to the pediatric aspects, become part of the conference, and the process of problem solving is enhanced for all present. The arrangement provides for peer education and for peer auditing of the quality of problem management.

Around conferences the physician consultant performs three functions:

1. Reviews all student health records after the major health assessment procedures of history, physical examination, and teacher's health observation of the interval comprehensive evaluations; reviews other records as problems are added to the problem list.
    The physician's reviewing check on the record means:
    a. Data base items checked have been reviewed for completeness.
    b. Additional data obtained on positive items in the data base have been reviewed for completeness.
    c. All medical problems evident in the data base are listed on the problem list.
    d. The medical content of the plan of management for each problem has been approved.
    This record review, greatly facilitated by the specific design of the Pennsylvania record, is best done on a group of 10 to 20 records by the consultant alone. New records can be reviewed in as little as 3 minutes, and some update records can be reviewed in less than a minute. In about 85 percent of cases the consultant will agree with the findings and plan of the nurse practitioner. In about 10 percent of cases the consultant may request additional data, add a new problem,

or suggest a minor change in management. In about 5 percent of records the consultant will request a case consultation.

2. Participates in regular case conferences with school nurse practitioners. Children are selected by the consultant following record review, or by the nurse practitioners for reasons ranging from unsureness of physical findings to lack of progress in carrying out a plan of management.

Freedom of discussion, sharing of present and past experiences, and use of the problem-oriented format (data, assessment, plan) help to make case conferences experiences in problem solving for the most difficult health cases in the school student population.

3. Performs follow-up functions decided in case conference. These are fairly infrequent, can be scheduled for appointment after the case conference, and may include checking a child for a specific finding made by the practitioner on physical examination, performing part of a physical or neurological examination, interviewing a child or mother, meeting with another school staff member, and attending a special conference of school and/or other agency personnel regarding a specific child or family.

It is in the physician consultant's role that the logic of the services subsystem comes together. The schedule for both interval and ongoing health assessments of the total student population reveals health problems; nurse practitioners, with additional time and paraprofessional assistance, work with students, parents, the families' sources of health care, and health and social agencies in the community and school in the process of problem management; students with the most unusual, difficult, and complicated conditions are sifted out of the process by nurse practitioner and/or physician consultant and receive directly, or indirectly through the practitioner, the services of the consultant.

This services subsystem follows the dictates of forward-looking pediatricians: "Pediatricians will have to abandon the assembly line approach, and spend more time with fewer patients who can benefit from their unique skills."[84] The school physician is provided with a structure that transforms him or her from the role of performing assessment tasks to the role of applying the unique knowledge set of the profession to the problems of children. That knowledge is concerned with "the nature of pathological processes: their etiology, manifestations, prognosis, effects upon physiological and psychological function and the growth and development of children."[29]

With such knowledge physicians can make immediate contributions to the analysis of data, to the assessment of the nature of problems, and to the formulation of plans, particularly the type and nature of diagnostic actions required to further the understanding of problems. The physicians (as a participant in a structured process of assessment and problem solving) becomes in effect a consultant available to the total school student population.[88] Certainly there are knowledge gaps[89] to be filled, as physicians, including pediatricians, are products of an academic world[90] that has concentrated on the "exotic" inpatient[91] and left the severe problems of the ambulatory and school worlds to flourish unseen. Physicians with basic knowledge, with eagerness to learn, and under requirements for continuing education, begin to fill their gaps regarding specific conditions once placed in a system that clearly presents the need and the challenge to do so.

Little has been written about the work of nonprofessionals in school health although the use of aides in health programs dates from the 1950's[92] and great interest was expressed in the whole field of paraprofessionals in the 1960's.[93] Studies have shown that in certain activities, such as communication of home care instructions, aides are as effective as physicians and nurses.[94]

One controlled study of clerical assistants to school nurses in 1966/67 in the Los Angeles school district showed their negative impact upon the nurses' follow-up activity measured by use of optimal referral patterns, care received by referred children, telephone contacts between nurse and parent, and time lag between referral and receipt of care.[95] Rejection of the role of the assistant by the nurses and problems in supervision were noted, as in other studies of professional acceptance of paraprofessionals.[93] The behaviors were probably related to the nurses' fear of job loss and to lack of supervisory skills.[95]

Such problems have not been a feature of the employment of health aide-technicians in the program in Pennsylvania, primarily because the school nurses are eager for their new practitioner role, which is impossible without the presence of an aide to perform the needed clerical, first aid, and screening test functions. The aide-technicians are selected for their basic intelligence and empathy with children; preservice Red Cross-type courses in first aid and home nursing, and also CPR are required; in-service training is given by the nurse practitioners in performance of all screening tests, recording of results, records, filing, telephone use, appointments, school functions and personnel, and an overview of the school health program.[96] Further details of the specific activities of the aide-technician are presented in the following discussion of the records.

Most school systems find that the change in staff roles can be made within current expenditures. In effect, the lesser number of physician hours required for consultation, against those formerly needed for physical examinations for the school health program, athletics, and working papers (when they are replaced by health histories or ongoing health monitoring or performance by the nurse practitioners), pays for the addition of aide-technicians to the program. School districts that in the past have paid physicians at a low rate or are pressed for funds have more difficulty, but in the experience in Pennsylvania have been able to find a mechanism.

It is worth noting the annual expenditures:

School nurse practitioner
    salary and fringe benefits, $20,000

Aide-technician @ 6 h/day
    × 200 days × $6/h (salary and fringe benefits) $7,200

Physician consultant @ 3 h/week
    × 40 weeks × $35/h (3 salary figures) $4,200

The total amount of $31,400 is equivalent to $31.40 per 1,000 students served, or $15.70 per 2,000 students served. Both amounts are below 1 percent of the total annual costs of school education per child.[97]

RECORDS

The services subsystem functions on a minimum of paperwork consisting of three basic elements: program control sheet, health record, and tickler file. Briefly, the program control sheet ensures that planned health assessments are received by the student; the health record contains the results of all assessments, is the repository of all health information on the student, and is the tool for solving health problems; the tickler file pulls the health record for problem-solving work at times required.

The program control sheet consists of a list of all assessment services, both interval and ongoing; it is kept by grade, listing all children in that grade and indicating those services to be received that year. The aide-technician maintains the program control sheet, using it for scheduling and to record service delivery. A simple tally of each column at the end of the year provides the basis for evaluation of the program's delivery of planned services. (See Appendix)

The student's health record, described in detail above, has been conceptualized as a document to accompany the student from school entry to departure, at which time the student should take the record as a means of continuing management of his or her own health care. There is no doubt that the record becomes bulky over time. One advantage of the problem-oriented system is that if a data base form of known questions has been completed, and if all problems present in it have been listed on the problem list, then the original form may be discarded. One practice is to discard the previous version, for example, the old teacher's health observation form, as a new one is inserted.

The student's health record is a confidential document and should be maintained in the same manner as a patient's hospital record, except that the client has access as requested. Thus the record is kept in a locked file to which only the school health staff have access; copies of part or all of the record may be shared with other agencies and professionals only with written permission of the client.

The Public School Code of Pennsylvania states: "All health records established and maintained pursuant to this act shall be confidential and their contents shall be divulged only when necessary for health of the child or at the request of the parent or guardian to a physician legally qualified to practice . . . in the Commonwealth."[98] It is worth noting the specificity of the Pennsylvania law in this matter simply because school administrators have in the past ignored the law and treated health records in the most cavalier of fashions; now that special laws govern education records, they again ignore the health law and, failing to understand the confidential nature of health records, often attempt to force parts of the record apart into classes of information defined by assessibility to parents, staff, or the public.

The question of who is the client with access to the health record is clearly answered as "the parent" until high school, where some students attain legal majority and some become "emancipated minors" in regard to health care because of marriage, pregnancy, motherhood, or certain conditions for which the law allows treatment without parental permission. All students could improve their skills in dealing with their own health care by working with health staff on their own problem-oriented record and taking it from school on graduation.

A suggested solution is to obtain parental permission to establish a new confidential health record accessible only to the student, upon entry to high school, transferring to it from the old record only certain routine documents, such as immunizations and screening tests. Upon graduation the original record is returned to the parent and the high school record is taken by the student. This policy assists school health to set as its major objective the optimum health of the student, it demonstrates respect for the wishes of the student, and yet it is compatible with the goal that students involve their parents in their health care.

The tickler file is basically a file box with dividers for each day or week in the year. Each health record contains a file card with the student's name and any other information that would lead to successful retrieval of the student's health record from its file. Before filing any health record, the aide notes the first date for planned action in the problem-oriented record. The student's file card is placed in the appropriate date of the tickler file. Each day or each week, the aide pulls the health records indicated in the tickler file for that date or week and presents them to the nurse practitioner, who simply has to turn to the plans in the progress notes to know the action required for that day or week.

STRUCTURE

The services subsystem must provide the structure necessary to ensure that services are performed as designed and that staff are functioning according to their roles. Nurse practitioners, in particular, have been shown to respond to their setting, or to the structural factors in that setting, and to modify the range of responsibilities assumed and thus the actual expression of the practitioner role.[99]

The most difficult change required of the nurse as a practitioner is to assume a new role, with different behavior, in relationships with physicians.[100] The difficulty involved becomes obvious when it is noted that physicians favorably disposed to delegation of certain patient-care tasks to nonphysicians infrequently give such tasks to the nurses in their own offices, whom they usually employ to preform services that could be more appropriately carried out by technician and aides.[101,102] It has been shown that, where physician and nonphysician practitioners work together, communication breaks down primarily because physicians do not respond to information about the patient generated by the nonphysician practitioner as they do to information generated by another physician or themselves.[80]

In hospital settings the major stumbling block to the nurse assuming an expanded role in "direct patient caretaking" is a structure that requires nurses to perform administrative and management tasks. Clerical and technical tasks in such settings need to be transferred to clerks and aides and certain middle management functions to administrative assistants.[103] In schools the failure of nurse practitioners to perform in the new role has, in some cases, been attributed to the school principal's desire for "a traditional nurse who was always available for first aid,"[104] a problem solved by employment of aides for that function.

It has been observed in Pennsylvania that school nurses trained as nurse practitioners will, without a newly structured services subsystem, revert to the functions of the old role; nurse practitioners without a background in school nursing will enter schools and essentially conduct a traditional clinic service for students attending the nurse's health office, thereby reflecting a clinical orientation to the individual patient and not a public health orientation to the total student population. The manifestations of this latter phenomenon were criticized by the American Academy of Pediatrics[105] without recognition that such failings are shared by all clinicians, including pediatricians, who enter health service systems without structure.

Pediatricians also have been found to respond to various organizational aspects of clinics in which they work. Work satisfaction is enhanced as their role is perceived as valued by the institution; staff conflict is reduced and performance and coordination improved when both pediatricians and other members of the staff have high levels of influence on clinic policy and function and also are in positions to influence each other.[106,107]

The quality of medical records was found to be significantly higher where nurses had major roles in screening, diagnosis, and treatment of patients.[107]

The structure of the services subsystem developed in Pennsylvania is clearly defined by certain elements designed to avoid some of the problems noted above.

The *program* of health assessment and problem management is defined by the records: the program control sheet and health record for assessment services and the health record and tickler file for problem management.

The *flow* of activities is initiated by the program control sheet, which defines the services to be received by each child from the nurse practitioner and aide-technician; results are entered into the health record and are immediately distilled into problems, with plans of management, as the nurse practitioner follows the dictates of the problem-oriented health record. Completion of the nurse practitioner's initial plans provides material for the regularly scheduled record review and case conferences with the physician consultant. Use of the problem-oriented health record and the tickler file provides the structure for the ongoing, cybernetic process of problem solving.

The *roles* of staff are defined by the records: the aide's scheduling and organizing by the program control sheet, screening by the program control sheet and health record, care of temporary problems by the health record's temporary problem list, and filing and organization of the nurse practitioner's time by the health record and tickler file. The nurse practitioner's roles in assessment and problem management are defined by the health record, and the physician consultant relies upon the well-designed health record to facilitate medical review of all records and consultation in problem solving of selected cases. Job descriptions for staff should reflect these functions structured around the records.

The staff structure removes interfering nonprofessional functions from the nurse practitioner and clearly establishes the high value of the physician consultant in care of the most difficult problems. Within the structure providing for an assessment and problem management services subsystem, the health staff have freedom to alter policy, procedure, specific services, roles, and methods; and in the case conferences and with the problem-oriented record,[108] they have means to influence each other, to communicate, to coordinate actions, and to ensure for themselves the quality of their services and the effectiveness of their care.

It is obvious that the school system must indicate its support of the program by provision of the usual items required by any group of professionals for efficient and effective function. These are minimal for the new services subsystem, usually being at the most, modification of what exists or provision of an item that was necessary for reasonable function under the old program: a health office or an area with provision for the taking of confidential history interviews and physical examinations; a waiting area, desk, direct-line phone, files, sink, and work area for the aide-technician to attend to scheduling, filing, and acute care; furnishing of the waiting area in an attractive manner, especially for adolescents, so that it can be used for group meetings; locked files for confidential health records to which only health staff have direct access and only health staff and parents (and later students) have a right; institution of sick-call hours in the school to control the flow of minor incidental illness to the health room, thus allowing nurses time to see parents and students by appointment and the aides to schedule and efficiently carry out screening tests; provision of a meeting room for periodic case conferences, (for 3 h once a month if the nurse shares the case conference with three other nurses and rotates the site), if the health room is too small; a soundproof room or portable soundproof booth for hearing screening to reduce the time for test performance and to improve results.

IMPLEMENTATION OF CHANGE

The process of institutional change, which is the point of attempting to institute a new services subsystem in school health, to be followed by new information and management subsystems, is slow. It consists of five phases as depicted in Figure 7–7.

Phase 1. Decision to Change; Planning for Change

The *goal* is change from the old input system of school health, with its lack of responsiveness to local needs, to installation of a purposive system, operated by the school district or school, which chooses

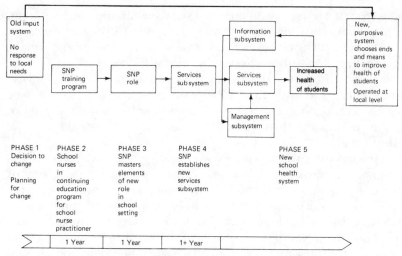

Figure 7–7.   (SNP = School Nurse Practitioner.)

both its ends and means and controls use of its resources in order to produce measurable improvement in the health status of the school student population. The *objectives* are development of the three subsystems of services, information, and management.

The *implementation strategy* is the training of nurses as nurse practitioners, around whom the roles of physicians and aides are orchestrated, in order to provide improved health assessment and problem management so that an effective and efficient services subsystem stimulates development of information and management subsystems.

Planning by school health and administrative staff includes a descriptive assessment of the current program along the lines suggested for occupational health programs;[109] definition of the interval and ongoing health assessments included in the new program; design and printing of records; development of job descriptions for new staff roles; provision of appropriate facilities, files, phones, etc., for the new activities; development of a training program for the aides and application to the school nurse practitioner education program.

In larger school districts, where school nurses may be educated in groups, planning must be directed to the transitional phase between the old and new program. Services to be delivered and those to be reduced or abolished must be agreed to and approval sought, if necessary, from state agencies. Staff roles must be defined, especially if other staff are extended to cover for those enrolled in courses.

Phase 2. School Nurse Practitioner-Training

The nurse practitioner course consists of didactic classwork, and clinical practice, usually arranged at the nurse's school, with a physician preceptor. The course may be full-time over approximately 16 weeks or part-time extending for a year.

Through coverage by another staff nurse or employment of an aide-technician, the school arranges for the acute care traffic in the health room not to interrupt the preceptored clinical practice sessions. At the end of this phase the nurse practitioner has firmly established skills in health history, interviewing, and physical examination including neurological assessment. The nurse practitioner has new knowledge in normal growth and development, family interactions, and identification and management of common pediatric problems.

The nurse practitioner is familiar with the assessment side of the problem oriented record and has had an introduction to the problem management side. Some of the effects of the new role on others have been experienced, and use of supervisory skills in relationships with the aide-technician has begun.

Phase 3. Mastery of Role

In the first year after completion of the course, the school nurse practitioner, with the aide-technician and the physician consultant, plans a program of services for the population, which is limited in volume especially in the number of complete interval health assessments. This phase recognizes the time it takes for the new office organization to go into effect, the early slowness of the new nurse practitioner in taking histories and doing physical examinations, and the greater initial use of the physician consultant by the nurse practitioner.

The slower pace ensures that all parties master use of the problem-oriented record, the problem-solving process, and conduct of the case conferences. In addition, nurse practitioners emerge at the end of the year confident of their supervisory skills and ability to manage delivery of the services subsystem for the student population under their care. During this phase the new nurse practitioner needs assistance in developing nursing skills from a nursing supervisor—either a member of the nurse practitioner education faculty, a school district supervisor who has taken the nurse practitioner course, or a nurse practitioner consultant from a department of health.

Phase 4. Services Subsystem; Program Evaluation

In the fourth phase nurse practitioners establish the new services subsystem for the student population under their care. The assessment services to be delivered are defined for the total population, and for subgroups within it, by the program control sheet; problem management is contained in the health record, and the effectiveness of problem solving is found in the number of problems resolved on the problem list page of the health record. Using this basic record system nurse practitioners control and evaluate the services subsystem under their management. The evaluation consists of:

1. Measurement of program performance
   a. Assessment services
      The numbers planned at the beginning of the year and the numbers actually delivered at the end of the year, with turnover of students to be served, are obtained by column tallies of the program control sheet.
   b. Acute, or health room, care
      A tally of a random sample of temporary problem lists in the health records, or
      Summaries of detailed encounter forms on all users of the health room for 1 or 2 random weeks per year.
   c. Staff activities and time studies
      The myriad activities of nurse practitioners, physician consultants, and aide-technicians and the use of time can be studied by time-activity logs maintained for 1 or 2 random weeks per year.
2. Quality of program activities
   a. Assessment services
      Various mechanisms, such as use of skilled observers,[110] and use of video and audio tape, are available to monitor the quality of nurse practitioner health history interviews and physical examinations. Nurse practitioner education programs should make their students familiar with these techniques that, used in practice, act to maintain the actuality and image of quality.
      The quality of the "specific interrogation" on positive findings on the data base forms can be checked in the process of record audit.
      The false-positive and false-negative findings of the nurse practitioner's physical examination can be checked against the physical examination of the physician consultant performed on the same group of children with appropriate blind techniques.
      Screening tests can be evaluated in similar fashion, for example, nurse practitioner performance of dental screening compared with examinations by a dentist to derive measures of sensitivity and specificity.[111]
   b. Problem management
      The audit of the problem-oriented record,[112] in

which data base, problem list, plan of management, and progess notes are systematically checked to ensure the quality of problem solving, is done internally by a peer group about twice a year, on a random sample of records, and by an audit group from the school district and/or nurse practitioner education program and/or the department of health on an annual basis.

3. Program effectiveness

The effectiveness of the services subsystem lies in its ability to resolve the health problems of children and thus measurably improve their health.

A review of the problem lists contained in a random sample of health records provides the following measures:

a. Number of health problems detected
b. Number of health problems resolved
   From which can be calculated:
c. Number of health problems detected per child
d. Number of health problems resolved per child
e. Percentage of health problems resolved

Also a classification of health problems detected can be made and used to standardize problem classification among staff.

The types of health problems not resolved can immediately provoke speculation concerning reasons; further study of difference between staff and schools can show whether staff problem-solving difficulties or community resource deficiencies are the reason.

4. Efficiency

Equipped with budget figures, measures of staff time use, and program output and effectiveness measures, one can make calculations of such items as the cost of various staff activities and program outputs and comparison of the costs of various aspects of the system compared with the old system or other delivery mechanisms.[113]

5. Consumer satisfaction

Special surveys can be designed to measure consumer satisfaction beyond that apparent from kept appointment rates, completed questionnaires, and program participation.[113,114]

Phase 5. Information and Management Subsystems; New System

The new school health system, with an operating services subsystem and emerging information and management subsystems, begins to operate, selecting both the ends and the means by which to increase the health of the population of students. On the basis of information generated by evaluation of the services subsystem, the nurse practitioner is able to program changes into next year's activities. These may be to alter the assessment schedule from groups with few problems to those with more; to reduce certain assessment services in order to increase problem-solving activities for those with severe problems; to form links with other problem-solving services, such as multidisciplinary teams for the handicapped;[23] to provide certain services (e.g., immunizations) in school where there is evidence of community lack; to put time into a preventive service (e.g., crisis counseling for children of divorcing parents discovered on health assessment to have high psychosomatic and psychoneurotic complaints) and to do this in conjunction with the school counselor and the local mental health agency and to measure the impact of intervention against the psychosomatic, psychoneurotic components of the health questionnaire.[115]

The services subsystem, by the fact of its comprehensive evaluation of the health status of the school student population, generates information where little previously existed. The record system, which makes simple evaluation of performances, quality, effectiveness, and efficiency possible, turns the data into an information system so that those in charge of services can use it for management purposes.

The services subsystem has also a direct impact on development of the management subsystem. Nurse practitioners and school physician consultants and aide-technicians, in their new roles, clearly show teachers and administrators that the school health program has grown in complexity, requiring managers with expertise in health care and health services to perform such functions as planning of assessment services, training of staff, and design and implementation of program evaluation. The wise administrator moves aside and places responsibility on the health staff to submit the annual program plan and budget for school health services for school board approval and, in places such as Pennsylvania with state reimbursement mechanisms, state approval.

The annual school health services program plan specifies:

1. Population of students and/or children of school age to be served
    a. By school
    b. By grade
    c. By school nurse/school nurse practitioner and other staff
2. Services
    a. Health assessment services to be provided, by number of children per grade and by school

    b. Problem management
    c. Acute care services to be provided
    d. Other preventive services to be delivered and health objectives to be attained
3. Staff categories, distribution, and job descriptions
4. Other resources required for program implementation, including:
    a. Facilities rental, renovation
    b. Equipment
    c. Locked-file cabinets (for confidential records)
    d. Supplies
    e. Records
    f. Postage, telephone
    g. In-service education
5. Records to be used for
    a. Clinical care
    b. Administration
    c. Evaluation
    and manuals describing the use of the records
6. Evaluation to be performed
7. Budget, specifying costs of
    a. Personnel
    b. Facilities
    c. Equipment and supplies
    d. Records
    e. Education
    f. Miscellaneous

It is clear that the services subsystems stimulates development of the information and management subsystems of the school health system. The next two chapters describe in greater detail the nature of those subsystems and emphasize that their incremental growth from a local services base may represent the best organizational approach at this time.

PROGRESS IN IMPLEMENTATION OF SERVICES SUBSYSTEM

Two areas of progress in development and implementation of the services subsystem in Pennsylvania will be discussed. One is concerned with applicability of the services subsystem to a special health problem area within school health, and the second records the spread of the systems change approach among the school districts of the state.
    1. In 1979/80, as part of the federal Supplemental Security In-

come program for disabled children, a team of school nurse practitioner, pediatric consultant, and aide-technician was developed in a special education center operating in the Berks County Intermediate Unit.[23] The team used the program records and roles of the services subsystem, as described, in the care of moderately and severely mentally retarded and/or multiply handicapped students. The assessments, problem lists, and plans of management were presented by the nurse practitioner to a multidisciplinary rehabilitation team consisting of developmental pediatrician, psychologist, social worker, classroom teacher, physical therapist, occupational therapist, speech therapist, parent, and other agency staff from time to time. The conferences were held at the child's school to enable school personnel to attend.[116]

The nurse practitioner–pediatric consultant assessments found significantly more health problems[117] per student (9.3), than did rehabilitation or multidisciplinary centers (5.5), school health services (3.2), or school psychological services (3.7), They developed plans for implementation by the practitioner and/or pediatrician in 42 percent of cases, 76 percent of which were unaltered after study by the team. In 3.5 months of school time the nurse practitioner had, as case manager, obtained execution of 49 percent of actions listed in the plans of management, resolution of 8 percent of problems, and use of 2.3 community resources and 1.4 special education services per child.

The multidisciplinary team, using the high degree of structure and content in the nurse practitioner's presentation, was able to perform an initial team evaluation in about 40 min per child. During that time the data presented resulted in addition of 1 problem per child, deletion or change in 0.4 problems per child, alteration of 24 percent of plans developed by the practitioner and pediatrician, and development of specific plans for 52 percent of problems.

A classification of health problems was made providing a crude but beginning nosology needed for further evaluation. Leading problem types were central nervous (with 2.4 problems per student), family and social (1.2), speech and communication (0.8), vision and eye (0.8), behavior (0.5), hearing and ear (0.5). The team made its contribution of additional problems in such functional areas as family and social, behavior, communication, posture, and feeding problems. The nurse practitioner and pediatrician, without team input, managed problems that constituted the substance of primary pediatric care; they required most team input in problems involving function.

Record audit revealed a high quality of problem management. The developmental pediatrician made the greatest number of inputs at team meetings (2.7 per child) and made most of the team's analytic and diagnostic inputs.

Team members and parents reported satisfaction with the program. Parent participation was 100 percent. Teachers were able to make immediate changes in classroom management. Parents received support in home management from team members, especially the nurse practitioner (as the aide-technician managed first aid). Private physicians were invited to all meetings, received reports, were kept informed by nurse practitioners, and gradually reported the sense that the school health program was in a partnership with them.

Two additional intermediate units developed similar programs within months, and within a year about half the intermediate units of the state indicated a desire for a similar program.[23]

2. Since early 1974, when the first school district in Pennsylvania sent three school nurses for nurse practitioner education, the number of involved school districts and trained school nurses has steadily grown. In 1980, 48 school districts representing 37 percent, or about 900,000 of the school student population of Pennsylvania voluntarily opted to change their school health system. The districts include Philadelphia, Pittsburgh, Erie, Lancaster, and Reading. About 230 school nurses graduated as nurse practitioners by the end of 1980. These changes indicate that school boards, nurse associations, unions, and parent groups are in agreement with the change.

The major problem has been and is the lack of school nurse practitioner education programs. The one federally funded pediatric nurse practitioner program at the University of Pittsburgh turned all its resources to education of the 50 school nurses of the Pittsburgh School District—accomplished in batches of 10. Four other programs are supported by the Pennsylvania Department of Health through a two-year grant from the Robert Wood Johnson Foundation. At maximum capacity the schools can educate about 100 nurses per year. This is of little comfort for the 2,000 school nurses in the state who desire to enter the program. The answer must lie in greater committment by government health agencies and professional schools to continuing education and further emphasis on development of self-teaching modules.

In both Philadelphia and Pittsburgh school nurses may enroll in master's programs to obtain practitioner skills, among others. A cadre of master's graduates may act as faculty associates who, with model or demonstration programs, can provide greater field nursing consultation and technical assistance to new practitioner graduates.

In many school districts—Pittsburgh is outstanding—the nurse practitioners have moved through the first four phases of program implementation and have, with a working evaluation mechanism, arrived at the point of developing the information and management subsystems envisioned as Phase V in development of the new school health system.

Chapter 8

INFORMATION SUBSYSTEM

To track to their sources the causes of disease, to correlate the vast stores of knowledge, that they may be quickly available for the prevention and cure of disease—these are our ambitions.

—William Osler*

Unfortunately a mathematical approach to the analysis and solution of problems in the health field is not yet feasible. The necessary facts and figures are not available: only bits and pieces are beginning to emerge . . . but the jig-saw puzzle has not yet taken form.

—Herman Hilleboe**

These two quotations define the struggles, ambiguities, and frustrations of attempting to describe, much less implement, an information subsystem for a school health services system. The truth is that we more clearly see where we want to be than understand the means necessary to arrive. In the words of Emily Dickinson:[1]

*Sir William Osler, 1849–1919, Canadian physician; professor at McGill, the University of Pennsylvania, Johns Hopkins, and Oxford; the most brillant and influential teacher of medicine of his times.

**"Public Health in the United States in the 1970's" *Amer. J. Public Health* *58*:1588,1968.

I never spoke with God
Nor visited in Heaven
Yet certain am I of the spot
As if the Checks were given.[1]

This disparity puzzles. Those outside school health sternly upraid it for lack of information systems, yet curiously these critics not to be found when school health turns to look for examples of such systems or even for specific consultant services. Even more intriguing than the lack of a tried-and-true path for school health is the lack of examples of health information systems in other comparable services, such as occupational health and ambulatory medical services. This chapter will describe a view of the ultimate goal of a school health information subsystem, a definition of a health information system, and the results of approaches taken in an attempt to find feasible and appropriate means to the goal.

GOAL

A school health system that has accepted as its mission improvement in the health status of the population of school students requires information on existing health status as the first step in rational development of services and further information to determine whether the services, when executed, are effective in improving health levels as desired. This concept has been expresed in the diagram of the school health system (Figure 8–1).

There are problems with this apparently simple and logical schema. The fact that no one has described an information system for such a health program presents difficulties for all: those without imagina-

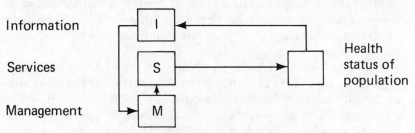

Figure 8–1   School Health Services System.

tion envision nothing, whereas those gifted in that respect concoct wildly different images from the same words.

One common misperception seems to be that an "information system" inevitably means a computer. This is not so; the methods used to collect, store, and analyze data are independent of the uses served by such data. Such conclusions can be forgiven, as articles apparently dealing with new systems for school health information[2-4] turn out to be descriptions of computerization of the current records of the usual input model of school health services.

DEFINITION OF HEALTH INFORMATION SYSTEM

Another misperception of the nature of a school health information system is that simple possession of data will immediately result in mastery of the system and an end to the purgatory of decision making based on few facts. The system is more than data and "far exceeds the bounds of a traditional health-statistics system."[5] The key word is information, and in the words of Tenney, "information is generally characterized as consisting of data with a purpose."[6] Thus an information system has been described by Murnaghan as "a system whose primary purpose is to select data pertaining to health services and transform them into the information needed for decision making."[7]

In the years 1970–1973 in the School District of Philadelphia, and 1973–1980 in the Pennsylvania Department of Health, work was done to determine the types of data needed by and available to the new school health services system. The traditional school health program was first examined to determine the level of current activities. Despite many complaints regarding paperwork and required weekly, monthly, and annual reports, very little data and almost no information were found. It was noted that the data at the school district level were "related more to activities performed than assessment of health status."[8] It was concluded that at the state level, "Health information subsystems to quantify health needs, and thus provide the basis for program planning and evaluation, are simply *not* found at the central nor local levels of the School Health Program."[9]

Other experience that tended to support this finding was that of the U.S. Bureau of the Census, which combed a number of small areas for health and other data to be included in a "social and health indicators system." The only information on health obtained from the Atlanta public schools was the number and percentage of children receiving physical examinations, by school;[10] in Los Angeles the number of children immunized was the only school-related health statistic identified.[11]

Attempts were then made by the school district of Philadelphia and Pennsylvania Department of Health to further describe and elaborate the concept of a health information subsystem for school health, beginning with information on the health status of the school student population.

HEALTH STATUS

The scope of an undertaking designed to comprehend the health status of a population group has been well described by Linder:

> A comprehensive program for disease prevention . . . requires access to a broad spectrum of health-related facts. . . . As the infectious diseases become of lesser numerical importance, those diseases more related to an increasingly complex environment, to shifts in the composition of the population, to changes in living habits due to urbanization, and to still other environmental, social, and economic factors all become major problems. The complicated and interrelated causal factors in these diseases demand scientific sophistication in the use of data and a variety of types of information not previously required in preventive medicine.[12]

Those who have attempted actual measurement of health status have found it a difficult and complex matter. The authors of a publication of the U.S. Department of Health, Education, and Welfare, *Baseline for Setting Health Goals and Standards*, concluded in 1976 that "The health of a population is difficult to measure. . . . There are too many questions which planners must ask, too many differences between national averages and local situations."[13]

There is no one measurement or index of health for a population group or community. There are, however, measures of other events or conditions, such as mortality, morbidity, age, air pollution, and lack of practicing dentists, that throw light on the health of the population group so affected. As Clark noted, "The validity of any measure of health is based upon observations that, where a particular value is found, certain *inferences* about health-related conditions, and at times the state of ill-health of the community generally, can be made"[14] (emphasis added).

The question for a school health system (whose goal is improvement in the health status of the population, or community, of school students) becomes one of selecting an array of measures from which inferences may be drawn regarding the health of the population of concern. As no precedents could be found in the literature for applying this approach to the population of school students, efforts made by others for other populations/communities were noted.

The National Health Planning and Resources Development Act sets forth in Section 1513 the types of data to be assembled and analyzed as a basic prerequisite for planning. The categories of measures can be viewed as follows:

1. *Health status,* and the determinants of that status, of the population of the health service area
2. *Health resources* as measured by the status of the health care delivery system including facilities and staff, use by the population, effect upon health
3. *Environmental,* including occupational and exposure factors affecting health

These categories match what others[14] described as commonly accepted groupings of measures:

Community health status
Community health services
Environmental health

It appears reasonable to include, for the school student population, a category for educational data to reflect environmental health factors in the students' occupational setting, indicate levels of educational function and dysfunction, measure health knowledge and behavior, and show the availability and use of school health services. Finally, in order that health measures move beyond administrative application to become inputs (with scientific meaning regarding the health status of the population of concern) to the health planning process, they must be expressed as rates or indices. "This requirement means that the collection of health statistics must, in most cases, be paralleled by a collection of data about the population . . . for such variables as age, sex, geographic area, and other variables by which health indices are to be estimated.[12] In other words, the measures discussed above are the numerators and population data are the denominators in calculations of rates of health or ill health.

Based on the above considerations, five categories of measures appear to be required to describe the health status of the school student population:

1. Measures of the *health status* of the population, that is, the occurrence of deaths, diseases, illnesses, accidents, disabilities, handicaps; for example, a school student population

may show rising number of deaths in home fires, high infant mortality rates among its pregnant teenagers, increasing rates of acquired handicap due to motor vehicle accidents, persistently high rates of dental caries, and lower immunization levels among medical assistance recipients.

2. Measures of *health resources* present in the community and their adequacy in maintaining and improving health; for example, a school student population may be in a community that lacks any or all of the following: water fluoridation, family planning services, publicly funded prenatal care and well-baby care, dentists who serve medical assistance recipients, and family social services.

3. Measures of conditions in the *environment*, including the school environment, that affect the health of the population; for example, school students may be adversely affected by private water sources, housing without plumbing, overcrowded housing, lead paint, asbestos tiles, air pollution, industrial and traffic emissions, nuclear reactors, economic recession, food advertising, traffic patterns, traffic in illegal drugs, gangs, lack of recreational facilities, unsafe school buses, poor gym equipment, chemicals, and unprotected machinery.

4. Measures from the processes of *education* that reflect aspects of the health status or health function of the student population; for example, students requiring special education, students qualified for school lunch programs, teacher observations of behavior, class and educational performance and function, absenteeism, dropout rates.

5. Measures describing the *population* of school students by demographic categories, such as age, sex, race, socioeconomic status, area of residence, family educational and occupational levels; for example, various services for a school student population planned on the basis of demographic descriptors include sickle cell anemia screening by race, vision screening by age, color vision screening by sex, nutrition screening by socioeconomic status, and lead screeening by certain parental occupations.

Linder could have been writing of school health when he noted "A comprehensive program for disease prevention embracing both chronic and communicable diseases requires *access* to a broad spectrum of health related facts and information necessarily collected by an array of data-gathering methods"[12] (emphasis added). The broad spectrum of facts required to quantify the health of the school student population is a daunting prospect for those working in school health systems that have little past or present experience with health information. The size of the undertaking diminishes when the implications of Linder's words are realized: that much data are already collected by an "array of data-gathering mechanisms" and therefore access to data rather than primary collection could satisfy many requirements of school health.

Establishment of a school health information system could logically begin with a description of the types of data required in each of the five categories and the likely sources of such data, as follows:

1. Health status
    a. The data would include mortality statistics; morbidity data, including such reportable diseases as T.B., lead poisoning, venereal disease, and other infectious diseases; data on conditions diagnosed and treated by medical care agencies; incidental illnesses in school; school absenteeism due to illness; handicapped and disabled children.

    Also data related to pregnancy: live births, infant mortality, maternal mortality, congenital defects, prematurity, illegitimacy, and inadequate prenatal care.

    Statistics on accidents, both in and out of school; dental caries and other dental problems; vision, hearing, and speech assessment results; anemia and sickle cell screening; developmental screening; child abuse; drug abuse, alcoholism.
    b. Sources of data would include state and local departments of public health, department of welfare, hospitals, clinics, children and youth projects, maternal and infant care programs, mental health and mental retardation programs, police departments, dental services, and various divisions of school districts, including school health, counseling, attendance, special education, research and evaluation, and health components of preschool programs.

    Sources of data may also include special studies, such as anthropometric, anemia, sickle cell, lead screening, speech screening, and teacher developmental screening, performed by any of the above agencies or by university, medical school, or other academic institution.
2. Health resources
    a. The data would include information on available services; types of services; determinants of service use, such

as hours, eligibility requirements, transportation patterns, and application and enrollment procedures; on conditions diagnosed; demographic data on providers and recipients of services; identified service deficiencies, such as lack of staff; service charges; recipient possession of means to pay for health services.

b. The sources of data may include state and local departments of public health, departments of welfare, public assistance programs, hospital survey committees, city planning agencies, health systems agencies, mental health and mental retardation programs, health and welfare councils, and federal health programs for children.

3. Environment

a. The data would include information on such community conditions as housing, lead paint, air and water pollution, street lighting, traffic patterns, safety hazards, rodents, gangs; location of such current or potential hazards as nuclear reactors, industrial sites, water holes, rail tracks; such school conditions as safety, sanitation, crowding, noise, ventilation, heat, light; and administrative practices related to safety, sanitation, nutrition, gangs, discipline.

b. The sources of data may include agencies or departments of the census, city planning, licenses and inspection, fire, welfare, and youth services; local and state departments of health; state environmental agency; departments of urban and regional planning at universities; division of research and evaluation of school districts; National Safety Council; federal Environmental Protection Agency and Occupational Safety and Health Administration; state and federal consumer protection agencies; consumer organizations; unions.

4. Education

a. The data would include information on academic achievement, standardized test scores, IQ, teacher assessment of behavior, special teacher screening of development and peer relationships, disciplinary referrals, suspensions, referrals to counselor, school absenteeism, self-referrals to school nurse, dropout statistics, special education placements, students qualified for school lunch programs.

b. The sources of data would include school districts and their divisions of research and evaluation, field opera-

tions, pupil personnel and counseling, special education, school health services; federal and other programs; parochial school administrative officers; private
school associations; federal and state departments of
education; intermediate units or regional education
agencies.
5. Population
   a. The data would include such descriptors as age, sex,
      race, religion, socioeconomic status, geographical area,
      employment, occupation, school, educational level,
      family status, welfare status.
   b. Sources of data may include the census, state and local
      departments of health, health and welfare agencies, the
      public and parochial school systems, city planning agen-
      cies, regional education agencies.

The School District of Philadelphia described and analyzed data
obtained in the above categories during the period 1970/71. This is the
only known written report by a school district on this subject, and the
authors regarded their results as "scanty and incomplete." One example of the problems they found was in the matter of mortality: "Contrary to what might be reasonably expected, complete data on the
deaths of children enrolled in Philadelphia's public, parochial and
private schools is not currently available." Death statistics were com-
piled by the department of health not by school student status but by
age, with considerable overlap of school and non-school attenders
among those one to four and fifteen to nineteen years old. The school
nurses maintained a list of student deaths containing more information about the actual circumstances of death but incomplete as to
number. Even so, the nurses' data, which included only school student
deaths brought to the attention of nurses, demonstrated some time
trends in causes of death, particularly rises in the percentage of deaths
due to homicide, suicide, and nontraffic accidents—all preventable.[8]
The following year a college student worked full-time for 3
months on the problem. All death certificates for a 12-month period
kept by the local department of health were reviewed. Each death
certificate in the age-group four to twenty one years old was checked
against school attendance records to determine school status at the
time of death. The school nurse was consulted for pertinent data from
the health record and for any information about the circumstances of
death; for example, some deaths classed as accidents on the death
certificate were strongly suggestive of suicides when further information, sometimes from eyewitnesses, was obtained.
Later, attempts to institutionalize the flow of mortality informa-

tion between the state department of health and school district ran into problems of confidentiality, labor shortage, movement of offices, computerization, and lack of interest, and to this date institutionalization has not been accomplished. This is, however, an extremely important example. In terms of health status, the mortality data of a population group are the very least one should possess. Mortality rates of school students are the lowest of all population groups, yet the age-group fifteen to nineteen was the only one to experience an increase during 1960–69 and over half the causes of death among students are preventable. Death data are routinely and completely collected using standardized terminology. A great deal of work is performed by computer operations in departments of health. Yet to draw from these data those entries pertinent to the school student population for the purposes of planning school health programs of a preventive nature, one would need to employ a person to travel to a small town on one side of the state and to review by hand all death certificates in order to copy those in certain age categories and send them to school districts for verification of attendance and attachment of additional information known to the school nurse. Following this the data would need to be collected, tabulated, and analyzed before inferences could be drawn.

If mortality data, the best and most complete health statistics extant, are not available for health planning purposes by public agencies with statutory responsibilities for preventive programs, then it is not too difficult to imagine the problems faced by school health when attempting to gain access to data of lesser quality and with less apparent health impact than mortality. It was found in Philadelphia that notifiable diseases and pregnancy could not be related to the student population; venereal disease statistics were grossly underreported; medical conditions seen by pediatric resources were available only as national rates; lead poisoning, child abuse, and drug abuse data were not available or not applicable to students; limited special studies of iron deficiency and nutrition were the only inputs for those problems; data generated by school health were useful in determining immunization levels and T.B. status but accidents statistics were unusable; and a special school health staff survey proved an excellent source of information, clearly revealing, for example, the magnitude of the problem of emotional disturbance.[8] Since then new mechanisms have been successfully developed to report and gather data on child abuse.[15,16] The success of school health–generated data compared with the frustrations of obtaining existing data from other sources is a theme that is picked up again below.

The Pennsylvania Department of Health worked with school districts other than Philadelphia in attempting to obtain access to sources of certain types of needed data. The school districts covered a major city in a county with a full health department, two medium-sized cities with contiguous school district and city boundaries, and a semirural school district covering a number of townships. Less progress was made than in Philadelphia. Some of the specific problems encountered were listed by the department. They included:

1. Conflict between school district boundaries and those of census tracts, minor civil divisions, counties, cities, regions, Standard Metropolitan Statistical Areas (SMSA).
2. Use of age-groupings, especially the fifteen-to-twenty-four-year category, that are not applicable to the school student population.
3. Lack of recording of school student—and occupational—status on health data.
4. Conflict between school year and calendar year.
5. Lack of morbidity data for the population generally, including data on accidents. The lack paradoxically closes official eyes to the need for data on those who are ambulatory but possibly malfuntioning. The lack of data creates the illusion that there is no problem and then that the services aimed at the problem do not exist. Thus when the opportunity to provide or share data arises, those laboring without data are not remembered.[17]

There were of course the general problems noted by others: lack of data quality, time lags between collection and retrieval, confidentiality barriers, and the overriding limitations of data collected to serve the purposes of other users.

Others confirm the difficulties encountered. The World Health Organization listed more than a score of different types of original sources of health data, most of which are records kept for such nonstatistical purposes as clinical records and administrative and financial reports and a few whose prime purpose is health data gathering.[18]

The Philadelphia Department of Health noted at the same time that the city's school district was attempting its mortality study:

At present, there is a multiplicity of sources of information on health and health related data. None of this information is coordinated. Each of the separate collections and compendiums exists as a separate entity within the confines of a separate agency, program, service, category or provider. Information which is needed for planning, management or evaluation must be obtained from multiple sources and is not always useful or complete as a

total entity. In many instances at present there is a lack of standardization for definitions, inclusions, exclusions, collection methods,
financial records and accounting techniques.[19]

Such a situation existing for the health department of one of the
nation's largest cities apparently justifies the thesis advanced by Glasser
"that the statistical system in this country is in reality a cottage industry.
. . [and] what exists is, for the most part, rather badly understaffed,
secondary in priority, and uneven in contribution."[5] It also means that
the situation is more complicated once one moves to areas smaller in
size than those covered by the official health statistics agencies, the state
and local departments of health. In the words of the federal government, the amount of health information "available on a small area basis
is severely limited at present."[13]

Partly for these reasons the U.S. Bureau of the Census undertook
a series of studies of social and health indicators for small geographic
areas or communities served by the Office of Economic
Opportunity.[10,11] The experience is pertinent to the struggles of
school health. Some of the salient points:

1. The purpose of these special studies was to design a system
    to monitor the health status of the population of small geo-
    graphic areas and to evaluate the impact of health services on
    that health status.
2. The data system included subject matters other than pure
    health.

    The level of well-being in a community can not be thoroughly
    examined unless and until health factors are placed in the context
    of the functioning of the community as a whole. Essentially, there
    are a host of other factors that need to be examined such as social
    pathological factors, which contribute to the stress in the com-
    munity; socioeconomic factors, which influence to a major extent
    the flow of social and health services by erecting barriers to the
    access of these services; the quality of housing; the effectiveness of
    the educational system; and resources distributed by the welfare
    systems as well as many other factors which contribute to social
    well-being which is inextricably related to health status.[10]

3. The inputs were data generated by state and county adminis-
    trative agencies.
4. The data were geocoded and, through computer programs,

spatial data summaries for census tracts of neighborhoods were produced. Collected over time, data gained a temporal dimension.

5. Problems were experienced in population estimating procedures for intercensal years, in order to provide denominator data. Using baseline census data, fluctuations year by year were calculated from birth and death records, housing permits, and demolition data. Still the method does not take into account subcomponents of the population or migration.

6. Obstacles to attainment of the numerator input to the system arose from its nature as data generated for administering local programs and included:

    a. Lack of organization of data
    b. Temporal discontinuity of data
    c. Spatial nonconformity, as agencies use different special geographic areas, for example, health district, catchment area
    d. Lack of reliability: clerical errors, missing records
    e. Access impeded by rigid confidentiality, property, or bureaucratic barriers
    f. Data not available in computer-readable form
    g. Need for large-scale clerical operations to prepare data for processing

Lest one be tempted to think that only health data present problems to those who would choose to gather them, the travails of Stodolosky and Lesser, in studying the learning patterns of disadvantaged children in New York City, confirmed that the problem is far more general. Seeking data on the social class and ethnic group of each child, they ran into legal restrictions that would not allow them to ask parents or school authorities directly about education or religion or even occupation. They were "forced" to use data gathered indirectly through 23 different community agencies and 4 sources of census and housing statistics. Interestingly, their "best single source of information was one of the largest advertising agencies in New York City, which had within its Component Advertising Division [which develops special marketing appeals for different ethnic groups] enormous deposits of information on the locations of the many cultural groups in New York City."[20]

Where have we arrived in considering the gathering of health status data for school health planning purposes? That it is a rational goal still holds. Part of the problem lies in obtaining access to relevant sources of data. What appears initially to resemble ordering items from a mail order catalog becomes something akin to picking over items on the city dump. Items of great interest can be found, but it takes time, patience, keen eyes, and imagination; and it will never be the way to furnish the whole house! It seems that special school health studies need to be done similar to those conducted by the U.S. Bureau of the Census on small geographic areas. These would delineate the nature, size, and complexity of the task and allow estimates of the personnel expertise and time required, the appropriate role of computers, and the variables imposed on school districts by size and administrative location. It is not reasonable, however, for school health to sit back and wait for the mail order catalog to be developed for it. In the first place, a flow of statistics into school health will not occur unless school health is asking for them, demanding them, showing how such statistics would be used and how services are suffering without them. Second, when one knows what is wanted and how to use it, odd pieces of data, like junk, can be gathered up and used. Third, enormously important pieces of health status data for school health, as outlined above, are derived from education sources: facts regarding the student population's morbidity, accidents, school health services provided and received, school environmental risks, school and classroom function and performance.

The promise is that nonschool data will constantly improve not only in coverage and retrievability but also in the "establishment of new routine sources" of data for "changing health needs"[21] such as accidents, mental health, therapeutic drug effects, and environmental impacts. The point is that school health may have to wait for certain data inputs but it cannot wait to develop an information system. Information is data collected for a purpose. If school health knows the purposes for which it will use data, it will be able to:

1. Develop a systematic way of using data generated from its own services
2. Stimulate sharing of data generated by other parts of the school system
3. Be alert to the collection and use of pieces of health status data as these become available
4. Describe for those in charge of statistics, data, and information operations the specific needs of school health

The next section describes such an information system, which begins with the actual operations of the school health services subsystem and an evaluation of these operations.

EVALUATION MODEL

Evaluation, derived from the latin *valere*, "to be worth," means the process of determining the worth or value of something.[22] Worth is context-dependent. The same item, action, service placed in a totally different context takes on different meaning.[23]

In seeking to conceptualize the various approaches to evaluation, Schulberg and Baker stated that two models stand out: (1) goal attainment and (2) system.[24] The goal attainment model simply looks at the achievement of goals; the system model includes goals but also concerns itself with establishing the social unit that is capable of achieving a goal.[25] A model of a system approach to evaluation has been designed (see Figure 8–2) and is described in detail below. The model owes much to Arnold, who conceptualized program evaluation and planning as parallels processes.[26]

The first products of a program or its services are the *activities* of the staff: the school nurse practitioner performs a physical examination on a child, meets with the mother for a health history interview, makes a referral to a child guidance clinic, develops a plan for classroom management of a disturbed child, counsels a parent on child management problems; the nurse's aide schedules a child for a vision screening, performs a hearing screening, enters data in records, maintains the tickler file and the nurse's appointment book, provides first aid for a cut finger. These activities must be performed at an accepted level of *quality* in order for subsequent evaluation measures to have any meaning. There are mechanisms available for assessment of the quality of screening tests, first aid, histories, and physical examinations, and

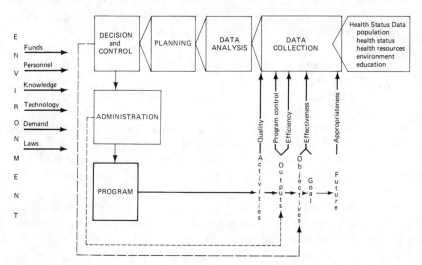

Figure 8–2.   Evaluation Within the School Health System.

the use of these establishes accountability of the program to children, parents, and community and removes the possibility of criticism from those who may be upset over expanded roles for aides or nurses.

It is patently obvious that such diverse staff members as a pediatric consultant, school nurse practitioner, and aide-technician have not assembled by chance but have been hired to perform certain activities that have been planned and are administered in order to produce certain outputs. Measurement of output places administration in the position of knowing if program activities are being performed as expected. Program outputs are, for example, the percentage of the target population on whom a health history was completed or a physical examination or screening test performed. Such data provide the means for *program control.*

Measurement of *outputs* also enables the *efficiency* of the program to be evaluated. For example, nurses may perform hearing screening at a high level of quality and may achieve an output of 98 percent screened of the target population. It may be known, from the work of others, that nurse's aides, well-trained, can reach similar levels of quality and output. If the nurses' salaries are three time those of the aides, then use of aides for hearing screening is more efficient.

A program's outputs are designed to achieve the program's objectives. Data on achievement of *objectives* are measures of the program's *effectiveness.* The objectives of a program may be: (1) to identify conditions of ill health or health problems among students (through health histories, physical examinations, and screening tests) and (2) to resolve health problems identified (through nursing case management activities) thus accomplishing the broader objective of reducing the level of health problems in the school student population.

Objectives are limited, measurable, and attainable portions of the program's *goal.* Goals are more statements of direction and intent, whose specific application at any time varies and is expressed in objectives. The effectiveness of a program in meeting its objectives is also a measure of its *effectiveness* in meeting its goal.

Programs, like everything else in this temporal world, move inexorably into their *future.* Programs that are superb in current time may be irrelevant if the environment changes. For example, health education teaching people wise decision making in the midst of a plethora of available foods may be inappropriate in a future of limited food and few choices, or a school health program aiming at optimal health of students in schools would need drastic rethinking if the future were "deschooled" and children learned at home in front of their own computer terminal. The *appropriateness* of present practice and goals to the constantly unfolding future needs to be included as part of program evaluation.

The ability of the program to understand its goal and objectives depends upon receiving some data on problems or needs. For a program whose goal is improvement in the health status of a population group, such as school students, there is a need, as discussed in detail in the previous section, for data to establish the health status of the population. Program objectives may be set on the basis of such data as decreased immunization levels, lack of dental care resources, presence of a new industry, increasing absenteeism.

Obtaining access to sources of health status data already collected in the broader community is, as noted, difficult or even impossible for school districts. Three measures can help to fill the gap until models are developed for which school health services can obtain access to such data. First, certain pieces of health status data can be picked up by the school health program that is alert to such data and their value. Second, the skilled observations by school nurses of the relatively small populations in their charge, the communities from which they come, and the schools to which they go are marvelously detailed data that if used may more than match the less comprehensive and less timely numerical collections of health status data to which access is sought. Third, program outputs may contain large amounts of information on the health status of the population not known to any other agency; for example, the use of a health history revealed, on 1,000 children entering kindergarten 7 times more health problems than did the previous program, which included only a physical examination.[27] The problems were types not formerly documented as health problems of that population of students: developmental, behavioral, family, and social. Such documentation of the health status of the group has implications for those required to plan programs whose objectives are improvement in such statistics.

The point of all the above activities, which result in data collection, is that some action follows. Schulberg and Baker noted that the goal attainment model of program evaluation measures the effectiveness or achievement of the program in meeting its objectives but leaves results dangling in space. "Nowhere is any indication found . . . of the manner in which the evaluator can insure closing the circle of the evaluation process." The system model of evaluation, however, concerned with "the degree to which an organization reaches its goals under a given set of conditions," is designed with feedback mechanisms so that the effectiveness of the program's activities and outputs are reported back and compared with desired performance.[24] Arnold described the data collected from evaluation as driving the planning process,[27] and Zemach took it a step further to become the major input to the "controller" of the system.[25]

Information is data with a purpose. In the model presented, data is collected and used by those in planning and decision-making capacities. Navarro presented data as the mortar of administration: "According to the flow of information, the major groups in the decision making process can be characterized as data collectors, data analyzers, and data users—the latter including the planners, . . . the administrators, and the decision makers."[28]

It is possible to show the clear connection between data collection and data use and thus the information flow between them:

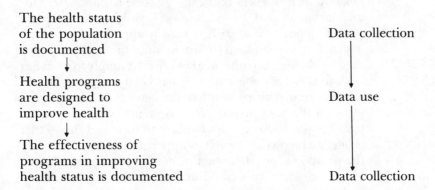

The health status of the population is documented	Data collection
↓	
Health programs are designed to improve health	Data use
↓	
The effectiveness of programs in improving health status is documented	Data collection

Data analysis is the function that links the two and provides the major intellectual function in the whole system. The essential nature of the intellectual function in data analysis is epidemiologic. If collected data on the health status of a population of students reveal certain conditions of disease or ill health, then the epidemiologic process enables one to search for causes so that preventive actions or programs can be planned.

Epidemiology is described as "the quantitative science of community and social medicine,"[29] as "a method of reasoning about disease phenomena in population groups",[30] and as "the study of the prevalence and dynamics of stages of health in populations;"[24] and although it is all these things their sum total is prized because it points the way to prevention. "The main practical application of epidemiology is disease prevention. Preventive measures based on knowledge of disease causation are the only insurance against 'widespread, uncritical programs for prevention based on untested information and on a mere desire to do something.'"[31]

White described a central, synthesizing, organizing role for epidemiology in health care organizations which serves to link the pieces of the model presented in these pages:[32]

1. He quoted the World Health Organization: "Health services information systems as they now exist are often ineffective and ineffecient despite the clear need for them. . . . [They]

need to be designed once again, starting from basic principles."[33] White believed "these principles are essentially epidemiologic in character."

2. Health services must not be confined to those conditions prevalent in the past. "The need for a theoretical framework that does not require all noxious agents to be physical, chemical or biological and that leaves room for such complex deleterious influences on health as noise pollution, jet fatigue, occupational stress, domestic violence, inadequate parenting and sexual strife is readily apparent."

3. The definition of health conditions or of the health status of the population also must not be confined simply to what has traditionally been measured. It has been said "that 'health statistics record births, deaths, marriages and divorces; people with the tears wiped off.' There are other sources of tears, anguish, distress, and failure to cope and thrive that challenge medicine, as well as opportunities for improving the prospects for attainment of man's full potential."

4. More sociologic data could be used as the numerator for such health status problems as "delinquency, social deviance, emotional deprivation, drug abuse, attempted suicide and loneliness" and demography turned to for denominator data. The epidemiologist can relate the two, and biostatisticians "develop the mathematical means for analysing and expressing the data objectively."

5. More data generated from health services need to be cycled back into the system in order to describe the health of the client population in greater complexity than that offered by mortality and limited morbidity data. In ambulatory systems, patients present with problems that are never "diagnoses" in language that fits the International Classification of Disease rubrics, that represent the earliest stages in the natural history of ill health, or that express limitations of functional capacity.

6. "Epidemiology provides the intellectual tools to enable all clinicians to examine, not only the natural history of disorders presented by their patients but also the natural history of medical care and the outcomes of that care. . . . Indeed, it can be argued that the medical practice of the future . . . [will be] responsible for the care of entire populations . . . to detect health problems at the earliest possible time and, when feasible, to prevent their occurrence."

7. "It is one of the tasks of epidemiologists to design these Health Information Systems so that clinical and administra-

tive decision-making can be based on a reliable flow of useful information."

8. A systems approach to evaluating the organization's response to the health status of the population served and "a cybernetic model that uses information about the health status and health care of populations as a basis for defining problems . . . and organizing services seems . . . a more useful sensing and intelligence device than the model usually conjured up when administrators invoke traditional vital statistics and morbidity statistics as a basis for determining health policy and planning services."

EXAMPLE OF MODEL

The approach taken by the Pennsylvania Department of Health to establish new school health programs always requires that the model be kept in mind even though all portions of the evaluation are not or cannot be carried out at the same time. That a total evaluation is not planned at the beginning of a new program and executed throughout is alien to the goal achievement model of program evaluation, based, as it is, on a time-limited research project. The system model maintains that all facets of evaluation are important but that in the real world everything cannot be done at once, and in agencies with fairly constant missions and resources—such as school districts and the school health services in them—everything does not have to be done at once.

In a research project planned, funded, put into operation for 1 to 2 years, and then terminated, everything possible must be done to obtain results before the project ends. In contrast is the school health services system, operating for 70 years, not threatened with immediate termination, and where most staff will be maintained in employment, but where a new program with different objectives, new outputs, broader activities, and new staff roles and relationships is in the process of being implemented. In the latter case it is more important that the momentum toward change be maintained, school nurses be educated as nurse practitioners, aides be hired and trained, interested physicians be recruited as consultants, records be printed, locked record files be purchased, the principals of schools be painstakingly reached and won over, health rooms be refurnished to provide confidential space for histories and physicals, and students and teachers learn to use sick-call hours instead of demanding indiscriminate access to the health room.

System change is slow. One desired end is an evaluation process, with all elements included, that forms the major part of the information subsystem by which the overall system is controlled. It is necessary to see the cybernetic nature of the school health system from the beginning and to understand the complete evaluation process desired so that, on the one hand, establishment of the evaluation system does not drain the resources of the system but, on the other hand, quiet accumulation of evaluation results may be used to drive the system forward. The 12-month cycle of activity in school health greatly aids this incremental cybernetic approach. Each year the school health services system of the school district reviews the evaluation of the past year's activities, determines where the system has arrived, notes the health status of the population, and prepares a plan for the coming year.

The first step in establishing the information and evaluation subsystem in Pennsylvania is the annual plan expressed as a contract between the school district and the Pennsylvania Department of Health. The contract expresses the goals and objectives of the program within a general understanding of the future, sets the outputs for the coming year, outlines the program staff and activities, and describes those evaluations of quality, program control, efficiency, and effectiveness that will be done. In terms of the system model (see Figure 8–3) the contract specifies:

> Management *decisions* regarding the direction and operation of the program. These are expressed in specifications regarding:

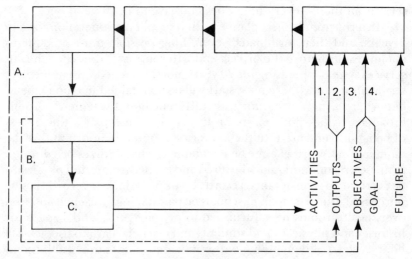

Figure 8–3.

A.   Objectives
B.   Outputs
C.   Program
Procedures to be performed in *evaluation* of the program.
These are expressed in specifications regarding:
1.   Quality of activities
2.   Program control of outputs
3.   Efficiency of outputs
4.   Effectiveness in achieving objectives

In terms of management decisions, the very existence of the contract recognizes that, in Pennsylvania, a new system of locally determined services has replaced the old centrally mandated operations. The *future* is thus open-ended, determined by the health needs of the school students in the districts and by the ability of the districts' school health services system to respond within the general mission of reducing hazards, improving health status, and providing anticipatory guidance.

The *goal* is to ensure optimal health in the student population so that the process of education may be optimally effective. The *objectives* (A) of the new school health service in its first years of operation in a school district recognize both the goal and the future of the system but also the incremental nature of implementation of the new program and the gradual nature of the process of system change. Thus objectives initially are set to achieve only part of the school's mission: to ensure the optimal attainable health of individual students as a means to increase the health and education levels of the population. The means are two: assessment procedures to find health problems, and problem management through the problem-oriented record to resolve problems. As problem management inevitably follows problem detection, it is necessary to specify in the contract only (i) the assessment schedule desired for the population (the periodic in-depth assessments of history and physical and the intercurrent monitoring assessments of questionnaire, screening tests, teacher observations, acute care, absenteeism, etc.) and (ii) the problem-oriented record to be used for problem resolution, for the objectives of the program to be clear.

The contract defines program *outputs* (B) as the number of children to be served by each assessment item as decided by each school nurse. This definition immediately places the school nurse practitioner in the management role specified in the job description as "management of the subsystem of the school health services program over which the School Nurse Practitioner has control." The projected number to be served (aim) is recorded on program control sheet kept by the nurse's aide-technician.

With program outputs described, further description of the *program* (C) and its projected activities and services is specified as necessary. Usually this includes:

> Population to be served: the number of children by grade and school, type of school, geographic location of school, distribution of school nurses by school
>
> Staff: the number of staff by categories, such as school nurse practitioners, school nurses, physician consultants, aides; the job descriptions of and qualifications for each staff category, which must be consistent with established standards
>
> Staff training: the number of staff, such as school nurses, to be sent for further training and the specifications of the course
>
> Facilities, etc: the particularities of the facilities, equipment, supplies, etc., to be provided in order that the outputs and objectives of the program can be met
>
> Budget: a budget providing details of all expenses projected for the coming year

The evaluation procedures to be followed are specified in the contract. An evaluation of the *quality* (1) of certain activities is needed if the school district is to assure both its community and the state department of health of the basic value of its health services. The history, physical examination, screening tests, and problem management are the most highly professional and technical areas, and a program found deficient in any of these would suffer great loss of public confidence.

The quality of the health history interview must be assessed by some observation, either direct or by video or audio tape, and rated according to an acceptable scale. The health history itself may be audited as part of the audit of the problem-oriented record where it can be ascertained that:

> All questions on the history questionnaire have been answered
>
> All positive answers have been subject to a specific interrogation
>
> All problems present in the data have been listed on the problem list

The quality of the physical examinations performed by the nurse practitioners may be audited by observation of the methodologies used, by spot checks of certain children, or by examinations of the same children by the nurse practitioner and a standard examiner, such as a pediatrics resident. The quality of screening tests may be assessed by observation of technique, spot checks of certain children, checks of reliability technique by repeating results on the same groups, and maintenance of acceptable false-positive rates.

The quality of problem management is assessed by use of the audit of the problem-oriented record in which

Completion of data base

Listing of all problems on the problem list

Initial plans of management

Progress notes

are reviewed in a standard fashion that reveals the logic of the problem-solving process used for a particular problem in its own particular circumstances. The results are not specified but the process is, thus allowing for resolution of a certain problem with the use of community resources in one instance and nonresolution of the same problem faced with a lack of community resources in another, or quick resolution of a child's vision problem with compliant middle-class parents and slow resolution with a retarded, overwhelmed single parent with meager financial resources.

Program control (2) is obtained for the nurse in the individual school(s) and for the director of the district's school health services primarily by use of the program control sheet. Children are listed by class, grade, and school at the beginning of the school year for receipt of assessment services according to the output projections of the school nurse. The aide maintains the program control sheet during the year, using it to schedule appointments with parents and children for assessments. At the end of the year the total of each column provides the accomplishments. The services delivered (final count) can be measured against those projected (aim count) and both can be measured against the total target population for such services. The gap between objectives and the capacity of the system's resources to deliver becomes a measurable quantity and thus subject to further planning refinements.

Additional information on program delivery can be obtained. For acute care no information is provided on the program control sheet beyond use of the temporary problem list to ensure that acute care data are entered into the ongoing monitoring of health status. Data on use of the health room for acute care (number; age, sex, and grade characteristics; visit duration; diagnosis; disposition) can be obtained during a random week of the year or can be done for a set of random days.

The activities of the school nurse practitioner are seen indirectly in the assessments performed, problem-oriented records kept, and aides supervised, but the full range of nursing activities cannot be appreciated from such indirect evidence. Time taken in telephone contacts, referrals, consultations, conferences, parent meetings, etc., in order to perform assessments and solve problems needs to be identified. One mechanism is a time chart kept for one or more random weeks per year, supplemented by a log of rarer activities such as faculty and community talks and presentations on the program. Similarly, a time chart kept by physicians for a random set of weeks reveals details of time use and activities performed.

Efficiency (3) in the production of activities is sought in this program. The new staff roles have been designed to ensure optimal utilization of professional time and expertise. That this is being maintained can be assessed by internal and external cost and output comparisons.

Effectiveness (4) of the program in meeting its objectives for improved health status is measured from the problem list. The number and type of problems found on a random sample of records, compared with a random sample from the old program, demonstrate the differences in problem assessment between the old and the new systems. The number, percentage, and type of problems resolved in the old and new programs provide a quantifiable measure of improvement in health status, for example, 0.25 problems per child resolved in old program compared with 1.75 problems per child resolved in new program is a sevenfold increase in health problem resolution.

SUMMARY

Information consists of data that have been selected, interpreted, and communicated for a purpose and thus have meaning for recipients. Information systems are arrangements for collection, analysis and, communication of information on a continuing and planned basis. Part of the system is concerned with program evaluation. Formulation of evaluation requirements during program planning allows for establishment of orderly, continuous arrangements for information collection and use. Such arrangements are called *management information systems.* However, as Schaefer clearly stated:

> No information system can be better than the management system it serves. Unless the management system, at its various levels from the supervision of work to the determination of broad, guiding policies, is based on clear ideas of what is needed and how it is to be

obtained, its information subsystem will be characterized by confusion, vagueness, inconsistency, irrelevancy and waste. This central fact is far more important than whether the information system operates with pencils and paper or with magnetic tape and cathode tube displays.[34]

Chapter 9

MANAGEMENT SUBSYSTEM

When the voices of children are heard on the green,
And laughing is heard on the hill,
My heart is at rest within my breast,
And everything else is still.

—William Blake, *Nurse's Song*

The school health services system is an organized effort at the state and local, or school district, levels to deliver health services to a population defined by its relationship to an institution known as the school. We can say with Fanshel and Bush that "to conceive of health services as a system is an analytical tool useful for rational planning"[1] and management. The school health services system has a structure organized for the purpose of delivering services. The system has functional relationships with its environment, particularly the health care system, the education system, and local community and community organizations.

"The major function of any health care system is to achieve an optimal level of health, for a defined population, through comprehensive health services."[2] This dominating view of the function of the school health services system is depicted in the diagram (Figure 8–1) used throughout this text. In this chapter the diagram will be slightly rearranged as in Figure 9–1. One could approach the operation of

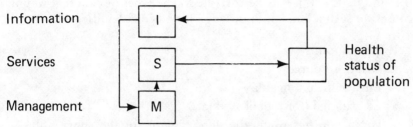

Figure 8–1. School Health Services System.

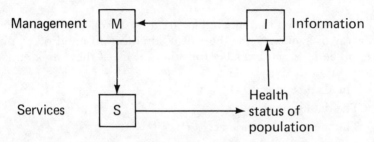

Figure 9–1. Rearranged View of School Health System

such a cyclic system from any point. It seems reasonable to begin at a point of cardinal importance, that, having been discussed in the previous chapter, will require but a few words of review: health status data (Figure 9–2).

Health Status Data. In operating a health system whose major function is to achieve an optimal level of health for a population group, a first task is that of knowing the health status of the population so that,

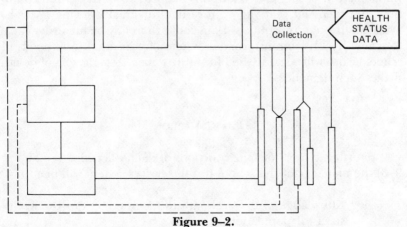

Figure 9–2.

if found deficient, it may be corrected. The types of data that would constitute such a body of knowledge have been identified as:

Health status
Health resources
Environmental health
Educational (for school students)
Population (to supply the denominator for the above numerators)

and it is considered that much data are already collected by a variety and array of agencies—for their own administrative and other purposes, to be sure, but available for others to use if they can identify:

The data required
The data source
The means to provide access

It has been demonstrated however, through hard experience that access to already collected data is difficult to obtain even for mortality statistics. Few models of data gathering for selected, small populations have been tried, and none for school health. It is not at all certain that current data collections contain much of value regarding the health status of school students as expressed by facts of morbidity, accidents, mental disease, disability and handicap, and functional disturbance.

The future may be brighter. Health status facts can be of importance even if gained slowly on a piecemeal basis. The scope of health status for which data are collected is likely to broaden beyond conditions prevalent 50 years ago. More data of great timeliness will be available through computers. Data could currently be made available to school health from its broader system of education. The needs of school health will be addressed in future data systems as school health makes such demands.

DATA COLLECTION

In order to carry out the functions of data collection, (see Figure 9–3) the manager of the school health services system will need:

1. Knowledge of data relevant to measurement of the health status of populations:
    a. Types of data collected

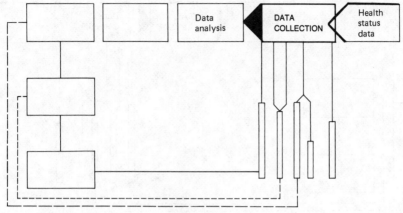

Figure 9–3.

    b.   Sources of collected data
    c.   Record linkage for possible future use
  2. Ability to decide on types of data to be collected, when, and in what form, weighing the population and its needs against data availability in a given community
  3. Skills in:
    a.   Collecting written formal and informal reports from other agencies
    b.   Manually processing data of other agencies
    c.   Computer programming to retrieve from data banks statistics in the form most useful to school health
  4. Skills in:
    a.   Describing the data needs of school health to those designing new information systems
    b.   Describing the data needs of school health to agencies with data to which school health desires access

DATA ANALYSIS

For what are the data collected? In what way will they be analyzed? What purposes will transform data into information? The first use of data is to provide a kind of pulse taking or monitoring or "bookkeeping"[3] of the health of the population. For this purpose statistics must be expressed as rates. Using these rates it is possible to look at disease occurrence in a population by noting variations in the rate of occurrence by characteristics of person, place, time; for example, the

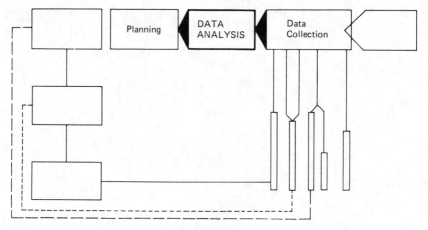

Figure 9–4.

rate of bus injuries rises over the years; there is a concentration of dermatitis in the ceramics class; the rate of drowning deaths is higher in males than in females. Statistical tests must be performed to decide whether the observed variations in rates between groups are statistically significant. The end result of expressing disease occurrence as rates and looking for significant variation between such groups of the population is a description of the distribution of disease in the population, or descriptive epidemiology. (See Figure 9–4).

The substance of epidemiology has to do with the occurrence, cause, and control of health disorders. "For these purposes enumeration is an essential first step. The study of the relation of these states of disordered health to society and habitat follows as a logical next step. To establish these relationships, we must discover the distribution of the enumerated disorders, that is, the way they vary in the population and the attributes and circumstances with which they are associated."[4]

Noting that a particular disease is not distributed randomly in the population but is distributed in association with other variables, the epidemiologist asks Why? and advances a hypothesis to account for the distribution; in effect, a cause is postulated. Further analysis is required to test the hypothesis. Usually further studies are designed and executed with further collection, recording, and analysis of data, often by sample and control groups.

The population study or survey is central to epidemiology. It gives the numerators, or cases of disease, meaning by relating them to the population from which they are drawn. "This procedure creates a standard of comparison, without which no conclusion can be reached on the abnormality or distinctiveness of any phenomenon . . . [It] is a general method that establishes the relation between two or more variables in a population in numerical terms."[4]

In investigation of hypotheses regarding relationships between variables[5] or the causes of conditions, knowledge of data types, sources, and means for access finds its second great use. Analytical epidemiology is made easier as variables of environment, education, health services, economic circumstances, etc., can be quantified and related to disease occurrence.

The final stage in epidemiologic analysis is reached when it is believed that the "cause" of the disease is understood. Proof of the hypothesis is sought in implementation of measures designed to reduce and prevent the cause or to alter the relationship between the person and environment in favor of the health of the former. Such action—planned and implemented as programs, described below—is an exercise in experimental epidemiology. All public health programs designed to prevent disease are in reality exercises in experimental epidemiology. If the program is evaluated negatively the hypothesis of disease causation has not been proven; a positive evaluation, showing improved health status from program activities, provides strong evidence that the hypothesis regarding the cause of the disease is correct.

The expertise needed to carry out data analysis functions includes:

1. Skills in:
   a. Reviewing raw data
   b. Tabulation of data
   c. Constructing rates
   d. Developing and using charts, graphs, maps and other data displays for descriptive and analytical purposes
   e. Performing tests of statistical significance on data
2. Knowledge of descriptive, analytical and experimental epidemiology theory and methods including research design, sampling techniques, case control and prospective studies.

PLANNING

If data collection delineates the existence of a health problem and data analysis suggests the cause, and thus the general nature of the solution, it is the role of planning to define the specific solutions that could be tried together with the advantages and disadvantages of taking each course of action or not taking it. "Planning is, in effect, anticipatory decision making."[2] It prepares, for the decision maker,

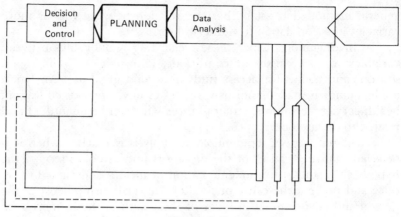

Figure 9–5.

pictures or models of the actions that could be taken in order to solve a problem—in this case to reduce a health status problem. (See Figure 9–5).

Planning requires knowledge of the total school health system and understanding of its goals. It comprehends the nature of the health status problem including the epidemiologic analysis that reveals the cause for which preventive services need to be developed. Tentative objectives are set, plus the outputs required and activities needed. The service capabilities of the school health system are known. Staff, consultants, the literature, and other sources are tapped for knowledge regarding types of services to meet objectives. Alternative services are weighed for their quality and efficiency, for cost-effectiveness and cost/benefit, for long-term and short-term advantages and disadvantages against other priorities. The effects on school health, the school district, and the community are weighed. The alternatives, with arguments for and against, are presented to the decision maker.

"The planner is concerned with organizational acceptance of planning, with implementation, with measurement, and feedback into the planning process."[2] In terms of expertise, "Planning requires a blend of scientific analysis, human judgement, and experience".[2] "Many of the requisites of the successful staff planner—flexibility, inclusiveness of thinking, deductive ability, intuitive perception, sensitivity to human considerations, and capacity to learn—depend as much on . . . emotional maturity as specific business experience or professional training."[6]

DECISION AND CONTROL

If planning is "anticipatory decision making," then the point of its activity is to give to the real decision makers blueprints or dry runs of

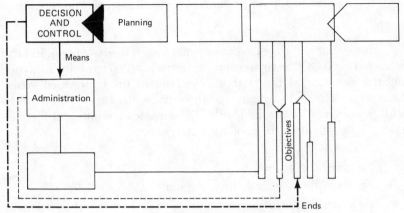

Figure 9–6.

actions about which decisions are required. As Schaefer said, "The outcome of planning is to distil policy and program alternatives and present them for decision."[7](see Figure 9–6). The decision maker has several alternatives; choice involves a comparison between alternatives and evaluation of their outcomes.[8]

In the school health system the decision maker performs the following functions in regard to:

1. Input:
   a. Receives input from planning regarding needs for action and alternatives available, and assesses its validity
2. Checking the system:
   a. Considers the direction and goals of the system
   b. Considers constraints and opportunities of the environment
   c. Considers nature of the staff and their ability to respond
   d. Obtains approval of those in power (e.g., school superintendent, school board, department of health) at both informal and formal levels, directly or through indirect political activity
3. Making decisions:
   a. Considers alternatives by weighing advantages and disadvantages of predicted outcomes
   b. Decides course of action
4. Supporting decisions:
   a. Decides strategy (e.g., cooperative agreements between community agencies, grant proposals, joint service delivery within school district, redeployment of school health staff to a new type of service) to accomplish/implement choice; all these strategies may require lead-

ership, public relations, constituency building, political support

Management is not only decision making, it is also control. In fact, it has been called "the profession of control."[2] It controls by influencing the behavior of the system in pursuit of predetermined goals. Control is exercised formally and informally. Because one is dealing with people it is intertwined with influence, leadership, and motivation. The elements of controlling a system are:

To know the system

To know the objectives of the system

To know the performance required of each part of the system, in both quality and quantity, and to be able to compare these against a standard

To be able to take corrective action for failure in performance

The skills needed for effective management are broad. The manager performs some of the following generally stated functions:

Management both formulates and implements *policies.*

The manager *decides* where the system is going (ends) and how it will get there (means) and controls the system enough to know it is moving toward its ends using the means decided.

School health is being redesigned as a purposeful system able to select its ends and means and thus display will. The will is exhibited through the manager, who is the agent of *change.* "Management is not a static concept; it is rather a dynamic process which takes place in a social and political world. Management both creates and controls change." "As a *process* management consists of a series of sequential or overlapping activities directed towards achieving organizational objectives. Management is a process of effectively integrating the efforts of a purposeful group whose members have at least one common goal." The skills involved in designing, instituting, and controlling the management process are "teachable, learnable and transferable." Management is the *"art* of getting things done with and through people"(Emphasis added).[2]

All systems are *political,* with authority in principal figures; symbolic ratification of collective decisions; and systems of command, of reward and punishment, and for enforcement of collective rules. *Conflict* arises in all systems, and its resolution is a management function. Sources of conflict may be in perception of appropriate objectives, technical authority versus hierarchical authority, role performed or perceived by organization, interdependence of personnel and functions, blocks to communication.

ADMINISTRATION

The decision maker or manager passes decisions to the administrator. The administrator implements policies and decisions, but does not usually formulate them; however, the administrator should be involved in such decision making to ensure that decisions reflect the realities of organizational life (see Figure 9–7). The administrator performs the following functions:

1. Program planning
   a. Defines and clarifies objectives set by the manager
   b. Establishes outputs to meet objectives
   c. Consults with staff, advisers, and literature to develop an approach to services that embodies the best of professional and technical knowledge and practice
   d. Describes the program, services, activities needed to deliver outputs
   e. Describes staffing pattern to provide services and supportive activities (including training) at acceptable levels of quality and as efficiently as possible
   f. Writes organization chart, job descriptions, position performance measures
   g. Develops records and forms
   h. Writes manuals
   i. Specifies facility, equipment, and supplies needed
   j. Writes planning flowchart
   k. Writes evaluation design for measurement of quality, program control, efficiency, effectiveness
   l. Develops budget for program

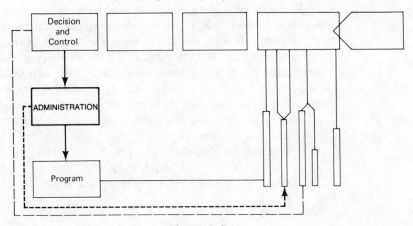

Figure 9–7.

2. Program implementation and operation
   a. Writes implementation flowchart (program evaluation review technique—PERT)
   b. Recruits and hires staff
   c. Establishes preservice and in-service training and program orientation
   d. Provides for supervision of quality of activities and quantity of outputs
   e. Provides for consultation in problem resolution
3. Operates program evaluation
   a. Quality: Measures of program performance as taken from supervisor observations, quantitative results (e.g., screening test failures), special observations, special tests or audits.
   b. Program control: Measures program performance against outputs planned, through use of program data on forms such as program control sheets or by special tallys or random counts.
   c. Efficiency: Outputs are measured per unit of input; calculations can be made by time sheets or budget to study internal efficiency. Comparisons between systems, for example, use of dentists compared with a team composed of a dental supervisor and dental technotheropists, requires up-to-date knowledge of other systems. Such input can be obtained from literature and/or special advisory committee composed of well-informed, nonthreatened professionals interested in the delivery of services.
   d. Effectiveness: Data generated from program activities and, in some instances, data collected from health status sources, for example, mortality, demonstrate changes in a problem following the introduction of the program.
   e. Appropriateness: Data regarding the future direction of programs must be gleaned from those with antennae beamed in that direction. Staff discussions, literature reviews, conferences, visitors to the program, and special advisory committees are some of the inputs to assist in this aspect of evaluation.
   f. Health status information: The provision of services to school students provides much data on:
      (i)   health conditions affecting the population
            dental
            medical
            behavioral
            functional

social
acute
chronic
handicapped
(ii)   health resources available for use and used; health problem resolved or not as a result
(iii)   environmental circumstances surrounding and causing health conditions
(iv)   educational aspects of health
class performance
gym performance
absenteeism
dropout rate
teacher observations of health and health behavior
acute conditions
accidents
use of special educational services: counseling, psychological, speech therapy, audiology, other therapies, special education, voc-tech
school environmental conditions
(v)   population: Demographic data on total child population of a community are available by age, race, sex, location of residence, occupation of parents, size of household, poverty and welfare status, school lunch assistance status

In conjuction with the data collectors the administrator can develop means to identify and collect these data and have them analyzed as a first step in more accurately describing the health status of the student population served. The skills and expertise needed by the administrator are reflected in an ability to perform the functions of program planning, operation, and evaluation as listed above.

PROGRAM

The program of services, the heart of the operation, has been described in Chapter 7 (see Figure 9–8).

EVALUATION

The brief description of the work of the administrator in establishing the evaluation system adds to the more lengthy discussion presented in the previous chapter. (see Figure 9–9).

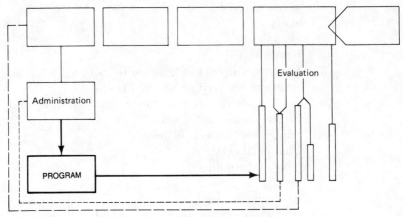

Figure 9–8.

Data Collection.   Data from the evaluation procedures and data describing the health status of the population are collected and stored by the data collection unit.

Data Analysis.   Health status data from the evaluation process are treated as described previously for health status data: rates are calculated, groups are compared, tests of statistical significance are performed, the distribution of diseases/problems in the population is described, and epidemiologic analyses are performed to arrive at the causes.

Evaluation data are analyzed relative to the expectations set for the program. Were the activities performed at the standard of quality required? Were the program's outputs as planned? Was the program as efficient as designed? Were objectives met? If the answers are yes,

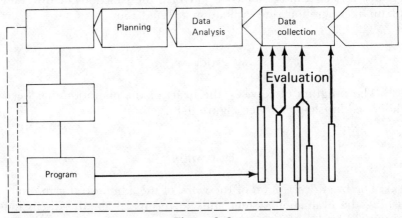

Figure 9–9.

the program can proceed unless population needs or system objectives change. If the answer to any of the evaluation questions is no, the data and situation must be analyzed to find the reason/cause.

The reasons may lie in invalid assumptions regarding the cause of the problem, intercurrent changes in the environment, an unrealistic plan, or inability of the system to follow the plan for external or internal reasons.[9] Once the reasons are found, the planners can deal with this service delivery issue as they deal with a health status issue and send alternatives for action to the decision maker.

Evaluation of an operating program provides information of importance for program control to the manager of the system. This can be done, as Zemach points out,[10] only if the evaluation is done within the system and not by an isolated, outside observer and is done over time as part of the dynamic operation of the system. Linked to the overall system, evaluation provides information to decision makers and can be altered by them to better reflect the needs of the system. All parts of the system, including the future toward which the system is moving, can be evaluated.

The organization of school health services in the school district is that of a rational, goal-oriented system. It is designed to be a purposeful system able to choose its ends as well as means. It is organized to be managed, and the central thread of management is information.

It is designed to achieve, as its major function, an optimal level of health in the population of students. As health is a dynamic variable, changing with the population and the environment, the school health system must be an adaptive, problem-solving organization constantly adjusting the use of its resources to prevent different health problems—or, as some have said, to be able to put together temporary service systems of diverse specialists linked by coordinating executives.

One of the interesting problems in the new school health is the change it requires in leadership and task patterns as chief school nurses move to administrative and management positions. These changes, noted in Table 9–1, have been described by Katz and Kahn[11] and modified by Katz[2] and this author.

Problems and Directions

There are unresolved political problems in the organization of public health services which the new school health system may avoid because of its heavy identification with the education delivery system. Schaefer saw health agencies struggling between state and local loci of control.[13] State control is grouped around programmatic areas whereas the local view is geographic: the specialist versus the generalist. A

Table 9–1.

Hierarchical level	Type of leadership process	Related task orientation	Related socioemotional orientation
Program or professional	Use of existing structure	Technical expertise Knowledge of rules	Concern with equity for subordinates
Administration	Extending, supplementing, and piecing out of structure	Insight into organizational problem Assessment of bargaining possibilities	Complex human relations skills in integrating group relations
Management (decision and control)	Origination and change of structure Formulation and implementation of new policy	System perspective Originality and creativity	Charisma: Symbolic Authoritarian Functional

third locus is the "ideology of regionalism" in which health administration is inherently weak, the region having no political or fiscal base. (In contrast is education, in which regional education agencies, or intermediate units in Pennsylvania, have been formed by legislative action pushing school districts into cooperation. At least in Pennsylvania, they perform as networks that coordinate agencies around their legally specified functions, e.g., special education, but also around their broader mandates to assist school districts.) The lack of integrating-coordinating functions is felt in public health, in which many agencies with health functions are organized along different local lines; for example, water drainage areas do not conform with the distribution of medical facilities and both have only an accidental relationship to the boundaries of cities, counties, or states.

Other problems have arisen with the growth of articulate special clienteles, unionization, specialization of providers, and relationships between government and voluntary effort. "What is striking about these problems is that they are not so much administrative in character as they are political. They have to do with the structuring of authority and power." Little help in resolving these problems can be derived from administrative theory.

Such theories cannot adequately orient executives for innovation, bargaining, modifying, planning under conditions of uncertainty.

They cannot raise the administrator beyond the level of coping with conflict—to dealing with it. . . . Consensus-building, constitutionalizing, bargaining, coalition-forming, compromise and trade-offs may sound strange in the lexion of community health administrators—but they are the keys to the future."[13]

A rational approach to delivery of school health services—one that places in local hands the responsibility to monitor needs and allocate resources for the best preventive outcome for a particular population group—brings school health, in mapping its own future, to a *terra incognito*. It looks logical, but it has never been tried, not in the field of school health and not in any other known health field. Occupational health services resemble school health but have also been bastions of limited clinical services. Local public health agencies in cities and counties come closest to the model of public agencies serving the measured health needs of the population. In reality, starved for money, they have accepted funds to provide specified inputs—services decided by others elsewhere; and they have not been able to develop information systems beyond the bare bones of vital statistics.

Various writers alluded to the need for something new. Something more local that fits, as Piel said, the facts that "the medical economy is a local one and medical services are rendered ultimately to the individual." Such "an entirely new kind of health agency would practice an entirely new kind of epidemiology that monitors the health of the population, assesses its needs, and fixes the denominators by which the distribution of resources is to be determined."[14]

White envisioned medical practices embracing the care of population groups and needing health information systems, established by epidemiologists, for the processes of clinical and administrative decision making.[15] Such a model could be used for populations defined by enrollment, such as school students. The data should be:

Population-based, that is, the denominator known or calculable

Problem-oriented, that is, describing the health problems of the population in such terms as "problems," "symptoms," "complaints," "disabilities," and "functional limitations," which amplify "diagnoses"

Person-specific, that is, within the system the individual identifiable so that specifics of assessment, problem list, plans, referrals, and outcomes can be linked

Provider-specific so that quality, efficiency, and outcomes can be measured

Period-specific so that changes over time can be studied

Practical in design, with the data system collecting only data with
some use in decision making

Hospitals now generate and store much data through various
computer uses yet have not been able to find ways to use the detailed
data from their records for preventive or population purposes. Hunt
suggested that an epidemiologist survey the numerator medical data
derived from the population served by a hospital. Without such a
resource "underutilization of clinical information for elucidating
cause-effect relationships" will continue.[16]

Currently no data base from which to examine national issues and
develop national policy for school health is available, yet using an
information system as described, school health could provide data on
type and volume of services, types of individuals served, health conditions found, and subsequent change in health status.[17]

TRAINING NEEDS

The work of managers of school health systems has been described
by others as being within the area of community medicine. The Royal
Commission on Medical Education in the United Kingdom wrote:

> The speciality practiced by epidemiologists and administrators of
> medical services . . . is concerned not with the treatment of indi-
> vidual patients but with the broad questions of health and disease
> in, for example, particular geographic and occupational sections
> of the community and in the communities at large. [It] embraces
> many activities and interests and includes doctors employed in
> different spheres partly because the health services have de-
> veloped in this country under several different authorities . . . the
> main elements in the professional education and training of the
> specialists in community medicine are already well recognized.
> Epidemiology, statistics, medical sociology, operational research
> and the organization of medical care and administration are the
> core subjects: Their assimilation requires academic instruction and
> preferably, even for doctors who expect to spend most of their
> working lives in professional practice, opportunity for some re-
> search experience.[18]

The functions of the specialist in community medicine in the reorga-
nized National Health Service in the United Kingdom have been
described as follows:

1. Information: development and provision of information, including design of information systems
2. Management: interpretation of information, epidemiological analysis, planning, management, evaluation of service effectiveness in meeting needs, viable alternatives
3. Services: provision of health services, advice and assistance to public and private agencies on planning and provision of services, coordination of preventive care services, staff development.[18]

The World Health Organization addressed the question of training programs in health planning and developed a schema of the levels of ability in health planning functions needed by policy makers, administrators, consultants, and others.[19] Skrovan et al. described an academic program to prepare public health nurses for the role of community nurse practitioner with skills in assessment of the health needs of communities and populations, social planning, and community development. A problem-oriented community record was used as a method for process evaluation of the community nurse practitioner. The authors viewed the program as a natural expansion of the role of the public health nurse.[20]

School nurses, engaged in a specialized aspect of public health nursing, also possess skills as health program managers. They move naturally toward the role of system manager, as outlined previously. They need additional skills, however, the problem is to determine the management skills already possessed and those requiring further development. In May 1980 the Pennsylvania Department of Health, in conjunction with the Wharton School of the University of Pennsylvania, conducted a workshop for 30 school nurse practitioners responsible for system management activities "to scan the environmental and role demands placed on the school nurse practitioner, to identify areas for further skill development."[21] A clear set of training priorities emerged: (1) skills in setting objectives and designing research or experimental programs were requested in order to more fully implement the epidemiologic core of the new system; (2) skills in conflict management, group dynamics, assertiveness, collegial relations, and creative problem solving were seen as assisting nurses to perform the management functions of the school health system where its emerging operations affect the larger systems of which it is a part.[21] Means are now under way to develop workshops and other continuing education programs to provide these skills.

Chapter 10

CONCLUSION

Upon this gifted age, in its dark hour,
Rains from the sky a meteoric shower
Of Facts . . . they lie unquestioned, uncombined.
Wisdom enough to leech us of our ill
Is daily spun, but there exists no loom
To weave it into fabric; . . .

> —Edna St. Vincent Millay, "Huntsman, What Quarry?"

This "gifted age" in which we live has transformed the lives of children. The miraculous lengthening of the average human life span which has occurred in the past century has been wrought by the saving of children. They have, in turn, changed the shape of our population and altered our perceptions of their health needs. Childhood has taken on a different meaning, as George Bernard Shaw noted: "A presumed long span of years is the precondition for taking life seriously."

There are two major tasks for those seriously concerned about the health of childhood: first, to be certain that longevity is maintained for the population generally and for at-risk subgroups within it; and second, to strive for optimal health for those living, so that having life they may have it more abundantly. In schools, where students need to be in optimal actual and potential health to engage in the work at hand,

and society has deemed that health services are necessary, the stakes for those who would seriously concern themselves with health services for schoolchildren are the future lives of the children and the future substance of society. This splendid challenge should invigorate our age. It would be a pity if we were overwhelmed by our ignorance of the health problems of children, our lack of historical perspective, and the nonresponsiveness of current health and education structures and came to resemble the picture painted by Somers and Somers: "We retreat from the idea of the tentativeness of our present knowledge, the impermanence of the institutional arrangements we know, and the inexorability of change. Thus, we deceive ourselves as to the nature of reality and raise our own barriers to understanding."[1]

I have described a new system of school health services that directly addresses the health status of the schoolchild population through development of a new type of health structure refashioned from the old. It is a local operation based primarily at the school and school district level. It has worked because someone at the local level—school nurse, superintendent, director of pupil services, physician, board member—has wanted it to work. It is not dependent upon approval or change by others, especially those in medicine or public health; in fact, the need for this approach has arisen because neither medicine nor public health is able to respond. The Carnegie Council on Children saw lack of medical interest in "our most neglected long-term health needs: chronic conditions, psychosocial and learning problems related to family stress and . . . prevention of crippling and handicapping conditions and the development of more healthful environments and behavior patterns," and perceived that societal structuring of medical practice and reimbursement encouraged this neglect.[2] The problems faced by public health agencies have been noted in previous pages: the lack of the core epidemiologic process; the deficient local structures for delivery of public health services; and the centralized, or state, orientation of public health administration, which is inimical to those struggling with local problems.

The new school health system draws together:

1. The health needs of children, which are undeniably impeding their education and are little understood and studied
2. Societal rationales for health services for students in their occupational role
3. School districts, which contain both schoolchildren with health problems and school health services
4. An accountable outcome of improvement in the health status of the student population
5. An epidemiologic internal process

The system requires operation of subsystems of information and management, both of which, in school health, can or will be found only at the local level. Information needed to operate a rational school health system becomes available only when gradually developed from locally centered activity.[3] System management functions, which combine professional and administrative content, are roles well filled by school nurses, who basically need only some additional epidemiologic skills.

This local model of services, information, and management subsystems would be appropriate for others responsible for small population groups, especially occupational health services and health maintenance organizations.

Although the actual selection of the ends and means of the local school health system cannot be done except by those responsible for local populations, the logic of the system opens it to mechanisms of public accountability. State and federal health agencies can set general standards to be used as reference points by the staff of school health services, school boards, funding agencies, parent and advocacy groups, and others concerned with quality. The standards mirror the internal process of the new school health system and resemble the audit of the problem-oriented record in clinical care:

1. Standards related to the content of the data base, or health information, on the population
2. Standards related to the process of problem analysis
3. Standards governing the plans chosen as appropriate for problems, for example, screening for developmental delay, or prevention of suicide
4. Standards governing implementation of plans and evaluation of results

Such standards complement the local process and fit with the approach of a constantly growing system in which evaluation, or performance measurement, is an ongoing process and not an attempt to measure effectiveness in meeting stated goals at only one point in time.[4]

The methods suggested in this book for achieving the transition from the old to the new system of school health have been found attractive and appropriate for a process of organizational development. It is attractive in and of itself to free nurses to function as their professional preparation and the law intended.[5] It is exciting to establish a structure within which the best that medicine has to offer can be provided. It is a portent of the central role of schools in delivery of health services to children to see varied professionals from many agencies attend schools for team meetings on multihandicapped students and to experience the enthusiasm for similar involvement from workers in the dental and mental health fields.

The proposed new system works. One sees school district administrators grasp the full potential of their health mission—and their capabilities. Nurses move from the old school nurse role to that of school nurse practitioner and then school health manager, completing the circle that began with the marvelous epidemiologic work of Florence Nightingale. The new school health system is a structure that can move into the future able to improve the health of students through action that is rational, purposive, and accountable, without creation of large bureaucracies or expenditures beyond current levels of investment.

The focus of the system is children and their health. Activity within the system spills over into the rest of society, stimulating professional school to establish courses (e.g., for school nurse practitioners and school nurse managers) and to see opportunities for research, for placement of students, and for demonstration of models of care. The possibility is that, in time, school health services will become the focus and stimulus in the community for advances in the health of the child of school age.

NOTES

Chapter 1

1. *Health in Schools,* Twentieth Yearbook, American Association of School Adminstrators, Washington, D.C., 1942.

2. B. Price, *School Health Services: A Selective Review of Evaluative Studies,* Children's Bureau, U.S. Department of Health, Education, and Welfare, Washington, D.C., 1957.

3. J. F. Rogers, *State-Wide Trends in School Hygiene and Physical Education,* Pamphlet 5, revised Ed., Office of Education, U.S. Dept. of the Interior, Washington, D.C., 1941.

4. A. S. Castile and S. J. Jerrick, *School Health in America: A Survey of State School Health Programs,* American School Health Association, Kent, Ohio, 1976.

5. A. S. Castile and S. J. Jerrick, *School Health in America: A Survey of State School Health Programs,* 2nd Ed., American School Health Association, Bureau of Health Education, Center for Disease Control, U.S. Department of Health, Education, and Welfare, 1979.

6. G. Scott, *Statistics of State School Systems, 1969-70,* Office of Education, DHEW Publication (OE) 74-11421, 1974.

7. E. S. Gendel, "Effective Interaction for School Health," presentation to School Health Section, American Public Health Association, Annual Meeting, October 20, 1965.

8.   N. B. Schell, "School Physicians: A Weakened Breed", *J. School Health 43*: 45–48, 1973.

9.   American Academy of Pediatrics, Committee on School Health, *School Health: A Guide for Health Professionals,* American Academy of Pediatrics, Evanston, Ill., 1977.

10. J. J. Hanlon, *Principles of Public Health Administration,* 5th Ed., Mosby, St. Louis, 1969.

11. American Academy of Pediatrics, Committee for the Study of Child Health Services, *Child Health Services and Pediatric Education,* Commonwealth Fund, New York, 1949.

12. G. A. Silver, *Child Health: American's Future,* Aspen Systems Corp., Germantown, Md., 1978.

13. A. Lynch, *Report on the School Health Program of the Department of Health, Commonwealth of Pennsylvania, September 1973–December 1974,* Harrisburg, 1975.

14. C. C. Wilson, ed., "School Health Services," 2nd Ed., National Education Association and the American Medical Association, Washington, D.C., 1964.

15. D. A. Cornely, "Health Services for Children," chap. 21 in *Maxcy-Rosenau Preventive Medicine and Public Health,* 10th ed. Ed., P. E. Sartwell, Appleton, New York, 1973.

16. K. D. Rogers, "School-Age Children," Chapter in *Ambulatory Pediatrics,* eds. M. Green, and R. J. Haggerty, Saunders, Philadelphia, 1968.

17. E. A. Crowley and J. L. Johnson, "Multiprofessional Perceptions of School Health: Definition and Scope," *J. School Health 47*: 398–405, 1977.

18. A. Lynch, "There Is No Health in School Health," *J. School Health* 47:410–413, 1977.

19. W. E. Schaller, "School Health at the Crossroads—An Introduction," *J. School Health* 47:393–394, 1977.

20. O. E. Byrd, *School Health Administration,* Saunders, Philadephia, 1964.

21. C. Mayshark, D. D. Shaw, and W. H. Best, *Adminstration of School Health Programs: Its Theory and Practice,* Mosby, St. Louis, 1977.

22. N. G. Hawkins, "Is There a School Nurse Role?", *Amer. J. Nursing* 71:744–751, 1971.

23. National School Health Conference, Resolution Submitted to Joseph A. Califano, Jr., May 12-13, 1977, Minneapolis, Minn., *J. School Health* 47:397–398, 1977.

24. D. S. Bryan, *School Nursing in Transition,* Mosby, St. Louis, 1973.

25. American Nurses' Association, *Functions and Qualifications for School Nursing,* New York, 1966.

26. L. A. Chilton, discussant, *School-Related Health Care,* Report of Ninth Ross Roundtable on Critical Approaches to Common Pediatric Problems, Ross Laboratories, Columbus, Ohio, 1978.

27. *The Pipeline,* Spina Bifida Association of America, March-April 1979, noted that the Office of Civil Rights for Region VII had defined intermittent catheterization as a "health" or "supportive" service under the Education of the Handicapped Act and not a medical service and thus should be provided by schools so that needy children could have the most normal daily schedule.

28. D. W. Clark and B. MacMahon, eds., *Preventive Medicine,* Little, Brown, Boston, 1967.

29. E. D. Kilbourne and W. G. Smillie, eds., *Human Ecology and Public Health,* Macmillan, London, 1969.

30. T. W. Lash and H. Sigal, *State of the Child: New York City,* Foundation for Child Development, New York, April 1976.

31. *A Child Health Plan for Raising a New Generation,* submitted by the Joint Child Health Planning Task Force of the North Carolina Pediatric Society and Chapter of the American Academy of Pediatrics, North Carolina Department of Human Resources, to the governor of North Carolina, 1979.

32. "Commentary: The Select Panel on Child Health,: *Clinical Pediatrics* 19:7–9, 1980.

33. P. Denton, J. S. Andrews, B. S. Levy, and B. Mitchell, "An Effective School-Based Influenza Surveillance System," *Public Health Reports,* 94:88–92, 1979.

34. J. B. Richmond, "Prevention: The Second Public Health Revolution," *Urban Health,* January-February 1980, pp. 30-32.

35. P. R. Nader, "Where School and Health Interact: The Child in His Family," paper prepared for Options for School Health, National School Health Conference, Galveston, Texas, June 20-23, 1976.

36. J. M. Lampe, "The School Physician of the Future," *J. School Health* 42:197–198, 1972.

37. "Demonstration, Research and Training in Comprehensive School Health," a proposal prepared for the Robert Wood Johnson Foundation by the University of Texas Medical Branch, March 1974.

38. P. R. Nader, A. Emmel, and E. Charney, "The School Health Services: A New Model," *Pediatrics 49:* 805–813, 1972.

39. P. R. Nader, "The School Health Service: Making Primary Care Effective," *Pediatric Clinics of North America 21:* 57–73, 1974.

40. P. J. Porter, R. L. Leibel, C. K. Gilbert, and J. A. Fellows, "Muncipal Child

Health Services: A Ten-Year Reorganization," *Pediatrics* 58:704–712, 1976.

41. H. K. Silver, "The School Nurse Practitioner Program: A New and Expanded Role for the School Nurse," *J. American Med. Assoc. 216*:1332–1334, 1971.

42. C. D. Schoenwetter, "The School Health Service: Review and Commentary," *Pediatric Clinics of North America 21*:75–80, 1974.

43. Report of the Court Committee on Child Health Services, Department of Health and Social Services, London, England, 16 December, 1976.

CHAPTER 2

1. For example, two short medical histories make no reference at all to school health services: Rogers, F. B., *A Syllabus of Medical History*, Little, Brown, Boston, 1962.
Wilcocks, C., *Medical Advance, Public Health and Social Evolution*, Pergamon Press, London, 1965.
The one book that appears promising is a history of school health education:
Means, R. K., *Historical Perspectives on School Health*, Charles B. Slack, Inc., Thorofare, N.J., 1975.

2. B. Ramazzini, *Diseases of Workers* (*De Morbis Artificum*, 1713), published under the auspices of the New York Academy of Medicine, Hafner Publishing Co., New York, 1964.

3. C. Thackrah, "The Effects of Arts, Trades and Professions, and of Civic States and Habits of Living, on Health and Longevity: with Suggestions for the Removal of Many of the Agents Which Produce Disease, and Shorten the Duration of Life," Longman et al., London, 1832, reprinted in A. Meiklejohn, *The Life, Works, and Times of Charles Turner Thackrah*, Livingstone, London, 1957.

4. S. Kurtz and W. Bridgewater, eds., *The Columbia Encyclopedia*, 3rd ed., Columbia University Press, New York, 1963: "The transformation of the United States into an industrial country took place largely after the Civil War and on the English model. The textile mills of New England had long been in existence, of course, but the boom period of industrial organization was from 1860 to 1890" (p. 1021).

5. Rogers, 1962.

6. C. F. Brockington, *A Short History of Public Health*, Churchill, London, 1956.

7. Papers published by the Board of Trade, Vol. IV, p. 382 ff. quoted in J. Kuczynski, *The Rise of the Working Class*, McGraw-Hill, New York, 1967.

8.   L. R. Villermé, *Tableau de l'Etat physique et moral de Ouvriers employés dans les Manfacutures de Coton, de Laine and de Soie*, vol. 1, Paris, 1840, p. 26, quoted from Kuczynski, 1967.

9.   *A Documentary History of American Industrial Society*, eds. J. R. Commons et al., vol. V., Cleveland, 1910, quoted in Kuczynski, 1967.

10. G. M. Trevelyan, *Illustrated English Social History: The Nineteenth Century*, vol. 4, Pelican Books, Harmondsworth, Middlesex, England, 1964.

11. G. M. Young, *Victorian England: Portrait of an Age*, 2nd ed., Oxford University Press, Oxford, 1953.

12. Wilcocks, 1965.

13. H. E. Sigerist, *The Great Doctors: A Biographical History of Medicine*, Doubleday, New York, 1958.

14. C. Woodham-Smith, *Florence Nightingale*, Penguin Books, Harmondsworth, Middlesex, England, 1955.

15. Some are honest on this point! "Many school administrators are at least partially confused in respect to the proper functions of a school nurse." (O. E. Byrd, *School Health Administration*, Saunders, Philadephia, 1964.)

16. F. Nightingale, *Notes on Nursing: What It Is and What It Is Not*, Harrison and Sons, London, 1859; facsimile reprint, G. D. Duckworth and Co., London, 1970.

17. C. F. Brockington, *The Health of the Community: Principles of Public Health for Practitioners and Students*, 3rd ed., Churchill, London, 1965.

18. C. Booth, *Life and Labour of the People of London 1889–1897*, quoted in Brockington, 1956.

19. M. MacMillan, *Life of Rachel MacMillan*, 1927, quoted in Brockington, 1956.

20. C. L. Anderson, *School Health Practice*, 4th ed., Mosby, St. Louis, 1968.

21. C. A. Beard, M. R. Beard, and W. Beard, *New Basic History of the United States*, Doubleday, Garden City, N.Y., 1960.

22. B. J. Stern, *American Medical Practice in the Perspectives of a Century*, Commonwealth Fund, New York, 1945.

23. J. C. Estrin, *American History Made Simple*, Doubleday and Co., Garden City, N.Y., 1956.

24. R. H. Bremmer, ed., *Children and Youth in America: A Documentary History, Vol. II: 1966–1932*, Harvard University Press, Cambridge, 1971.

25. W. G. Smillie, *Public Health: Its Promise for the Future: A Chronicle of the Development of Public Health in the United States, 1607–1914*, Macmillan, New York, 1955.

26. F. R. Butts and L. A. Cremin, *A History of Education in the American Culture*, Holt, New York, 1953.

27. J. C. Furnas, *The Americans: A Social History of the United States, 1587–1914,* Putnam, New York, 1969.

28. J. J. Hanlon, *Principles of Public Health Administration,* Mosby, St. Louis, 1969.

29. R. H. Shryock, "The Health of the American People: An Historical Survey," *Proc. Amer. Philos. Soc. 90*:251–258, 1946.

30. G. C. Whipple, *State Sanitation: A Review of the Work of the Massachusetts State Board of Health,* Harvard University Press, Cambridge, 1917, quoted in *A Guide to the Study of the United States of America,* Library of Congress, Washington, D.C., 1960.

31. B. G. Rosenkrantz, *Public Health and the State: Changing Views in Massachusetts, 1842–1936,* Harvard University Press, Cambridge, 1972.

32. B. W. Kunkle, *Milestones to Health in Pennsylvania,* Pennsylvania Department of Health, undated; about 1966.

33. E. Yost, *American Women of Nursing,* J. B. Lippincott Co., Philadelphia, 1955, quoted in *A Guide to the Study of the United States of America,* Library of Congress, Washington, D.C., 1960.

34. R. M. West, *History of Nursing in Pennsylvania,* Pennsylvania State Nurses Association, undated; about 1932.

35. R. J. O'Sullivan, "Sanitary Superintendent of the Public Schools of New York," *Sanitarian 1*:368–370, 1873.

36. A. Viele and W. H. B. Post, "Report on School-Buildings," *Third Annual Report of the Board of Health of the City of New York,* New York, 1873, quoted in Bremner, 1971.

37. New York Medico-Legal Society, *Report of Special Committee on School Hygiene, New York, 1876,* quoted in Bremner, 1971.

38. D. F. Lincoln, "Sanitation in the Public Schools of Massachusetts," *Report of the Massachusetts State Board of Health 9*:227, 1878.

39. *Fourth Annual Report of the Department of Health of the Commonwealth of Pennsylvania, 1909,* Part I, Harrisburg, Pa.

40. S. W. Newmayer, *Medical and Sanitary Inspection of Schools for the Health Officer, the Physician, the Nurse and the Teacher,* Lea and Febiger, Philadelphia, 1924.

41. L. P. Ayres and M. Ayres *School Buildings and Equipment,* The Cleveland Foundation, Cleveland, 1916, quoted in Bremner, 1971.

42. A. Nemir, "The School Plant and Healthful School Living," chapter in H. Medovy, ed., "School Health Problems," *Pediatric Clinics of North America 12*:1085–1097, 1965.

43. C. Harrington and M. Richardson, *A Manual of Practical Hygiene,* Lea and Febiger, Philadelphia, 1914.

44. C. F. Bolduan, "Over a Century of Health Administration in New York City," *Public Health Monographs 13*, Vol 2, Part 1, March 1916.

45. L. R. Struthers, *The School Nurse*, Putnam, New York, 1917.

46. M..M. Roberts, *American Nursing—History and Interpretation*, Macmillan, N.Y., 1954.

47. L. L. Rogers, "A Year's Work for the Children in New York Schools," *Amer. J. Nursing IV*: 181–184, 1903–1904.

48. New York City, Department of Health, Annual Report, 1903.

49. A. Garside, *The Development of School Nursing in Philadelphia*, School District of Philadelphia, mimeo, undated.

50. J. S. Baker, "The Medical Inspection and Examination of School Children in New York City," *Ann. Gynecology and Pediatry XIX*, 450–451, 1906.

51. J. Baker, *Fighting for Life*, 1939, pp. 148–151, quoted in Bremner, 1971.

52. C. V. Chapin, *The Medical Inspection of Schools in Providence*, Ansonia, Conn., 1909, quoted in Bremner, 1971.

53. H. L. Blumgart, "Caring for the Patient," *New England J. Medicine 270*: 449–456, 1964.

54. T. M. Rotch, "Iconoclasm and Original Thought in the Study of Pediatrics," *Transactions of the American Pediatric Society lll*: 6–9, 1891, quoted in Bremner, 1971.

55. W. M. Schmidt, "The Development of Health Services for Mothers and Children in the United States," *Amer. J. Public Health 63*: 419–427, 1973.

56. J. H. Berkowitz, *Free Municipal Clinics for School Children: A Review of the Work of the School Children's Nose and Throat Clinics in New York City*, New York City Health Department, Reprint Series, #41, February 1916.

57. M. Terris, "Evolution of Public Health and Preventive Medicine in the United States," *Amer, J. Public Health 65*: 161–169, 1975.

58. P. A. Corning, *The Evolution of Medicare from Idea to Law*, Research Report 29, Office of Research and Statistics, Social Security Administration, U.S. Department of Health, Education, and Welfare, 1969.

59. B. Price, "School Health Services: A Selective Review of Evaluative Studies," *Children's Bureau*, U.S. Department of Health, Education, and Welfare, Washington, D.C., 1957.

60. R. K. Means, *Historical Perspectives on School Health*, Charles B. Slack, Thorofare, N.J., 1975

61. American Public Health Association, *Keystones for Public Health in Pennsylvania*, New York, 1948.

62. D. B. Nyswander, *Solving School Health Problems—The Astoria Demonstration Study*, Commonwealth Fund, New York, 1942.

CHAPTER 3

1. A. N. Myerstein, "The Value of Periodic School Health Examinations," *Amer. J. Public Health 59*:1910–1926, 1969.

2. D. A. Cornely, "Health Services for Children," chap. 21 in *Maxcy-Rosenau Preventive Medicine and Public Health*, 10th ed., ed. P. E. Sartwell, Appleton, New York, 1973.

3. A. F. North, quoted by K. Lessler, "Health and Educational Screening of School-Age Children—Definition and Objectives," *Amer. J. Public Health 62*: 191–198, 1972.

4. D. F, Lincoln, "School Hygiene," *Sanitarian 3*:193–202, 1875, quoted in W. G. Smillie, *Public Health: Its Promise for the Future. A Chronicle of the Development of Public Health in the United States, 1607–1914*, Macmillan, New York, 1955.

5. F. J. W. Miller, S. D. M. Court, E. G. Knox, and S. Brandon, *The School Years in Newcastle-upon-Tyne, 1952–62, Being a Further Contribution to the Study of a Thousand Families*, Oxford University Press, London, 1974.

6. R. J. Haggerty, K. J. Roghmann, and I. B. Pless, *Child Health and the Community: Results from the Rochester Child Health Studies 1966–71*, Wiley, New York, 1975.

7. D. P. McCormick, "Pediatric Evaluation of Children with School Problems," *Amer. J. Diseases Children 131*: 318–322, 1977.

8. M. Rutter et al., "A Tri-axial Classification of Mental Disorders in Childhood," *J. Child Psychol. Psychiatry 10*:41–61, 1969.

9. B. MacMahon, T. F. Pugh, and J. Ipsen, *Epidemiologic Methods*, Little, Brown, Boston, 1960.

10. M. Susser, *Causal Thinking in the Health Sciences: Concepts and Strategies of Epidemiology*, Oxford University Press, London, 1973.

11. R. Ross, *The Prevention of Malaria*, 2d ed., Dutton, New York, 1910, cited in M. Susser, 1973.

12. P. J. Graham, *Epidemiological Approaches in Child Psychiatry*, Academic Press, London, 1977.

13. W. Malenbaum, "Progress in Health: What Index of What Progress?" *Annals Amer. Acad. Political Soc. Science 393*:109–121, January 1971.

14. J. B. Amadio, J. Mueller, and R. Casey, "Measuring the Benefit of Public Health Services," *Public Health Currents 18* (4), August 1978.

15. R. J. Haggerty, "Changing Lifestyles to Improve Health," *Prev. Med. 6*:276–289, 1977.

16. M. Hurster, "The Identification of Value Orientations of Sixth Graders,

with Specific Reference to Health Concepts in the School Health Education Study Curriculm," *Amer. J. Public Health 62*: 82–85, 1972.

17. C. E. Lewis, M. A. Lewis, A. Lorimer, and B. B. Palmer, "Child-Initiated Care: The Use of School Nursing Services by Children in an 'Adult-Free' System," *Pediatrics 60*:499–507, 1977.

18. M. Weisenberg, S. S. Kegeles, and A. K. Lund, "Children's Health Beliefs and Acceptance of a Dental Preventive Activity," *J. Health Social Behavior 21*: 59–74, March 1980.

19. D. F. Duncan, "Mental Health and Health Education: An Emerging Partnership," *Urban Health*, May 1979, pp. 12–13.

20. C. I. Cohen and E. J. Cohen, "Health Education: Panacea, Pernicious or Pointless?: *New England J. Medicine 299*: 718–720, 1978.

21. P. M. Densen, D. B. Ullman, E. W. Jones, and J. E. Vandow, "Childhood Characteristics as Indicators of Adult Health Status," *Public Health Reports 85*: 981–996, 1970.

22. H. E. Hilleboe, "Modern Concepts of Prevention in Community Health," *Amer. J. Public Health 61*: 1000–1006, 1971.

23. A. R. May, J. H. Kahn, and B. Cronholm, *Mental Health of Adolescents and Young Persons*, Public Health Papers No. 41, World Health Organization, Geneva, 1971.

24. World Health Organization, *Human Development and Public Health*, Technical Report Series, 485, Geneva, 1972.

25. G. Caplan, *Principles of Preventive Psychiatry*, Basic Books, New York, 1964.

26. G. Caplan, *Social Support Systems and Community Mental Health*, Behavioral Publications, New York, 1974.

27. Cambridge Research Institute, *Trends Affecting the U.S. Health Care System*, U.S. Department of Health, Education, and Welfare, 1976.

28. J. B. Richmond, "The Needs of Children," *Daedalus*, Winter 1977, pp. 247–259.

29. Children's Defense Fund of the Washington Research Project, Inc., *Children Out of School in America*, Washington, D.C., 1974.

30. School District of Philadelphia, *Report of Head Start Health Services, 1971–73*.

31. Foundation for Child Development, *National Survey of Children: Summary of Preliminary Results*, New York, 1977. The study consisted of interviews with 2,200 children age seven to eleven and more than 1,700 of their parents.

32. E. Mumford, "Promises and Disaffections in Mental Health Programs in Schools," *Psychology in the Schools VII*: 20–28, 1970.

33. Public School Code, Commonwealth of Pennsylvania, Article XIV, "School Health Services," Section 1401. Definitions (24 P.S. § 14-1401 et seq.).

34. University of Pittsburgh, Law School, *Public Health Laws of Pennsylvania*, 1958.

35. S. W. Newmayer, *Medical and Sanitary Inspection of Schools for the Health Officer, the Physician, the Nurse and the Teacher*, Lea & Febiger, Philadelphia, 1924.

36. F. R. Butts and L. A. Cremin, *A History of Education in the American Culture*, Holt, New York, 1953.

37. School District of Philadelphia, *1978 Survey of Philadelphia High School Graduates, Classes of 1974, 1976 and 1978*, Report 7908, May 1979.

38. Center for Disease Control, "Enforcement of a State's Immunization Law for Entering School Children—Detroit," *Morbidity and Mortality Weekly Report, January 6, 1978*, DHEW Publication (CDC) 77-8017, Atlanta, Ga.

39. I. F. Litt and M. I. Cohen, "Prisons, Adolescents, and the Right to Quality Medical Care: The Time Is Now," *Amer, J. Public Health 64*: 894–897, 1974.

40. H. James, *Children in Trouble: A National Scandal*, Pocket Books, New York, 1969. Based on a series of articles appearing weekly in the *Christian Science Monitor*, March 31 to July 7, 1969.

41. J. G. Bachman, S. Green, and I. D. Wertanen, "Youth in Transition, Volume III, Dropping Out—Problem or Symptom?" Excerpts reported in *The Effects of Dropping Out*, U.S. Senate, Select Committee on Equal Educational Opportunity, August 1972.

42. A. S. Compton, "Health Study of Adolescents Enrolled in the Neighborhood Youth Corps," *Public Health Reports 84*: 585–596, 1969.

43. W. G. Smillie, "The Period of Great Epidemics in the United States," in *The History of American Epidemiology*, ed. F. H. Top, Mosby, St. Louis, 1952.

44. S. Shapiro, E. Schlesinger, and R. Nesbitt, *Infant, Perinatal, Maternal & Childhood Mortality in the United States*, Harvard University Press, Cambridge, 1968.

45. National Center for Health Statistics, *Advance Report, Final Mortality Statistics 1974*, Vol. 24, No. 11, 3 February 1976.

46. M. G. Kovar, "Some Indicators of Health-Related Behavior Among Adolescents in the United States," *Public Health Reports 94*: 109–118, 1979.

47. National Center for Health Statistics, *Mortality Trends: Age, Color, and*

Sex, United States, 1950–69, Vital and Health Statistics, Series 20, No. 15, 1973.

48. School District of Philadelphia, Division of School Health Services, *Annual Report 1970–1971,* 1971.

49. Philadelphia Department of Public Health, *Annual Statistical Report, 1969.*

50. National Center for Health Statistics, *Five Leading Causes of Death at Various Ages, United States, 1960.*

51. Youth Conservation Services, personal communication, staff members, city of Philadelphia, 1971.

52. T. W. Lash and H. Sigal, *State of the Child: New York City,* Foundation for Child Development, New York, 1976.

53. L. Bender, "Children and Adolescents Who Have Killed." *Amer. J. Psychiatry 116:* 510–513, 1959.

54. W. M. Easson and R. M. Steinhilber, "Murderous Aggression by Children and Adolescents," *Arch. Gen. Psychiatry 4:* 27–35, 1961.

55. G. M. Duncan, S. H. Frazier, F. M. Litin, A. M. Johnson, and A. J. Barron, "Etiological Factors in First-Degree Murder," *J. Amer. Medical Assoc. 168:* 1755–1758, 1958.

56. R. E. Gould, "Suicide Problems in Children and Adolescents," *Amer. J. Psychotherapy 19:* 228–246, 1965.

57. L. Morgan, "On the Rise: Teenage Suicides," *Philadelphia Inquirer,* June 15, 1980.

58. H. Jacobziner, "Attempted Suicides in Adolescents," *J. Amer. Medical Assoc 191:* 101–105, 1965.

59. J. M. Toolan, "Depression and Suicide," chap. 20 in *American Handbook of Psychiatry,* 2d ed., vol. II, ed. S. Arieti, Basic Books, New York, 1974.

60. R. D. Rohn, R. M. Sarles, T. J. Kenny, B. J. Reynolds, and F. P. Heald, "Adolescents Who Attempt Suicide," *J. Pediatrics 90:* 636–638, 1977.

61. A. Schrut, "Suicidal Adolescents and Children," *J. Amer. Medical Assoc. 188:* 1103–1107, 1964.

62. H. M. Connell, "Attempted Suicide in School Children," *Medical J. Australia 1:* 686–690, 1972.

63. H. C. Faigel, "Suicide Among Young Persons: A Review of Its Incidence and Causes, and Methods for Its Prevention," *Clinical Pediatrics 5:* 187–190, 1966.

64. J. C. Schoolar, *Current Issues in Adolescent Psychiatry,* Brunner/Mazel, New York, 1973.

65. J. Jacobs, *Adolescent Suicide,* Wiley-Interscience, New York, 1971.

66. National Safety Council, *Accident Facts*, Chicago, 1975.

67. Insurance Institute for Highway Safety, *Status Report 11*:8, May 1976, quoted in Pizzo and Aronson (see note 68).

68. P. Pizzo and S. S. Aronson, "Concept Paper on Health and Safety Issues in Day Care," prepared for U.S. Department of Health, Education, and Welfare, Federal Interagency Day Care Requirements, September 1976.

69. T. Ehrenpreis, *Prevention of Childhood Accidents in Sweden*, The Swedish Institute, Palmeblads Trycheri A. B. Goteborg, 1973.

70. H. E. C. Millar, *Approaches to Adolescent Health Care in the 1970s*, Public Health Service, DHEW Publication (HSA) 75-5014, 1975.

71. National Center for Health Statistics, Vital and Health Statistics, Series 10, No. 105, 1971–72.

72. F. Grosso et al., *An Analysis of Reported Student Accidents in the Public School Systems of the Town of Greenwich, Connecticut, 1976–1978*, Department of Epidemiology and Public Health, Yale University School of Medicine, New Haven.

73. National Safety Council, *Accident Facts*, Chicago, 1978.

74. C. J. Johnson, A. P. Carter, V. K. Harlin, and G. Zoller, "Student Injuries Due to Aggressive Behavior in Seattle Public Schools during the School Year 1969–1970," *Amer. J. Public Health 64*: 904–906, 1974.

75. R. A. McFarland, "The Epidemiology of Industrial Accidents in the U.S.A.," chap. 19 in *Epidemiology: Reports on Research and Teaching, 1962*, ed. J. Pemberton, Oxford University Press, London, 1963.

76. S. P. Baker, "Determinants of Injury and Opportunities for Intervention," *Amer. J. Epidemiology 101*:98–102, 1975.

77. D. W. Hight, H. R. Bakalar, and J. R. Lloyd, "Inflicted Burns in Children: Recognition and Treatment," *J. Amer. Medical Assoc. 242*: 517–520, 1979.

78. L. S. Robertson, "Crash Involvement of Teenaged Drivers When Driver Education Is Eliminated from High School," *Amer. J. Public Health 70*: 599–603, 1980.

79. J. L. Bass and K. A. Mehta, "Developmentally-Oriented Safety Surveys," *Clinical Pediatrics 19*: 350–356, 1980.

80. P. Husband, "Environmental Factors Cause Accident Proneness," *Practitioner 211*: 335, 1973.

81. E. R. Padilla, D. J. Rohsenow, and A. B. Bergman, "Predicting Accident Frequency in Children," *Pediatrics 58*: 223–226, 1976.

82. A. F. Schaplowsky, "Community Injury Control—A Management Approach," *Amer. J. Public Health 63*: 252–254, 1973.

83. A. B. Bergman, Testimony before the Department of Labor, and Health, Education, and Welfare Subcommittee of the House Committee on Appropriations, June 16, 1971.

84. C. G. Schiffer and E. P. Hunt, *Illness Among Children,* Public Health Service Publication 2074, U.S. Department of Health, Education, and Welfare, 1963.

85. National Center for Health Statistics, *Current Estimates from the Health Interview Survey, United States, 1973,* Vital and Health Statistics, Series 10, No. 95, DHEW Publication (HRA) 75-1522, 1975.

86. G. S. Parcel, S. C. Gilman, P. R. Nader, H. Bunce, "A Comparison of Absentee Rates of Elementary Schoolchildren with Asthma and Nonasthmatic Schoolmates," Pediatrics, 64: 878–881, 1979.

87. National Center for Health Statistics, *Acute Conditions: Incidence and Associated Disability, United States, July 1974–June 1975,* Vital and Health Statistics, Series 10, No. 114, U.S. Department of Health, Education, and Welfare, February 1977.

88. J. A. Lakin, S. Anselmo, and H. C. Solomons, "Development of a Minor Illness Inventory for Children in Day Care Centers," *Amer. J. Public Health 66*: 487–488, 1976.

89. National Center for Health Statistics, Selected reports from the 1973 Health Interview Survey, Vital and Health Statistics, Series 10.

90. T. E. Minor et al., "Greater Frequency of Viral Respiratory Infections in Asthmatic Children as Compared with Their Non-asthmatic Siblings," *J. Pediatrics 85*: 472–477, 1974.

91. National Center for Health Statistics, *Examination and Health History Findings Among Children and Youths, 6–17 Years, United States,* Vital and Health Statistics, Series 11, No. 129, U.S. Department of Health, Education, and Welfare, November 1973.

92. *Health Status of Children: A Review of Surveys, 1963–1972,* DHEW Publication (HSA) 78-5744, 1978.

93. C. V. Blonde et al., "Physician-Diagnosed Abnormalities in Black and White Children in a Total Community," *Public Health Reports 94*: 124–129, 1979.

94. D. B. Nyswander, *Solving School Health Problems—The Astoria Demonstration Study,* The Commonwealth Fund, New York, 1942.

95. State of Maine, Department of Health and Welfare, *A Down East School Health Program: The Maine School Health Demonstration 1947–1953,* 1955.

96. School District of Philadelphia, *Annual Report 1970–71, Division of School Health Services,* 1971.

97. A. Lynch, *Report on the School Health Program of the Department of Health,*

Commonwealth of Pennsylvania, September 1973–December 1974, Pennsylvania Department of Health, 1975.

98. K. D. Rogers and G. Reese, "Health Studies—Presumably Normal High School Students," *Amer. J. Diseases Children 109*: 9–27, 1965.

99. J. P. Bendel, S. T. Halfon, and P. Ever-Hadani, "Absenteeism in Primary School: Poverty Factors and Ethnicity," *Amer. J. Public Health 66*: 683–685, 1976.

100. D. E. Roberts, D. Basco, C. Slome, J. H. Glasser, and G. Handy, "Epidemiologic Analysis in School Populations as a Basis for Change in School Nursing Practice," *Amer. J. Public Health 59*: 2157–2167, 1969.

101. D. Basco, S. Eyers, J. H. Glasser and D. E. Roberts, "Epidemiologic Analysis in School Populations as a Basis for Change in School Nursing Practice—Report of a Second Phase of a Longitudinal Study," *Amer. J. Public Health 62*: 491–497, 1972.

102. L. E. Hinkle, N. Plummer, and L. H. Whitney, "The Continuity of Patterns of Illness and the Prediction of Future Health," *J. Occupational Medicine 3*: 417–423, 1961.

103. J. H. Glasser, "A Stochastic Model for Industrial Illness Absenteeism," *Amer. J. Public Health 60*: 1936–1944, 1970.

104. R. W. Tuthill, C. Williams, G. Long, and C. Whitman, "Evaluating a School Health Program Focused on High-Absence Pupils: A Research Design," *Amer. J. Public Health 62*: 40–42, 1972.

105. National Center for Health Statistics, unpublished data from the Hospital Discharge Survey and the Health Interview Survey.

106. National Center for Health Statistics, unpublished data from the Health Interview Survey.

107. The National Health Examination Survey of children in 1963–1965 did not include any questions about psychological or psychiatric care. These findings were compared with the Health Examination Survey of youths conducted during 1966–1970.

108. F. A. North and Z. Blockstein, *Schools as Providers of Health Services: Estimates Based on a Household Survey*, Department of Epidemiology and Pediatrics, University of Pittsburgh, 1976.

109. S. Isaacs, "Some Notes on the Incidence of Neurotic Difficulties in Young Children," *British J. Educational Psychology 2*: 71–90, 1932.

110. A. Long, "Parents' Reports of Undesirable Behavior in Children," *Child Development 12*: 43–62, 1941.

111. P. Crowther, "A School Mental Health Program," *Mental Hygiene 5*: 400–404, 1968.

112. W. K. Bentz and A. Davis, "Perceptions of Emotional Disorders Among

Children as Viewed by Leaders, Teachers, and the General Public," *Amer. J. Public Health 65*: 129–132, 1975.

113. W. G. Morse, "The Crisis Teacher" in *Mental Health at School*, National Institute of Mental Health, U.S. Department of Health, Education, and Welfare, 1973.

114. E. M. Bower, "The Emotionally Handicapped Child and the School: Present Research Plans and Directions," *Exceptional Children 26*: 232–242, 1960.

115. *Helping Teachers Understand Children*, Commission on Teacher Education, American Council on Education, Washington, D.C. 1945.

116. M. M. Lawrence, *The Mental Health Team in the Schools*, Behavioral Publications, New York, 1971.

117. E. L. Cowen, M. A. Trost, R. P. Lorion, D. Dorr, L. D. Izzo, and R. V. Isaacson, *New Ways in School Mental Health: Early Detection and Prevention of School Maladaptation*, Human Sciences Press, New York, 1975.

118. A. M. Marmorale and F. Brown, *Mental Health Intervention in the Primary Grades*, Community Mental Health Journal Monograph Series, No. 7, Behavorial Publications, New York, 1974.

119. M. B. Ahmed and E. L. Young, "The Process of Establishing a Collaborative Program Between a Mental Health Center and a Public Health Nursing Division," *Amer. J. Public Health 64*: 880–885, 1974.

120. D. A. Trauner, "Learning Disabilities: An Overview," *Continuing Education*, March 1980, pp. 84–86.

121. G. E. Gardner and B. M. Sperry, "School Problems—Learning Disabilities and School Phobia," chap. 7 in *American Handbook of Psychiatry*, 2d ed., vol. II, ed. S. Arieti, Basic Books, New York, 1974.

122. B. A. Freeman and C. Parkins, "The Prevalence of Middle Ear Disease Among Learning Impaired Children," *Clinical Pediatrics 18*: 205, 1979.

123. P. H. Wender and L. Eisenberg, "Minimal Brain Dysfunction in Children," chap. 8 in *American Handbook of Psychiatry*, 1974 (see note 121).

124. A. E. Bell, D. S. Abrahamson, and K. N. McRae, "Reading Retardation: A 12-Year Prospective Study," *J. Pediatrics 91*: 363–370, 1977.

125. D. C. Leighton, "Measuring Stress Levels in School Children as a Program-Monitoring Device," *Amer. J. Public Health 62*: 799–806, 1972.

126. M. B. McConville, C. C. Boag, and A. P. Purohit, "Three Types of Childhood Depression," *Canad. Psychiatr. Assoc. J. 18*: 133, 1973.

127. H. James, *Children in Trouble: A National Scandal*, Pocket Books, New York, 1970, based on articles appearing weekly in the *Christian Science Monitor*, March 31 to July 7, 1969.

128. L. T. Wilkins, *Delinquent Generations*, A Home Office Research Unit Report, Her Majesty's Stationery Office, London, 1960.

129.   J. M. Martin, J. P. Fitzpatrick, and R. E. Gould, *Analyzing Delinquent Behavior*, U.S. Department of Health, Education, and Welfare, 1968.

130.   L. E. Ohlin, *A Situational Approach to Delinquency Prevention*, U.S. Department of Health, Education, and Welfare, 1970.

131.   E. M. Lemept, *Instead of Court: Diversion in Juvenile Justice*, National Institute of Mental Health, Chevy Chase, Md., 1971.

132.   D. O. Lewis and S. S. Shanok, "Medical Histories of Delinquent and Nondelinquent Children," *Amer. J. Psychiatry 134*: 1020, 1977.

133.   J. F. Short, "Delinquent Gangs: An Answer to the Needs of the Socially Disabled," chapter in *The Mental Health of the Child. Program Reports of the National Institute of Mental Health*, ed. J. Segal, National Institute of Mental Health, Rockville, Md., 1971.

134.   J. G. Rogers, "Runaway Kids: How One City Handles the Problems," *Parade Magazine*, October 7, 1973.

135.   M. A. Butters, "Yesterday's Runaways Becoming Children's Bureau's Self-Referrals," *Indianapolis Star*, March 5, 1972.

136.   H. G. Birch, "Malnutrition, Learning, & Intelligence," *Amer. J. Public Health 62*: 773–784, 1972.

137.   D. B. Jelliffe, *The Assessment of the Nutritional Status of the Community*, World Health Organization, Geneva, 1966.

138.   H. P. Chase and H. P. Martin, "Undernutrition and Child Development," *New England J. Medicine 282*: 933–939, 1970.

139.   C. J. Sells, "Microcephaly in a Normal Population," *J. Pediatrics 59*: 262–265, 1977.

140.   W. A. Weinberg, S. G. Dietz, E. C. Penick, and W. H. McAlister, "Intelligence, Reading Achievement, Physical Size, and Social Class," *J. Pediatrics 85*: 482–489, 1974.

141.   R. Martin, R. Karp, T. Sewell, J. Manni, and A. Heller, "Relationship of Height, Weight and Other Anthropometric Measures to Academic Achievement in Black, Inner-City Kindergarten Children," unpublished paper, Thomas Jefferson University, Philadelphia, 1979.

142.   *Health Status of Children: A Review of Surveys 1963–1972*, U.S. Department of Health, Education, and Welfare, Publication (HSA) 78-5744, 1978.

143.   S. A. Topp, J. Cook, W. W. Holland, and A. Elliott, "Influence of Environmental Factors on Height and Weight of School Children," *Brit. J. Preventive Social Medicine 24*: 154–162, 1970.

144.   R. Karp et al., "Effects of Rise in Food Costs on Hemoglobin Concentrations of Early School Age Children, 1972–1975," *Public Health Reports 93*: 456–459, 1978.

145.   R. Mack, F. Johnston, and D. Paoloni, "Bone Age, Blood Pressure, and Body Composition in Adolescents of High and Low Infant Relative Weight," paper presented the Annual Meeting of the American Public Health Association, Miami Beach, October 20, 1976.

146.   R. J. Karp, M. Nuchpakdee, J. Fairoth, and J. M. Gorman, "The School Health Service as a Means of Entry into the Inner-City Family for Identification of Malnourished Children," *Amer. J. Clinical Nutrition 29*: 216–218, 1976.

147.   D. E. Hardenbergh, "Who's Picking Up the Check for Pennsylvania's School Lunches?", *Evaluation 1*(3): 65–69, 1973.

148.   E. N. Todhunter, "School Feeding from a Nutritionist's Point of View," *Amer. J. Public Health 60:* 2302–2306, 1970.

149.   American Academy of Pediatrics, *School Health: A Guide for Physicians,* Evanston, Ill. 1972.

150.   J. W. Knutson, "Prevention of Dental Disease, in *Preventive Medicine,* eds. D. W. Clark and B. MacMahon, Little, Brown, Boston, 1967.

151.   J. J. Hanlon, *Public Health Administration,* Mosby, St. Louis, 1969.

152.   W. B. Davis, "Dental Health in Children," in *Ambulatory Pediatrics,* eds. M. Green and R. J. Haggerty, Saunders, Philadelphia, 1968.

153.   W. J. Pelton and J. M. Wisan, eds., *Dentistry in Public Health,* Saunders, Philadelphia, 1955.

154.   G. M. Stein et al., "Experiences in Establishing a 'Tooth Keeper' Preventive Dentistry Program for Elementary School Students," *J. Soc. Preventive Dentistry,* July-August 1974, p. 46.

155.   T. T. Craig, ed., *Comments in Sports Medicine,* American Medical Association, Chicago, 1973.

156.   D. P. Rice and K. M. Danchik, "Health Services Access and Utilization by Children," *Urban Health,* January-February 1980, pp. 26–27.

157.   *Trends Affecting the U.S. Health Care System,* U.S. Department of Health, Education, and Welfare, January 1976.

158.   National Center for Health Statistics, *Decayed, Missing, and Filled Teeth Among Youths 12–17 Years, United States,* Vital and Health Statistics, Series 11, No. 144, 1975.

159.   World Health Organization, *Health Problems of Adolescence: Report of a WHO Expert Committee,* Technical Report Series, No. 308, Geneva, 1965.

160.   *Youth: Transition to Adulthood,* Report of the Panel on Youth of the President's Science Advisory Committee, Office of Science and Technology, Executive Office of the President, U.S. Government Printing Office, June 1973, 0-504-826.

161.   E. R. McAnarney and W. J. McAveney, "The Adolescent and the

Pediatrician—A Future Marriage," Abstract, Ambulatory Pediatric Association Annual Meeting, 1975.

162. I. F. Litt, S. C. Edberg, and L. Finberg, "Gonorrhea in Children and Adolescents: A Current Review," *J. Pediatrics 85*: 595–607, 1974.

163. American School Health Association, 1969, quoted in Litt, Edberg, and Finberg, 1974.

164. *11 Million Teenagers: What Can Be Done About the Epidemic of Adolescent Pregnancies in the United States?*, Alan Guttmacher Institute, New York, 1976.

165. H. M. Wallace, E. M. Gold, H. Goldstein, and A. C. Oglesby, "A Study of Services and Needs of Teenage Pregnant Girls in the Large Cities of the United States," *Amer. J. Public Health 63*: 5–16, 1973.

166. A. S. Compton, "Health Study of Adolescents Enrolled in the Neighborhood Youth Corps," *Public Health Reports 84*: 585–596, 1969.

167. A. J. Salisbury and R. B. Berg, "Health Defects and Need for Treatment of Adolescents in Low-Income Families," *Public Health Reports 84*: 705–711, 1969.

168. D. E. Fiedler, D. M. Lang, and J. M. Carlson, "Pathology in the Healthy Female Teenager," *Amer. J. Public Health 63*: 962–965, 1973.

169. M. I. Cohen et al., "Health Care for Adolescents in a Traditional Medical Setting," Youth, Health and Social Systems Symposium, Washington, D.C., April 1974; adapted and quoted by Millar, 1975 (see note 70), and further adapted by this author.

170. I. F. Litt and M. I. Cohen, "End of An Epidemic?" *J. Pediatrics 86*: 293–294, 1975.

171. H. I. Abelson, P. M. Fishburne, and I. Cisin, *National Survey on Drug Abuse: 1977. Main Findings Vol. 1,* National Institute on Drug Abuse, DHEW Publication (ADM) 78-618, 1977.

172. C. D. Johnston, J. G. Bachman, and P. M. O'Malley, *Drug Use Among American High School Students: 1975–1977,* National Institute on Drug Abuse, DHEW Publication (ADM) 78-619, 1977.

173. "Alcohol Consumption: An Adolescent Problem," American Academy of Pediatrics, *Pediatrics 55*: 557–559, 1975.

174. M. E. Chafetz, "Adolescent Drinking and Parental Responsibility," *Newsletter of the Parents' Council of Washington,* Vol. 2, October 1974.

175. E. E. Lee, G. M. Shimmel, R. Fishman, "Emerging Trends of Alcohol Use and Abuse Among Urban Teen-agers," paper delivered at the School Health Section, American Public Health Association 102nd Annual Meeting, New Orleans, 23 October 1974.

176. "Reports Teen Abusing Alcohol May Abuse Other Drugs," *Pediatric News,* Vol. 10, No. 10, October 1976, p. 51.

177. I. F. Litt, S. C. Edberg, and L. Finberg, "Gonorrhea in Children and Adolescents: A Current Review," *J. Pediatrics 85*: 595–607, 1974.

178. K. Hein, A. Marks, and M. I. Cohen, "Asymptomatic Gonorrhea: Prevalence in a Population of Urban Adolescents," *J. Pediatrics 90*: 634–635, 1979.

179. "Teen Fertility Rises; Number of Births Falls," *The Nation's Health,* June 1980, p. 10.

180. J. F. Jekel, J. T. Harrison, D. R. E. Bancroft, N. C. Tyler, and L. V. Klerman, "A Comparison of the Health of Index and Subsequent Babies Born in School-Age Mothers," *Amer. J. Public Health 65*: 370–374, 1975.

181. M. Collins, "Review of Female Adolescent Development," *Clinical Pediatrics,* June 1980, p. 437.

182. L. V. Klerman, J. F. Jekel, J. B. Currie, I. W. Gabrielson, and P. M. Sarrel, "The Evolution of an Evaluation: Methodological Problems in Programs for School-Age Mothers," *Amer. J. Public Health 63*: 1040–1047, 1973.

183. J. B. Currie, J. F. Jekel, L. V. Klerman, "Subsequent Pregnancies Among Teenage Mothers Enrolled in a Special Program," *Amer. J. Public Health 62*: 1606–1611, 1972.

184. A. Foltz, L. V. Klerman, and J. F. Jekel, "Pregnancy and Special Education: Who Stays in School?" *Amer. J. Public Health 62*: 1612–1619, 1972.

185. *American Medical News,* May 6, 1974, quoted paper on psychological considerations in adolescent pregnancy by M. Rosenthal and E. Rothchild, at Case Western Reserve University School of Medicine.

186. H. Hansen, G. Stroh, and K. Whitaker, "School Achievement: Risk Factors in Teenage Pregnancy," *Amer. J. Public Health 68*: 753–759, 1978.

187. I. W. Gabrielson, L. V. Klerman, J. B. Curril, N. C. Tyler, and J. F. Jekel, "Suicide Attempts in a Population Pregnant as Teen-agers," *Amer. J. Public Health 60*: 2289–2301, 1970.

188. B. J. Stern, "The Health of Towns and the Early Public Health Movement," *Ciba Symposium 9*: 871, 1948.

189. E. L. Baker et al., "Lead Poisoning in Children of Lead Workers: Home Contamination with Industrial Dust," *New England J. Medicine 296*: 260–261, 1977.

190. H. L. Needleman et al., "Deficits in Psychologic and Classroom Performance of Children with Elevated Dentine Lead Levels," *New England J. Medicine 300*: 689–695, 1979.

191. J. S. Koopman, "Diarrhea and School Toilet Hygiene in Cali, Columbia," *Amer. J. Epidemiology 107*: 412–420, 1978.

192. M. McCann, *Health Hazards Manual for Artists*, Foundation for the Community of Artists, New York, 1975.

193. School Health Program, Department of Health, Commonwealth of Pennsylvania, *Hazardous Materials and Media in the Art Class*, February 1975.

194. "Chemist Tours School Labs on Safety Crusade," *The Evening News*, Harrisburg, Pa., November 27, 1978.

195. J. Gordon, J. B. Saratsiotis, D. R. Berzon, and F. Bennett, "Classroom Ecology and Safety," *Amer. J. School Health 42*: 178–181, 1972.

196. A. Lynch, "The Special Health Needs of the Walter Biddle Saul High School of Agricultural Sciences," mimeo, School District of Phildelphia, May 25, 1972.

197. C. Mangel, "How Good Are Organized Sports for Your Child?", *Look*, June 1, 1971.

198. M. R. Zavan, "Poisoning from Pesticides: Diagnosis and Treatment," *Pediatrics 54*: 332–336, 1974.

199. T. W. Lash and H. Sigal, *State of the Child: New York City*, Foundation for Child Development, New York City, 1976.

200. P. J. Landrigan et al., "Increased Lead Absorption with Anemia and Slowed Nerve Conduction in Children Near a Lead Smelter," *J. Pediatrics 89*: 904–910, 1976.

201. E. L. Baker et al., "A Nationwide Survey of Heavy Metal Absorption in Children Living Near Primary Copper, Lead and Zinc Smelters," *Amer. J. Epidemiology 106*: 261–273, 1977.

202. V. Benko, "Arsenic in Hair of Professionally Non-Exposed Population," in *Collected Studies of Health Effects of Air Pollution on Children*, Vol. 3, U.S. Public Health Service, Washington, D.C., 1969.

203. *A Report to the 1976 Legislature on Health Effects of Air Pollution Pursuant to Assembly Concurrent Resolution No. 45, 1975*, State of California Health and Welfare Agency, Department of Health.

204. Z. Blockstein, "Results of the Health Effects Committee Questionnaires: Athletic and Gym Activities of Parochial and Public Schools During High Air Pollution Levels," Graduate School of Public Health, University of Pittsburgh, unpublished paper, November 1974.

205. A. F. Williams, "Observed Child Restraint Use in Automobiles," *Amer. J. Diseases Children 130*: 1311–1317, 1976.

206. *Youth Camp Safety and Health: Suggested State Statute and Regulations*, U.S. Department of Health, Education, and Welfare, Publication (CDC) 75-8300, 1975.

207. W. A. Bleyer, "Surveillance of Pediatric Adverse Drug Reactions: A Neglected Health Care Program," *J. Pediatrics 85*: 308–310, 1975.

208. M. S. McIntire and E. Sadeghi, "The Pediatrician in Disasters," *Clinical Pediatrics 16*: 702–705, 1977.

209. A. Freud and D. Burlingham, *War and Children*, Medical War Books, London, 1943.

210. H. Blaufarb and J. Levine, "Crisis Intervention in an Earthquake," *Social Work 17*: 16–19, 1972.

211. R. Barker, *Ecological Psychology*, Stanford University Press, Stanford, Calif. 1968.

212. T. R. Lee, "On the Relation Between the School Journey and Social and Emotional Adjustment in Rural Infant Children," *Brit. J. Educational Psychology 27*: 101–114, 1957.

213. D. Canter and P. Stringer, *Environmental Interaction: Psychological Approaches to Our Physical Surroundings*, International Universities Press, New York, 1975.

214. L. Finberg, "Interaction of the Chemical Environment with the Infant and Young Child," *Pediatrics 53*: 831–836, 1974.

215. L. Baumgartner, "Some Phases of School Health Services," *Amer. J. Public Health 36*: 629–635, 1946.

216. R. W. Miller, "How Environmental Effects on Child Health Are Recognized," *Pediatrics 53*: 792–799, 1974.

217. J. B. Richmond, "The Needs of Children," *Daedalus*, Winter 1977, pp. 247–259.

218. V. R. Iglehart, D. Conner, and C. H. Sinnette, "A Comprehensive School Health Program in Harlem: A Retrospective View," *J. School Health 47*: 88–93, 1977.

219. Edward Livingston Trudeau, pioneer chest physician: "*Guerir quelquefois/Soulager souvent/Consoler toujours.*"

220. H. K. Silver and P. R. McAtee, "A Descriptive Definition of the Scope and Content of Primary Health Care," *Pediatrics 56*: 957–959, 1975.

221. R. L. Kane, "Primary Care: Contradictions and Questions," *New England J. Medicine 296*: 1410–1411, 1977.

222. D. MacCarthy, "Communication Between Children and Doctors," *Developmental Medicine Child Neurology 16*: 279–285, 1974.

223. H. Foye, R. Chamberlain, and E. Charney, "Content and Emphasis of Well-Child Visits," *Amer. J. Diseases Children 131*: 794–797, 1977.

224. National Center for Health Statistics, *Health Care Coverage: United States, 1976*, Advance Data, No. 44, September 20, 1979.

225. J. G. Cauffman, E. L. Petersen, and J. A. Emrick, "Medical Care of School Children: Factors Influencing Outcome of Referral from a School Health Program," *Amer. J. Public Health 57*: 60–73, 1967.

226. I. W. Gabrielson, L. S. Levin, and M. D. Ellison, "Factors Affecting School Health Follow-up," *Amer. J. Public Health 57*: 48–59, 1967.

227. J. G. Cauffman, M. I. Roemer, and C. S. Shultz, "The Impact of Health Insurance Coverage on Health Care of School Children," *Public Health Reports, 82*: 323–328, 1967.

228. D. P. Slesinger, R. C. Tessler, and D. Mechanic, "The Effects of Social Characteristics on the Utilization of Preventive Medical Services in Contrasting Health Care Programs," *Medical Care XIV*: 392–404, 1976.

229. M. Schour and R. L. Clemmens, "Fate of Recommendations for Children with School-Related Problems Following Interdisciplinary Evaluation," *J. Pediatrics 84*: 903–907, 1974.

230. M. T. Campbell, A. H. Garside, and M. E. C. Frey, "Community Needs and How They Relate to the School Health Program: S.H.A.R.P.—The Needed Ingredient," *Amer. J. Public Health 60*: 507–514, 1970.

Chapter 4

1. C. F. Brockington, *The Health of the Community: Principles of Public Health for Practitioners and Students*, 3rd ed., J. & A. Churchill, Ltd., London, 1965.

2. Department of Education, Commonwealth of Pennsylvania, *Goals for Quality Education*, 1973.

3. World Health Organization, *Human Development and Public Health*, Technical Report Series, 485, 1972.

4. American Academy of Pediatrics, Committee on School Health, "School Health Policies," *Pediatrics 24*: 672–682, 1959.

5. *Health Characteristics of Low-Income Persons*, DHEW Publication (HSM) 73 - 1500, July 1972.

6. M. R. Greenlick et al., "Comparing the Use of Medical Care Services by a Medically Indigent and a General Membership Population in a Comprehensive Prepaid Group Practice Program," *Medical Care X*: 187, 1972.

7. School District of Philadelphia, Division of School Health Services, *Annual Report 1970–1971*, 1971.

Chapter 5

1. S. J. Baker, "The Medical Inspection and Examination of School Children in New York City," *Annals of Gynecology and Pediatry XIX*: 450–451, 1906, quoted in R. H. Bremner, ed., *Children and Youth in America: A Documentary History*, Harvard University Press, Cambridge, 1971.

2. S. J. Baker, *Fighting for Life*, Macmillan, New York, 1939, quoted in Bremner, 1971.

3. L. R. Struthers, *The School Nurse*, Putnam, New York, 1917.

4. M. E. Chayer, *School Nursing*, Putnam, New York, 1931.

5. P. Henderson, "The Health of the School Child," chap. 29 in *The Theory and Practice of Public Health*, ed. W. Hobson, Oxford University Press, London, 1965.

6. R. Perlman, "Social Planning and Community Organization: Approaches," in *Encyclopedia of Social Work*, 16th issue, vol. II, ed. R. Morris, National Association of Social Workers, New York, 1971.

7. M. Foucault, *The Birth of the Clinic: An Archaeology of Medical Perception*, Pantheon Books, New York, 1973.

8. S. Levey and N. P. Loomba, *Health Care Administration: A Managerial Perspective*, Lippincott, Philadelphia, 1973.

9. A. Lynch and G. W. Allan, "Role of a State Health Department in Upgrading School Health Services," presented, School Health Section, American Public Health Association, 103rd Annual Meeting, Chicago, November 18, 1975.

10. Committee on Administrative Practice, American Public Health Association, *Keystones of Public Health in Pennsylvania*, New York, 1948.

11. *School Health Services*, a report of the Joint State Government Commission to the General Assembly of the Commonwealth of Pennsylvania, Session of 1955.

12. School of Hygiene and Public Health of Johns Hopkins University, *Reports of a Study of Health Needs and Resources of Pennsylvania*, 1961.

13. D. B. Nyswander, *Solving School Health Problems: The Astoria Demonstration Study*, Commonwealth Fund, New York, 1942.

14. K. D. Rogers, "School-Age Children," in *Ambulatory Pediatrics*, eds. M. Green and R. S. Haggerty, Saunders, Philadelphia, 1968.

15. *A Program Audit Report on the School Health Services Program 1911–1970 in Pennsylvania*, Division of Program Audit, Budget Bureau, Office of Administration, Governor's Office, Commonwealth of Pennsylvania, July 23, 1970.

16. A. Lynch, *Report on the School Health Program of the Department of Health, Commonwealth of Pennsylvania, September 1973–December 1974*, Harrisburg, 1975.

17. B. Bullough and V. L. Bullough, *The Emergence of Modern Nursing*, Macmillan, New York, 1964.

18. K. D. Rogers, "School-Age Children," chapter in M. Green and R. J. Haggerty, eds., *Ambulatory Pediatrics*, Saunders, Philadelphia, 1968.

19. R. M. Thorner and Q. R. Remain, *Principles and Procedures in the Evaluation of Screening for Disease,* Public Health Monograph, No. 67, U.S. Department of Health, Education, and Welfare, 1961.

20. Vision-testing machines are not necessary to high-quality vision programs. See *Report of the Fact-finding Committee on Vision Screening in the School Health Program,* Pennsylvania Department of Health, Harrisburg, March 1975.

21. Screening for sickle cell trait was often done without arrangements for appropriate genetic, vocational, and family and personal counseling for those discovered to be positive.

22. Scoliosis treatment methods have not been subject to controlled clinical trials to establish their effectiveness. The basis for screening, to improve the health outlook for those with the condition, cannot be shown to exist.

23. Rules & Regulations, Department of Health, Commonwealth of Pennsylvania, "School Nurse Service," P. S. 28§23.51-23.79, adopted January 26, 1962.

24. C. W. Humes, "Who Should Administer School Nursing Services?", *Amer. J. Public Health 65*: 394–396, 1975.

25. Department of Education, Commonwealth of Pennsylvania, *Recommendations of the Citizens Commission on Basic Education,* 1973.

26. M. J. E. Senn, "The Role, Pre-requisites and Training of the School Physician," in "Symposium on School Health Problems," *Pediatric Clinics of North America 4*: 1039–1056, 1965.

27. L. Frels, "National Survey—School Nurse Certification," *J. School Health 44*: 340–341, 1974. As of January 1973, 19 states had a mandatory school nurse certification requirement; in 9 states certification was permissive; 4 were studying the feasibility of such a requirement.

28. School District of Philadelphia, Division of School Health Services, *Annual Report 1970–1971.*

29. R. Morgan and M. L. Balog, *Pennsylvania's Nurses: 1972 Inventory of Registered Nurses,* Bureau of Nursing, Pennsylvania Department of Health, Harrisburg.

30. University of the State of New York, New York State Department of Education, *Nonprofessional Assistants in the School Health Program,* Albany, ca. 1972.

31. School District of Philadelphia, *Report of the Head Start Health Program, 1971–1973.*

32. M. L. Shetland, "An Approach to Role Expansion—The Elaborate Network," *Amer. J. Public Health 61*: 1959–1964, 1971.

CHAPTER 6

1. *Recommendations of the Pennsylvania School Health Program Advisory Committee*, chairperson, K. D. Rogers, Department of Health, Commonwealth of Pennsylvania, February 10, 1973.

2. A. Lynch, *Report on the School Health Program of the Department of Health, Commonwealth of Pennsylvania, September 1973–December 1974*, 1975.

3. R. K. Watts, ed., "Toward a Comprehensive School Health Policy for New York State," working paper, Interagency Task Force on School Health, Governor's Health Advisory Council, Albany, February 24, 1978.

4. A. Lynch and G. W. Allan, "Role of a State Health Department in Upgrading School Health Services," presented, School Health Section, American Public Health Association, 103rd Annual Meeting, Chicago, November 18, 1975.

5. S. Lynch, "Evaluating School Health Programs," "in Health Services: The Local Perspective," ed. A. Levin., *Proc. Academy Political Science 32*: 89–105, 1977.

6. A. Lynch, "There Is No Health in School Health," *J. School Health 47*: 410–413, 1977.

7. B. P. Baxter, personal communication, Division of School Health, Pennsylvania Department of Health, June 30, 1980.

CHAPTER 7

1. E. Switzer, "Preventive Medicine Guide: How to be Healthy at Any Age," *Family Circle, 4*: 137–144, 1975.

2. A. M. Harvey, J. Bordley, III, and J. A. Barondess, eds., *Differential Diagnosis: The Interpretation of Clinical Evidence*, 3rd ed., Saunders, Philadelphia, 1979.

3. A. F. North, "The Physical Examination," in *Ambulatory Pediatrics*, eds. M. Green and R. J. Haggerty, Saunders, Philadelphia, 1968.

4. H. K. Silver, C. H. Kempe, and H. B. Bruyn, *Handbook of Pediatrics*, 7th ed., Lange Medical Publications, Los Altos, Calif., 1967.

5. F. J. De Castro and U. T. Rolfe, *The Pediatric Nurse Practitioner*, Mosby, St. Louis, 1972.

6. A. Yankauer, "An Evaluation of the Effectiveness of the Astoria Plan for Medical Service in Two New York City Elementary Schools," *Amer. J. Public Health 37*: 853–859, 1947.

7. R. A. Sturner, R. H. Granger, E. H. Klatskin, and J. B. Ferholt, "The Routine Well Child Examination: A Study of Its Value in the Discovery of Significant Psychological Problems," *Clinical Pediatrics 19*: 251–260, 1980.

8. A. Lynch, "Use of Health History and Problem-Oriented Medical Record to Upgrade School Health Care and Staff Roles," presented, School Health Section, American Public Health Assoc., Annual Meeting, New Orleans, October 23, 1974. Summary: "Use of Health History in Upgrading School Health Care," *Pennsylvania's Health 36*: 16, Spring 1975.

9. A. Lynch, "The Role of the Health History in Re-establishing the Value of School Health Services," presented, American School Health Association, Annual Meeting, New York, October 13, 1974. Abstract ED 110195, "Resources in Education," December 1975.

10. J. H. Menkes, "On Failing in School," *Pediatrics 58*: 392–393, 1976.

11. G. G. Shapiro, G. W. Bierman, C. T. Furukawa, and W. E. Pierson, "Allergy Skin Testing: Science or Quackery?" *Pediatrics 59*: 495–498, 1977.

12. Division of School Health, Department of Health, *Reports of the School Health Program of the Penn Manor School District, Lancaster County, Pennsylvania, 1974–1975 and 1975–1976,* Harrisburg.

13. A. L. Cochrane, P. J. Chapman, and P. D. Oldham, "Observers' Errors in Taking Medical Histories," *Lancet 1*: 1007–1009, 1951.

14. G. S. Kilpatrick, "Observer Error in Medicine," *J. Medical Education 38*: 38–43, 1963.

15. K. Brodman, A. J. Erdmann, I. Lorge, and H. G. Wolfe, "The Cornell Medical Index: An Adjunct to Medical Interview," *J. Amer. Medical Assoc. 140*: 530–534, 1949.

16. N. G. Alexiou and G. Wiener, "Reliability of a Self-Administered Health Questionnaire for Secondary School Students (Adolescents)," *Amer. J. Public Health 58*: 1439–1446, 1968.

17. N. G. Alexiou, G. Wiener, M. Silverman, and T. Milton, "Validity Studies of a Self-Administered Health Questionnaire for Secondary School Students," *Amer. J. Public Health 59*: 1400–1412, 1969.

18. A. J. Erdmann, "Experiences in Use of Self-Administered Health Questionnaire," *A.M.A. Arch. Indust. Health, 19*: 79/339-84/344, 1959.

19. J. H. Abramson and L. Terpolsky, "Cornell Medical Index as a Health Measure in Epidemiologic Studies: A Test of the Validity of a Health Questionnaire," *Brit. J. Preventive Social Medicine 19*: 103–110, 1965.

20. K. Brodman, A. J. Erdmann, I. Lorge, and H. G. Wolff, "The Cornell

Medical Index—Health Questionnaire: II. As a Diagnostic Instrument," *J. Amer. Medical Assoc. 145*: 152–157, 1951.

21. School District of Philadelphia, *Pre-kindergarten Head Start Health Services, Achievement of Program Objectives in Program Proposal 1972–1973,* January 1973.

22. J. A. Willoughby and R. J. Haggerty, "A Simple Behavior Questionnaire for Preschool Children," *Pediatrics 34*: 798–806, 1964.

23. A. Lynch, *Evaluation of the Function and Impact of a Multidisciplinary Rehabilitation Team upon the Health and Education of Children Enrolled in Special Education, Interim Report, April 1979–February 1980,* report to Berks County Intermediate Unit, Reading, Pa., 1980.

24. C. Singer-Brooks, "Of What Value Are Health Inventories Filled Out by Parents?", *Amer. J. Public Health 42*: 661–664, 1952.

25. A. Lynch, *A Method to Improve the Health Evaluation of School Children,* report on the Pilot Health Program 1972–73 of the Division of School Health Services of the School District of Philadelphia, vol. I, 1974.

26. Bristol Township School District, *Use of Health History Questionnaire in Ninth Grade 1976–1977,* report to Division of School Health, Pennsylvania Department of Health, Harrisburg.

27. M. F. Gutelius, A. D. Kirsch, S. MacDonald, M. R. Brooks, and T. McErlean, "Controlled Study of Child Health Supervision: Behavioral Results," *Pediatrics 60*: 294–304, 1977.

28. A. G. Morris, R. London, and J. Glick, "Educational Intervention for Preschool Children in a Pediatric Clinic," *Pediatrics 57*: 765–768, 1976.

29. Z. Blockstein, *Number and Type of Problems Found in the Old School Health Records and Psychologist's Notes Compared with the School Nurse Practitioner's Assessment of Disabled Children,* report to Allegheny Intermediate Unit and Division of School Health, Pennsylvania Department of Health, Harrisburg, October 1979.

30. E. Moult and A. Lynch, *Report of Initial Assessment of Health Status of Handicapped-Disabled Students in Allegheny Intermediate Unit #3, March–June 1979, for Supplemental Security Income-Disabled Children's Program, Pennsylvania Department of Health,* Harrisburg, November 1979.

31. A. Bridges and L. A. Sarig, Berks County Intermediate Unit, oral report to Division of School Health, Pennsylvania Department of Health, Harrisburg, January 1980.

32. L. Breslow and A. R. Somers, "The Lifetime Health-Monitoring Program: A Practical Approach to Preventive Medicine," *New England J. Medicine 296*: 601–608, 1977.

33. L. A. Barness, *Manual of Pediatric Physical Diagnosis,* 4th ed., Year Book Medical Publishers, Chicago, 1972.

34. J. H. Menkes, "On Failing in School," *Pediatrics 58*: 392–393, 1976.

35. M. Kinsbourne, "School Problems," *Pediatrics 52*: 1973.

36. K. D. Rogers and G. Reese, "Health Studies—Presumably Normal High School Students. I. Physical Appraisal," *Amer. J. Diseases Children 108*: 572–600, 1964.

37. W. K. Frankenburg and B. W. Camp, eds., *Pediatric Screening Tests*, Charles C. Thomas, Springfield, Ill., 1975.

38. National Center for Health Statistics, *NCHS Growth Charts, 1976*, Monthly Vital Statistics Report, Vol. 25, No. 3, Supp. (HRA) 76-1120, Health Resources Administration, Rockville, Md., June 1976. *National Health Survey: Blood Pressure Levels of Children 6–11 Years*, DHEW Publication (HRA) 74-1617, Washington, D.C., December 1973.

39. A. F. Roche, "Growth Assessment of Handicapped Children," *Public Health Currents 19*, (6), November - December 1979.

40. H. Knobloch, F. Stevens, A. Malone, P. Ellison, and H. Risenberg, "The Validity of Parental Reporting of Infant Development," *Pediatrics 63*: 872–878, 1979.

41. C. D. Schoenwetter, "The School Health Service: Review and Commentary," *Pediatric Clinics of North America 21*: 75–80, 1974.

42. L. Eisenberg, E. J. Landowne, D. M. Wilmer, and S. D. Imber, "The Use of Teacher Ratings in a Mental Health Study: A Method for Measuring the Effectiveness of a Therapeutic Nursery Program," *Amer. J. Public Health 52*: 18–28, 1962.

43. R. W. Chamberlain, "The Use of Teacher Checklists to Identify Children at Risk for Later Behavioral and Emotional Problems," *Amer. J. Diseases Children 130*: 141–145, 1976.

44. A. M. Ritter, "Using a Teacher's Health Observation Form to Evaluate School Child Health," *J. School Health 46*: 235–237, 1976.

45. K. D. Rogers and G. Reese, "Health Studies—Presumably Normal High School Students. III. Health Room Visits," *Amer. J. Diseases Children 109*: 50–64, 1965.

46. R. F. Woolley, M. Warnick, R. L. Kane, and E. Dyer, *Problem-Oriented Nursing*, Springer, New York, 1974.

47. L. L. Weed, *Medical Records, Medical Education and Patient Care*, Year Book Medical Publishers, Chicago, 1971.

48. R. A. Kane, "Look to the Record," *Social Work 19*: 412–419, 1974.

49. L. Weed, "The Problem-Oriented Record—Its Organizing Principles and Its Structure," National League for Nursing, League Exchange No. 103, *Problem-Oriented System in a Home Health Agency—A Training Manual*, New York, 1975.

50. H. K. Walker, "The Problem-Oriented Medical Record: An Introduction," chap. 2 in *Applying the Problem-Oriented System*, eds., H. K. Walker, W. J. Hurst, and M. F. Woody, Medcom Press, New York, 1973.

51. *Problem-Oriented Medical Record System and Medical Record Management Guidance*, U.S. Department of Health, Education, and Welfare, Public Health Service, Bureau Community Health Services, Rockville, Md., 1978.

52. G. S. Lang and K. J. Dickie, *The Practice-Oriented Medical Record*, Aspen Systems Corp., Germantown, Md., 1978.

53. H. M. Tufo, W. M. Eddy, H. C. Van Buren, R. E. Bouchard, J. C. Twitchell, and L. Bedard, "Implementing a Problem-Oriented Practice," chap. 3 in Walker, Hurst, and Woody, *Applying the Problem-Oriented System*, 1973.

54. H. K. Silver, "The School Nurse Practitioner," *Pediatrics 65*: 641–643, 1980. "There are probably less than 750 full-time doctors specializing in school health in the approximately 88,000 schools in the United States."

55. P. M. Andrews and A. Yankauer, "The Pediatric Nurse Practitioner: Growth of the Concept," *Amer. J. Nursing 71*: 504–506, 1971.

56. E. Levine, "What Do We Know About Nurse Practitioners?", *Amer. J. Nursing 77*: 1799–1803, 1977.

57. R. Roemer, "The Nurse Practitioner in Family Planning Services: Law and Practice," *Family Planning/ Population Reporter 6*: 28–34, 1977.

58. H. K. Silver, "The School Nurse Practitioner Program: A New and Expanded Role for the School Nurse," *J. Amer. Medical Assoc. 216*: 1332–1334, 1971.

59. American Nurses' Association and American School Health Association, *Recommendations on Educational Preparation and Definition in the Expanded Role and Functions of the School Nurse Practitioner*, American Nurses' Association, Kansas City, Mo., 1974.

60. H. K. Silver, J. B. Igoe, and P. R. McAtee, "The School Nurse Practitioner: Providing Improved Health Care to Children," *Pediatrics 58*: 580–584, 1976.

61. California School Nurses Organization, "Definitions of School Nursing," *The School Nurse*, Spring 1978.

62. *Extending the Scope of Nursing Practice, A Report of the Secretary's Committee to Study Extended Roles for Nurses*, U.S. Department of Health, Education, and Welfare, Washington, D.C., 1971. See also: T. E. Adamson, "Critical Issues in the Use of Physician Associates and Assistants," *Amer. J. Public Health 61*: 1765–1779, 1971.

63. B. Bullough, *The Law and the Expanding Nursing Role*, Appleton, New York, 1975.

64. J. P. Connelly and A. Yankauer, "Allied Health Personnel in Child Health Care," *Pediatric Clinics of North America 16*: 921–927, 1969. "It is probable that delegation to nurses under physician supervision can be made of virtually any medical procedure. . . . This has already been accomplished with respect to nurse anesthetists without the benefit of any special statute."

65. L. Kahn, "The Influence of Funding òn the Future of Pediatric Nurse Practitioner Programs," *Pediatrics 64*: 106–110, 1979.

66. J. M. Scott, "Federal Support for Nursing Education to Improve Quality of Practice," *Public Health Reports 94*: 31–35, 1979.

67. L. Hochheiser, "Nurse Practitioner Research Conference," University of Connecticut Health Center, Farmington, Conn., 1974.

68. "Guidelines on Short-Term Continuing Education Programs for Pediatric Nurse Associates," A Joint Statement of the American Nurses' Association, Division on Maternal and Child Health Nursing Practice, and the American Academy of Pediatrics, *Amer. J. Nursing 71*: 509–512, 1971.

69. F. E. McLaughlin, H. G. Johnson, S. J. Anderson, M. M. Lemmons, J. R. Gibson, and P. J. Larson, *Clinical Judgments of Nurses and Physicians in the Assessment and Management of Essential Hypertension*, Nursing Research Grant, # Nu - 00528, U.S. Department of Health, Education, and Welfare, ca. 1977.

70. W. O. Spitzer, "Pediatric Nurse Practitioners," *New England J. Medicine 298*: 163–164, 1978.

71. D. Levinson, "Roles, Tasks and Practitioners," *New England J. Medicine 296*: 1291–1293, 1977.

72. E. D. Cohen, M. G. Crootof, K. Goldfarb, M. M. Keenan, and M. Triffin, *An Evaluation of Policy-Related Research on New and Expanded Roles of Health Workers*, Yale University School of Medicine, New Haven, 1974.

73. B. Duncan, A. N. Smith, and H. K. Silver, "Comparison of the Physical Assessment of Children by Pediatric Nurse Practitioners and Pediatricians," *Amer. J. Public Health 61*: 1170–1176, 1971.

74. C. C. Henriques, V. G. Virgadamo, and M. D. Kahane, "Performance of Adult Health Appraisal Examinations Utilizing Nurse Practitioners–Physician Teams and Para-medical Personnel," *Amer. J. Public Health 64*: 47–53, 1974.

75. P. J. Johnson, A. L. Jung, and S. J. Boros, "*A New Expanding Nursing Role*," *Perinatology-Neonatology 3*: 34–36, 1979.

76. J. L. Schwartz, "Economic Feasibility and Patient Diagnostic Mix of Family Nurse Practitioners," *Public Health Reports 94*: 148–155, 1979.

77. S. Greenfield, A. L. Komaroff, T. M. Pass, H. Anderson, and S. Nessim, "Efficiency and Cost of Primary Care by Nurses and Physician Assistants," *New England J. Medicine 298*: 305–309, 1978.

78. L. S. Linn, "Patient Acceptance of the Family Nurse Practitioner," *Medical Care 14*: 357–364, 1976.

79. C. E. Lewis and T. K. Cheyovich, "Who Is a Nurse Practitioner? Processes of Care and Patients' and Physicians' Perceptions," *Medical Care 14*: 365–371, 1976.

80. D. W. Simborg, B. H. Starfield, and S. D. Horn, "Physicians and Non-Physician Health Practitioners: The Characteristics of Their Practices and Their Relationships," *Amer. J. Public Health 68*: 44–48, 1978.

81. J. E. Ott, V. Moore, and R. D. Krugman, "Clinical Competence of Child Health Associates in Practice Settings," Department of Pediatrics, University of Colorado Medical Center, Denver, Colo., presented at Ambulatory Pediatrics Association Annual Meeting, 1975.

82. J. C. Horroks and F. T. DeDombal, "Diagnosis of Dyspepsia from Data Collected by a Physician's Assistant," *Brit. Medical J. 16*: 421–423, 1975.

83. E. C. Perrin and H. C. Goodman, "Telephone Management of Acute Pediatric Illnesses," *New England J. Medicine 298*: 130–135, 1978.

84. A. B. Bergman, "Pediatric Education—For What?" *Pediatrics 55*: 109–113, 1975.

85. C. E. Lewis, A. Lorimer, C. Lindeman, B. B. Palmer, and M. A. Lewis, "An Evaluation of the Impact of School Nurse Practitioners," *J. School Health 44*: 331–335, 1974.

86. N. A. Hilmar and P. A. McAtee, "The School Nurse Practitioner and Her Practice: A Study of Traditional and Expanded Health Care Responsibilities for Nurses in Elementary Schools," *J. School Health 43*: 431–441, 1973.

87. A. Lynch, *Report on the School Health Program of the Department of Health, Commonwealth of Pennsylvania, September 1973–December 1974*, Harrisburg, 1975.

88. N. B. Schell, "School Physicians: A Weakening Breed," *J. School Health 43*: 45–48, 1973.

89. J. M. Lampe, "The School Physician of the Future," *J. School Health 42*: 197–198, 1972.

90. E. McAnarney, P. R. Nader, R. F. Coleman, S. Goldstein, and S. B. Friedman, "The Pediatrician in an Innovative Public School Health Program," *Clinical Pediatrics 10*: 86–89, 1971.

91. H. Moghadam, "The Rare and the Plentiful—A Dilemma in Pediatric Manpower," *Canad. Medical Assoc. J. 110*: 497–498, 1974.

92. L. B. Callan, "A Conceptual Framework for Consideration in the Utilization of Health Aides," *Amer. J. Public Health* 61: 979–987, 1971.

93. C. Grosser, W. E. Henry and J. G. Kelly, eds., *Nonprofessionals in the Human Services*, Jossey-Bass, San Francisco, 1971.

94. J. G. Cauffman, W. A. Wingert, D. B. Friedman, E. A. Warburton, and B. Hanes, "Community Health Aides: How Effective Are They?", *Amer. J. Public Health 60*: 1904–1909, 1970.

95. H. B. Randall, J. G. Cauffman, and C. S. Shultz, *Effectiveness of Health Office Clerks in Facilitating Health Care for Elementary School Children*, U.S. Public Health Service Grant # PH-108-66-97, Los Angeles city schools, October 1967.

96. A detailed training program for school health aides has been developed by the Department of Health, Greenwich, Conn. 1980.

97. National Statistics Bureau, U.S. Department of Education, personal communication, August 1980: in 1976/77 education expenditures for day school students in public schools averaged $1,816 per student with a range of $1,218 (Arkansas) to $3,890 (Alaska).

98. Public School Code, Article XIV. School Health Services, Section 1409. "Confidentiality, Transference and Removal of Health Records," March 10, 1949, P.L. 30, as amended July 15, 1957, P.L. 937, (24 P.S.§1409) Commonwealth of Pennsylvania.

99. A. Yankauer, S. Tripp, P. Andrews, and J. P. Connelly, "The Outcomes and Service Impact of a Pediatric Nurse Practitioner Training Program—Nurse Practitioner Training Outcomes," *Amer. J. Public Health 62*: 347–353, 1972. Also consult J. Lewis, H. Bailit, and L. Hochheiser at the University of Connecticut Health Center, Farmington, Conn.

100. P. M. Andrews, "The Pediatric Nurse Practitioner; The Concept, Her Role and Responsibilities—Part II," *Public Health Currents 12*, January–February 1972.

101. A. Yankauer, J. P. Connelly, P. Andrews, and J. J. Feldman, "The Practice of Nursing in Pediatric Offices—Challenge and Opportunity," *New England J. Medicine 282*: 843–847, 1970.

102. A. Yankauer, J. P. Connelly, and J. J. Feldman, "Task Performance and Task Delegation in Pediatric Office Practice," *Amer. J. Public Health 59*: 1104–1117, 1969.

103. J. P. Connelly and A. Yankauer, "Health Manpower: The Problem and the National Scene," *Clinical Pediatrics 7*: 245–249, 1968.

104. "Nurse practitioners go to schools: Aim is expertise between that of traditional school nurse and doctor," *Medical World News*, September 8, 1975.

105. Committee on School Health, American Academy of Pediatrics, "School Nurse Practitioner," *Pediatrics 65*: 665–666, 1980.

106. C. A. Nathanson and M. H. Becker, "Control, Structure and Conflict in Outpatient Clinics," *J. Health Social Behavior 13*: 251–262, 1972.

107. C. A. Nathanson and M. H. Becker, "Doctors, Nurses, and Clinic Records," *Medical Care 11*: 214–223, 1973.

108. E. Brunetto and P. Birk, "The Primary Care Nurse—The Generalist in a Structured Health Care Team," *Amer. J. Public Health 62*: 785–794, 1972.

109. P. Serafini, "Nursing Assessment in Industry," *Amer. J. Public Health 66*: 755–760, 1976.

110. L. Aiken and J. L. Aiken, "A Systematic Approach to the Evaluation of Interpersonal Relationships," *Amer. J. Nursing 73*: 863–867, 1973.

111. *Sensitivity and Specificity of Dental Screening Performed by School Nurse Practitioners,* report of Penn Manor School District to Pennsylvania Department of Health, Harrisburg, 1975. In 100 cases the nurse practitioners had zero false positives and a false negative rate of 8 percent, or sensitivity 92 percent and specificity 100 percent.

112. H. M. Tufo et al., "Audit in a Practice Group," chap 4 in *Applying the Problem-Oriented System,* eds. H. K. Walker, H. J. Hurst, and M. F. Moody, Medcom Press, New York, 1973.

113. Spitzer, 1978 (see note 70) described a "strategy of evaluation" for pediatric nurse practitioners with a sequence of studies as follows: definition of need, establishment of safety or efficacy, demonstration of quality of care, proving of efficiency in use, satisfaction on the part of consumers and providers, and degree to which functions are transferred to new providers.

114. J. W. Hughes, A. M. Ritter, and M. Young, *Parent Perceptions of the Nurse Practitioner Program at the Penn Manor School District,* Report to the Pennsylvania Department of Health, Harrisburg, 1976.

115. S. H. Woolf, Lower Dauphin School District, communication to Pennsylvania Department of Health, 1979.

116. D. P. McCormick, "Pediatric Evaluation of Children with School Problems, *Amer. J. Diseases Children 131*: 318–322, 1977.

117. M. Kappelman, P. Roberts, R. Rinaldi, and M. Cornblath, "The School Health Team and School Health Physician: New Role and Operation," *Amer. J. Diseases Children 129*: 191–195, 1975.

CHAPTER 8

1. *The Complete Poems of Emily Dickinson,* ed. T. H. Johnson, Little, Brown, Boston, 1960, No. 1052.

2. S. Johansen and J. E. Orthoefer, "Development of a School Health Information System," *Amer. J. Public Health 65*: 1203–1207, 1975. Describes computer control of school nursing records.

3. D. J. Hosking, "The Computer Assisted School Health Program (CASH): A Field Unit's Viewpoint," *Canad. J. Public Health 64*: 521–536, 1973. Redesigned school nurse records were computerized with little saving of nurse time devoted to clerical work.

4. L. J. Rosner, *Systems Study of School Health Records*, report and renewal proposal for Health Services Demonstration grant, Health Services and Mental Health Administration, U.S. Department of Health, Education, and Welfare, 1969–1971. A demonstration of the feasibility of an automated record system for the Bureau of School Health Services of the NYC Health Department.

5. J. H. Glasser, "Health-Information Systems: A Crisis or Just More of the Usual?", *Amer. J. Public Health 61*: 1524–1530, 1971.

6. J. B. Tenney, "Information for Developing National Statistics on Ambulatory Medical Care," *Medical Care,* Supplement, *XI* (2): 87–95, 1973.

7. J. H. Murnaghan, "Health Services Information Systems in the United States Today," *New England J. Medicine 290*: 603–610, 1974.

8. School District of Philadelphia, Division of School Health Services, *Annual Report 1970–1971,* 1971.

9. A. Lynch, *Report on the School Health Program of the Department of Health Commonwealth of Pennsylvania, September 1973–December 1974,* Pennsylvania Department of Health, Harrisburg, 1975.

10. *Social and Health Indicators System: Atlanta: Part 2,* Bureau of the Census, Social and Economic Statistics Administration, U.S. Department of Commerce, 1973.

11. *Social and Health Indicators System: Los Angeles,* Bureau of the Census, Social and Economic Statistics Administration, U.S. Department of Commerce, 1973.

12. F. E. Linder, "Sources of Data on Health in the United States," chap. 5 in *Preventive Medicine,* eds. D. W. Clark and B. MacMahon, Little, Brown, Boston, 1967. It is appropriate to recall that Florence Nightingale, who played a major role in the development of health statistics in England, noted in 1860, "The material exists but it is inaccessible."

13. *Papers on the National Health Guidelines: Baselines for Setting Health Goals and Standards,* DHEW Publication (HRA) 76-640, 1976.

14. D. W. Clark, "A Vocabulary for Preventive Medicine," chap. 1 in *Preventive Medicine,* eds. D. W. Clark and B. MacMahon, Little, Brown, Boston, 1967.

15. A. Lynch "Child Abuse in the School-Age Population," *J. School Health* *45*: 141–148, March 1975.

16. A. Lynch and C. A. Krall, "Role of Schools in Reporting and Management of Child Abuse," presented at Maternal and Child Care Section, American Public Health Association, 103rd Annual Meeting, Chicago, November 17, 1975.

17. A. Lynch and W. A. Miller, "Health Information Systems for School Health Services," presented at Statistics Section, American Public Health Association, 103rd Annual Meeting, Chicago, November 19, 1975.

18. World Health Organization, Expert Committee on Health Statistics, WHO Technical Report Series, No. 53, Geneva, 1952, p. 6.

19. Philadelphia Department of Public Health, *Proposal for Performance of Work for the Planning and Development of an Experimental Health Services Delivery System in the City of Philadelphia, Pennsylvania,* May 1971.

20. S. S. Stodolosky and G. Lesser, "Learning Patterns in the Disadvantaged," *Harvard Educational Review 37*: 546–593, Fall 1967.

21. K. Uemura, "Collection of Data from Established Sources," in *Data Handling in Epidemiology,* ed. W. W. Holland, Oxford University Press, London, 1970.

22. *Webster's New Universal Dictionary of the English Language* 2d ed., The Publisher's Guild, New York, 1970.

23. E. G. Mishler, "Meaning in Context: Is There Any Other Kind?", *Harvard Educational Review 49*: 1–19, February 1979.

24. H. C. Schulberg and F. Baker, "Program Evaluation Models and the Implementation of Research Findings," *Amer. J. Public Health 58*: 1248–1255, 1968.

25. K. Zemach, "Program Evaluation and System Control," *Amer. J. Public Health 63*: 607–609, 1973.

26. M. F. Arnold, "Evaluation: A Parallel Process to Planning," chap. 16 in *Administering Health Systems: Issues and Perspectives,* eds. M. F. Arnold, L. V. Blankenship, and J. M. Hess, Aldine-Atherton, Chicago, 1971.

27. A. Lynch, "Use of Health History in Upgrading School Health Care," *Pennsylvania's Health 36*: 16, Spring 1975.

28. V. Navarro, *National and Regional Health Planning in Sweden,* DHEW Publication (NIH) 74-240, 1974. Navarro also included regulators as one of the groups in the decision-making process. Regulators assure implementation of the plan by administrators, checking implementation against standards and indicators defined by the plan, such as the budget.

29. R. R. Frerichs and R. Neutra, "Letters to the Editor, Re: 'Definitions of Epidemiology'," *Amer. J. Epidemiology 108*: 74–75, 1978.

30. D. E. Lilienfeld, "Definitions of Epidemiology," *Amer. J. Epidemiology 107*: 87–90, 1978.

31. M. Greenburg, *Studies in Epidemiology: Selected Papers of Morris Greenberg*, Putnam, New York, 1965.

32. K. L. White, "Contemporary Epidemiology," *International J. Epidemiology 3*: 295–303, 1974.

33. World Health Organization, *Organizational Study on Methods of Promoting the Development of Basic Health Services*, Official Records of the World Health Organization No. 206, Geneva, 1973.

34. M. Schaefer, *Evaluation/Decision-Making in Health Planning and Administration*, University of North Carolina at Chapel Hill, HADM Monograph Series, No. 3, 1973.

Chapter 9

1. S. Fanshel and J. W. Bush, "A Health-Status Index and Its Application to Health Services Outcomes," *Operations Research 18*: 1021–1066, 1970.

2. S. Levey and N. P. Loomba, *Health Care Administration: A Managerial Perspective*, Lippincott, Philadelphia, 1973.

3. J. J. Hanlon, *Principles of Public Health Administration*, Mosby, St. Louis, 1969.

4. M. Susser, *Causal Thinking in the Health Sciences. Concepts and Strategies of Epidemiology*, Oxford University Press, London, 1973.

5. B. MacMahon, T. F. Pugh, and J. Ipsen, *Epidemiologic Methods*, Little, Brown, Boston, 1960. Also note: L. Thomas, Editorial, "Biostatistics in Medicine," *Science 198*, November 18, 1977: "Perhaps the greatest advance in medicine and public health in the past decade has been the acceptance of the role of scientifically designed trials in the testing of hypotheses . . . the acceptance of the principles involved indicates a revolution in medical thinking."

6. M. C. Branch, *Planning—Aspects and Application*, Wiley, New York, 1966.

7. M. Schaefer, *Evaluation/Decision-Making in Health Planning and Administration*, University of North Carolina at Chapel Hill, HADM Monograph Series, No. 3, 1973.

8. S. Eilon, "What Is a Decision?", Selection 10 in Levey and Loomba, 1973.

9. M. F. Arnold, "Evaluation: A Parallel Process to Planning," chap. 16 in *Administering Health Systems: Issues and Perspectives*, eds. M. F. Arnold, L. V. Blankenship, and J. M. Hess, Aldine-Atherton, Chicago, 1971.

10. R. Zemach, "Program Evaluation and System Control," *Amer. J. Public Health 63*: 607–609, 1973.

11. D. Katz and R. L. Kahn, *The Social Psychology of Organizations*, Wiley, New York, 1966.

12. D. Katz, "Patterns of Leadership," chap. 8 in *Handbook of Political Psychology*, ed. J. N. Knutson, Jossey-Bass, San Francisco, 1973.

13. M. Schaefer, "Current Issues in Health Organization," *Amer. J. Public Health 58*: 1192–1199, 1968.

14. G. Piel, "Improving the Nation's Health: Joint Leverage for Economic and Social Adjustment," chap. 3 in *Social Economics for the 1970's*, ed. G. F. Rohrlich, Dunellen Co., New York, 1970.

15. K. L. White, "Contemporary Epidemiology," *International J. Epidemiology 3*: 295–303, 1974.

16. V. R. Hunt, "Use of Hospital Records to Monitor Morbidity and Mortality of Certain Diseases," paper prepared for Hospital Research and Educational Trust, Chicago, 1976.

17. National Center for Health Statistics, *The Nation's Use of Health Resources*, DHEW Publication (HRA) 77-1240, 1976.

18. Royal Commission on Medical Education (Todd Report), 1968, quoted in S. Palmer and D. G. Gill, *Public Accountability and Peer Review in Health Care Delivery in the United States and the United Kingdom*, John E. Fogarty International Center for Advanced Study in the Health Sciences, DHEW Publication (NIH) 77-1429, 1977.

19. World Health Organization, *Training in National Health Planning*, Technical Report Series, No. 456, Geneva, 1970.

20. C. Skrovan, E. T. Anderson, and J. Gottschalk, "Community Nurse Practitioner: An Emerging Role," *Amer. J. Public Health 64*: 847–853, 1974.

21. T. Gilmore, L. Hirschhorn, and P. McGinity, *Program Planning and Management Skills for School Nurse Practitioners*, report of a training needs identification workshop for the Division of School Health Services, Pennsylvania Department of Health, Harrisburg, June 26, 1980.

CHAPTER 10

1. H. M. Somers and A. R. Somers, *Doctors, Patients, and Health Insurance: The Organization and Financing of Medical Care*, Brookings Institution, Washington, D.C., 1961.

2. K. Keniston and The Carnegie Council on Children, *All Our Children: The American Family Under Pressure*, Harcourt, New York, 1977.

3. W. H. Stewart, "The Challenging Need for Assessment," in *Assessing the Effectiveness of Child Health Services,* Fifty-sixth Ross Conference on Pediatric Research, Ross Laboratories, Columbus, Ohio, 1967, pp. 9–23.

4. H. L. Blum, "Research into the Organization of Community Health Agencies: An Administrator's Review," *Milbank Memorial Fund Quarterly 44*: 52–93, July 1966.

5. R. E. Numeroff, "Expanded Nurse Role from the Perspective of the New Medicine," *HCM Review,* Summer 1978, pp. 45–51.

APPENDIX

Name _____ First Name _____ Initial _____ School District _____

STUDENT'S HEALTH RECORD

CONFIDENTIAL

- TO BE KEPT UNDER LOCK & KEY
- TO BE USED BY HEALTH STAFF ONLY

Figure A–1.   Record Folder

Left Side of Record (Data Base):

TEMPORARY PROBLEM LIST
Acute Self-Limited Problem List

DATE	PROBLEM	DISPOSITION

Figure A–2. Temporary Problem List

INFORMATION FOR MEDICAL EMERGENCIES

Last name_____ First name_____ Middle name_____ Date of birth_____
Parents or Guardians:
                    Mother   Father   Guardian (relationship)

Name_____

Home address_____

Phone_____

Work place_____
Phone_____

Person looking after child during day/after school:

Name_____
Address_____
Phone_____

Relative/friend to contact in emergency when above people cannot be contacted:

Name_____
Address_____
Phone_____

Doctor to be notified:

Name_____   In an emergency, if a choice is possible, which
Address_____   hospital would you perfer for your child?
Phone_____   _____

I give permission to the staff of the_____ School District to transport,
or to make arrangements for the transportation of, my child to emergency medical care,
and to sign permission for medical treatment declared immediately necessary by the
physician, in the event that the persons listed above cannot be contacted.

_____   _____   _____
    Witness   Date   Signature of Parent/Guardian

Figure A–3. Information for Medical Emergencies

SPECIAL HEALTH NEEDS

Between now and the time when the School Nurse will have an appointment with you to take
a full health history of your child, it would be helpful to have the following information
so that the school can immediately meet any special health needs of your child.

Has you child ever had any serious illnesses or operations?   No   Yes
What?_____ When?_____
Is your child going to a hospital, clinic or doctor now?   No   Yes
What for?_____ Where?_____
Apart from vitamins, is your child taking any medicines, tablets or drugs? No   Yes
What?_____ What for?_____
Does your child need to take any medicines, tablets, or drugs at school?   No   Yes
What?_____ What for?_____
Is your child allergic to anything, such as foods, plants, insects, medicines? No Yes
What?_____
Has your child had any convulsions or fits or seizures in the past year?   No   Yes

How many?_____ Treatment_____   No   Yes
Does your child need a special diet or have any food problem?   No   Yes
Give details_____
Does your child have any special health needs or problems the school   No   Yes
should know? What?_____

Figure A–4.   Special Health Needs

PARENT PERMISSION FORM
(MODIFIED SCHOOL HEALTH PROGRAM)
(ELEMENTARY)

TO: THE PARENTS OF _____   _____

                            Student's Name   Home Room

I understand that the information I give is important in aiding the health and education of my child.

I understand that the information will be kept confidential by the school health staff and will be shared with other professionals in the school only when the School Nurse Practitioner or the School Physician believes that it is in the best interest of my child's health and education.

Copies of this health record will be sent to other agencies who request it only with my written consent.

Permission for Examinations and Tests

I give permission for my child to receive medical and dental examinations, and/or screenings as provided by the School Health Services of the   School District.

I understand that the   School District has obtained approval from the Pennsylvania Department of Health to provide a Modified School Health Program of expanded health services.

I further understand that I will be informed, in writing, of any abnormal results of examinations and screenings given my child.

I give permission for the following: Health History
                                         Physical Examination
                                         Dental Examination
                                         Screening for: - Growth
                                                      - Vision
                                                      - Color Vision
                                                      - T. B.
                                                       - Hearing
                                                      - Development
                                        Teacher Assessment of Health & Progress
                                        (Delete items not to be given)

Signature of Parent/Guardian_____

Date _____

Figure A–5.   Permission Form

MODIFIED SCHOOL HEALTH PROGRAM
(CERTIFICATE OF IMMUNIZATION FOR SCHOOL ATTENDANCE)

TO THE PARENT: Please have completed by your physician either Section A, Section B, or Section C, whichever is appropriate for your child. For additional information, call the school nurse.

Due Date: September 1, 1980

Name of Pupil_____ M _____ F _____ Birth Date _____

Name of Parent or Guardian _____

Address _____

Home Phone _____ Work Phone _____

* * * * * * * * * * * * * * * * * * * *

IMMUNIZATION RECORD Section A

The above named pupil has been immunized against:
Immunization Dates

1. Diphtheria-Tetanus-Pertussis #1_____ #2_____ #3_____ First Booster_____
   Second Booster 4-6 years of age optimum protection_____

2. Oral Polio (Sabin) #1_____ #2_____ #3_____
   Second Booster 4-6 years of age optimum protection_____

3. Measles Vaccine (Rubeola)_____ or had disease_____

4. German Measles Vaccine(Rubella)_____

5. Mumps Vaccine_____

Signed_____ Date_____
                    Physician

Physician's Address_____

* * * * * * * * * * * * * * * * * * * *

IMMUNIZATION PLAN Section B

The above named pupil is in the process of being immunized against:
Immunization Dates

1. Diphtheria-Tetanus-Pertussis #1_____ #2_____ #3_____ First Booster_____
   Second Booster 4-6 years of age optimum protection_____

2. Oral Polio (Sabin) #1_____ #2_____ #3_____ First Booster_____
   Second Booster 4-6 years of age optimum protection_____

3. Measles Vaccine (Rubeola)_____ or had disease_____

4. German Measles Vaccine (Rubella)_____

5. Mumps Vaccine_____

Signed_____ Date_____
                    Physician

Physician's Address_____

* * * * * * * * * * * * * * * * * * * *

MEDICAL EXCLUSION Section C

This is to certify that immunization of the above named pupil is medically contraindicated at this time. (Temporary exclusion from above immunization program.)

Signed_____ Date_____
                    Physician

Physician's Address_____

* * * * * * * * * * * * * * * * * * * *

RELIGIOUS EXCLUSION Section D

If there are objections to the above immunization program based on religious grounds, a statement should be made, dated, signed, and attached to this form and returned to the school nurse.
* * * * * * * * * * * * * * * * * * * *

Reviewed: 1. For follow-up_____
                              Date

          2. Approved_____   _____
                              Date   School Nurse

Figure A–6. Certificate of Immunization

STUDENT'S HEALTH HISTORY

1. Pregnancy and Birth

Put a circle around the answer.

1. Did the mother have any illness during the pregnancy? — No Yes

2. Did the mother take any medicines or drugs (other than iron or vitamins) during the pregnancy? — No Yes

3. Was the mother or the family under any unusual strain during the pregnancy? — No Yes

4. Did the baby come on time? — Yes No

5. Was it a difficult birth? — No Yes

6. What was the baby's birth weight? — _____

7. Did the baby have any trouble while in hospital? — No Yes

8. How many days did the baby stay in hospital? — _____

2. Early Childhood History

1. Would you describe the baby as average, quiet or active? — _____

2. Did the baby have any special problems in the first six months? — No Yes

3. How old was the baby when breast feeding stopped? — _____

4. How old was the child when bottle-feeding was stopped? — _____

5. At what age did the child sit alone without support? — _____

6. At what age did the child walk alone without support? — _____

7. At what age did the child begin to say two or three words together? — _____

8. Can the child use the toilet without help now? — Yes No

9. If the child has stopped wetting the bed, at what age did he or she stop? — _____

3. Health History

1. Has the child ever been in hospital or had an operation? — No Yes
   When?   What for?   Name of hospital
   _____

2. Has the child had any other illnesses, accidents, broken bones, or fractured bones? — No Yes
   When?   What was the problem?
   _____

3. Where is the child usually taken when he is sick? Give the names of doctors or hospitals _____
   _____

4. Is the child attending a hospital or clinic at present? — No Yes
   Where?   What for?
   _____

5. Is the child taking any medicines, tablets or vitamins now? — No Yes
   What for?_____

6. Has the child ever been seen by a dentist? — No Yes
   Name of dentist _____

7. Does the family have some way to help pay for medical expenses? — Yes No
   What: Blue Cross, Union, D.P.A. (white card), Medical Assistance (green card), Medicare, Other _____
   _____

Figure A–7. Student Health History

4. Family Health History

1. Circle any of the following diseases that this child's parents, grandparents, aunts, uncles, brothers, sisters, have had:

    allergy, asthma, cancer, drug or alcohol addiction, diabetes, heart disease, nervous breakdown, seizures, tuberculosis, lead poisoning, mental retardation, sickle cell anemia, sickle cell trait, other inherited or family diseases.

2. FAMILY MEMBERS
   (Note any special relationships such as step-parent, adopted, foster-child, etc.)

Relationship	Age	Name	State of Health	Occupation or School	Grade reached in school
Mother					
Father					
Brothers					
Sisters					

3. Have any members of the family died? (not miscarriages)   No   Yes

4. How many members of the family live in the same house as the child?   _____

5. Are there any family problems such as problems with housing, employment, food, etc.?   No   Yes

6. Who mostly looks after the child during the day? _____

_____

5. Health History — Continued

1. Check ☑ any of the following illnesses the child has had:

   "red" measles ☐   German or "3 day" measles ☐
   mumps ☐   chicken pox ☐
   whooping cough ☐   pneumonia ☐
   rheumatic fever ☐

                                             Put a circle around
                                                the answer.

2. Has the child had more than six colds or throat infections, with a fever, a year?   No   Yes

3. Has the child had any trouble with ears or hearing?   No   Yes

4. Has the child had any trouble with eyes or seeing?   No   Yes

5. Has the child had any trouble with teeth?   No   Yes

6. Has the child ever had a convulsion or fit?   No   Yes

7. Has the child ever had a fainting spell?   No   Yes

8. Does the child complain of headaches?   No   Yes

9. Has a doctor ever said the child had a heart murmur?   No   Yes

10. Does the child have trouble keeping up with other children?   No   Yes

11. Do any foods disagree with the child?   No   Yes

12. Does the child often have diarrhea?   No   Yes

13. Has constipation ever been much of a problem for this child?   No   Yes

14. Has the child ever had worms or parasites?   No   Yes

Figure A–7.   Student Health History (Continued)

15. Have you ever seen blood in the child's stools (bowel movements)?   No   Yes

16. Has the child ever had yellow jaundice or trouble with the liver?   No   Yes

17. Does the child complain of belly aches?   No   Yes

18. Does the child have any problem with passing water (urination)?   No   Yes

19. Does the child have any skin problems?   No   Yes

20. Has the child ever had eczema or allergy?   No   Yes

21. Has the child ever had asthma or wheezing?   No   Yes

22. Has the child ever had an allergy or reaction to any medicines or injections?   No   Yes
    What was the medicine or injection? _____
    _____

23. Does the child seem to have trouble breathing through the nose?   No   Yes

24. Does the child snore at night?   No   Yes

25. Has the child ever complained of pain in the arms or legs?   No   Yes

26. Has the child ever had swelling of any joints or limping?   No   Yes

27. Has there ever been any trouble with the child's blood?   No   Yes

28. Has the child ever eaten paint or plaster or anything else which is
    not food?   No   Yes

29. Does the child have any trouble sleeping?   No   Yes

30. How does the child put himself or herself to sleep? _____
    _____

31. Has the child ever had a skin test for T.B. (tuberculosis)?   Yes   No
    Was the result normal?   Yes   No

32. What does the child usually eat for:

Breakfast	Lunch	Supper	Snacks

How many snacks a day? _____

Put a circle around any of the following things which worry you about the child:

1. Bedwetting

2. Wetting during the day

3. Thumbsucking

4. Stammering or stuttering

5. High strung or easily upset?

6. Too restless

7. Shy

8. Sad or sulky

9. Feelings easily hurt

10. Wanting too much attention

11. Wanting too much comfort or
    support from parent

12. Day dreams

13. Nightmares

14. Temper tantrums

15. Contrary or stubborn

16. Disobedient

17. Lying

18. Selfish in sharing

19. Jealous of brothers and sisters

20. Fighting with other children

21. Purposely destroys things

22. Feeding

23. Bowels

24. Any other problems not mentioned? What?
    _____

Figure A–7.   Student Health History (Continued)

6. Current Functioning of the Child

1. How would you describe the child as a person? _____
    _____
    _____

2. How does the child get along with brothers and sisters? _____
    _____
    _____

3. How does the child get along with neighborhood friends? _____
    _____
    _____

4. How does the child feel about coming to school? _____
    _____
    _____

5. What does the child like to do? _____
    _____
    _____

6. What kinds of things scare or worry the child? _____
    _____
    _____

7. What are some of the things the child does that upset you or make you angry? _____
    _____
    _____

8. What do you do to discipline the child?   How does he or she react? _____
    _____
    _____

9. What are some of the things the child does which please you or make you proud? _____
    _____
    _____

Figure A–7.   Student Health History (Continued)

INTERVAL OR UPDATE HEALTH HISTORY

Student Name_____ Date of Birth_____

Address_____

Grade_____ School_____

Date _____ *To be completed by Parent/Guardian*

Put A Circle Around Answer

1. Has your child been in good health in the past year?   Yes   No
   If no, please explain _____

   _____

2. Has your child had any of the following in the past years:—

   a)   any illness lasting more than three (3) days   No   Yes

   b)   any severe injuries or accidents?   No   Yes

   c)   any fractures or broken bones?   No   Yes

   d)   any sprains or strains?   No   Yes

   e)   any time in hospital?   No   Yes

   f)   any operations?   No   Yes

   g)   any drugs or treatments prescribed by a physician or clinic?   No   Yes

   If yes to any of the above please explain _____

   _____

   _____

3. a)   Is your child under the care of a physician or clinic now?   No   Yes

   b)   Is your child taking any drugs or treatments or medications now?   No   Yes

   If yes to either of the above please explain _____

   _____

   _____

4. In the past year have you noticed that your child has any of the following
   problems:—

   a)   has trouble with eyes or seeing   No   Yes

   b)   has begun to wear glasses   No   Yes

   c)   has begun to wear contact lenses   No   Yes

   d)   has trouble with ears or hearing   No   Yes

   e)   has trouble with allergy   No   Yes

   f)   has trouble with asthma or breathing   No   Yes

   g)   has trouble with eating or with weight gain or loss   No   Yes

   h)   has trouble with sleeping   No   Yes

   I)   has trouble keeping up with the activities of
        his/her friends   No   Yes

   j)   has trouble with class work   No   Yes

Figure A–8.   Interval or Update Health History

k)   has trouble with school   No   Yes

l)   has trouble with the family   No   Yes

m)   has problem with general development and
     maturity   No   Yes

If yes to any of the above please explain _____

_____

_____

5.   a)   Has your child seen a dentist in the past year?   Yes   No

     b)   How would you describe the state of your child's teeth —

	Circle Those Which Apply		
Teeth Missing	None	Some	All
Teeth Decayed (cavities)	None	Some	All
Teeth Filled	None	Some	All

6.   Has your child had any immunizations in the past year?   No   Yes

     If yes please explain _____

_____

     Has your child received the following immunizations —

          three (3) or more doses of Diphtheria and Tetanus   Yes   No

          three (3) or more doses of Polio   Yes   No

          one (1) dose of Measles   Yes   No

          one (1) dose of Rubella (German Measles)   Yes   No

7.   Has any member of the family developed any serious health problem
     in the past year?   No   Yes

     If yes, please explain _____

_____

_____

8.   Do you think your child is fit to participate in all school sports, athletics
     and gym?   Yes   No

     If no, please explain _____

_____

9.   Do you have any concerns regarding your child which you would like to dis-
     cuss with a nurse or physician?   No   Yes

     If yes, the School Nurse Practitioner will contact you to set up an appoint-
     ment.

Figure A–8.   Interval or Update Health History (Continued)

PEDIATRIC-NEUROLOGIC EXAMINATION

4. DATE OF EXAM.	Mo.	Day	Year	5. AGE OF CHILD	Yrs.	Mos.

9. HEAD CIRCUMFERENCE _____ cm.

10. BLOOD PRESSURE *(right arm)*

_____ Systolic _____ Diastolic

11. HEAD – SHAPE AND CONTOUR
☐ Normal   ☐ Other *(describe)*

12. FACIES
☐ Normal   ☐ Other *(describe)*

13. EYES – STRUCTURE – EXTERNAL EXAMINATION *(lids, cornea, sclera, conjunctiva, iris)*
☐ Normal   ☐ Other *(describe)*

14. EARS – SIZE, SHAPE, AND POSITION
☐ Normal   ☐ Other *(describe)*

15. EARS – OTOSCOPIC EXAMINATION
☐ Normal   ☐ Other
                            ☐ Unable to evaluate because of cerumen

16. DENTITION
☐ Normal   ☐ Other *(describe)*

17. NOSE, MOUTH AND PHARYNX
☐ Normal   ☐ Other *(specify)*

18. NECK *(abnormalities of cervical vertebrae including "short neck" should be noted under spine)*
☐ Normal   ☐ Other *(specify)*

19. THYROID
☐ Normal   ☐ Other *(specify)*

20. THORACIC WALL
☐ Normal   ☐ Other *(specify)*

21. LUNGS
☐ Normal   ☐ Other *(specify)*

24. HEART

NONE 0	FINDING 1	*(describe)*
☐	☐	Murmur
☐	☐	Thrill
☐	☐	Abnormal Rate *(< 70 or > 110 at rest)*
☐	☐	Irregular Rhythm *(exclude sinus arrhythmia)*
☐	☐	Enlargement
☐	☐	Cyanosis *(associated with heart disease)*
☐	☐	Other *(describe)*

25. RADIAL AND FEMORAL PULSES, BILATERALLY
☐ Normal   ☐ Other *(specify)*

26. ABDOMEN

NONE 0	FINDING 1	*(describe)*
☐	☐	Wall Abnormality *(include hernia and specify site)*
☐	☐	Palpable Spleen _____ cm. below costal margin
☐	☐	Palpable Liver _____ cm. below costal margin
☐	☐	Palpable Kidney
☐	☐	Other *(specify, include abdominal masses)*

27. GENITALIA

NONE 0	FINDING 1	*(describe)*
☐	☐	Cryptorchidism
☐	☐	Hypospadias
☐	☐	Other *(specify)*

28. LYMPH NODES
☐ Normal   ☐ Other *(describe)*

29. SKIN *(exclude mongolian spots and stork bites, describe skin abnormality in detail)*

NONE 0	FINDING 1	*(describe)*
☐	☐	Vascular Nevi-Portwine
☐	☐	Vascular Nevi-Strawberry
☐	☐	Pigmented nevi
☐	☐	Café-au-lait spots *(approximate size and number)*
☐	☐	Eczema
☐	☐	Cyanosis *(other than cardiac)*
☐	☐	Scars *(specify location and extent)*
☐	☐	Vitiligo
☐	☐	Other *(describe)*

30. SPINE *(include scoliosis and kyphosis)*

NONE 0	FINDING 1	*(describe)*
☐	☐	Dimple *(specify site)*
☐	☐	Sinus *(include suspect, specify site)*
☐	☐	Other *(include overlying skin changes)*

Figure A–9.   Pediatric-Neurologic Examination

33. MUSCULOSKELETAL SYSTEM

NORMAL   OTHER (describe)
0   8

☐ ☐ Shoulder Girdle
☐ ☐ Pelvic Girdle
☐ ☐ Upper Extremities
☐ ☐ Lower Extremities
☐ ☐ Neck and Trunk (include Torticollis)

34. OPHTHALMOSCOPIC EXAM (discs, lens, media, macula, vessels, retina. Be sure to test pupils before mydriatic is used)

A. Right

☐ Normal   ☐ Other (describe)

B. Left

☐ Normal   ☐ Other (describe)

C. Mydriatic

☐ Used

☐ Not Used

35. PALPEBRAL FISSURES

NONE   FINDING (describe)
0   1

☐ ☐ Ptosis
☐ ☐ Asymmetry without Ptosis
☐ ☐ Other (specify)

36. PUPILS (size, shape and equality)
☐ Normal   ☐ Other (specify)

37. REACTION TO LIGHT (direct and consensual)
☐ Normal   ☐ Other (specify)

38. VISUAL FIELDS (confrontation)
☐ Normal   ☐ Other (specify)

39. REACTION TO ACCOMMODATION
☐ Normal   ☐ Other (specify)

42. EYE MUSCLES (III, IV & VI Cranial)

43. POSITION OF EYES AT REST

A. Without Glasses
1. UNCOVERED
☐ Normal   ☐ Other
☐ Unable to Evaluate

2. COVERED
☐ Normal   ☐ Other
☐ Unable to Evaluate

B. With Glasses   ☐ Glasses Not Worn
1. UNCOVERED
☐ Normal   ☐ Other
☐ Unable to Evaluate

2. COVERED
☐ Normal   ☐ Other
☐ Unable to Evaluate

44. WEAKNESS OR PARALYSIS OF INDIVIDUAL EYE MOVEMENTS

45. Right Eye   **46. Left Eye**
☐ None (normal movements)   ☐ None (normal movements)
☐ Other (describe)   ☐ Other (describe)
☐ Unable to Evaluate (explain) ☐ Unable to Evaluate (explain)

47. CONVERGENCE
☐ Normal   ☐ Other (describe)

48. CONJUGATE GAZE, TO FOLLOW
☐ Normal   ☐ Other (describe)

49. CONJUGATE GAZE, TO COMMAND
☐ Normal   ☐ Other (describe)

50. NYSTAGMUS (describe any nystagmus under comments)
☐ None
☐ Central Only
☐ Only on Directed Gaze
☐ Latent Only (specify which eye is uncovered)
☐ Other (describe)

51. FIFTH MOTOR NERVE
☐ Normal   ☐ Other (describe)

Figure A–9.   Pediatric-Neurologic Examination (Continued)

54. FIFTH SENSORY NERVE

☐ Normal   ☐ Other (describe)

55. SEVENTH MOTOR NERVE

LOWER MOTOR NEURON

☐ Normal   ☐ Other (describe)

SUPRANUCLEAR

☐ Normal   ☐ Other (describe)

56. EIGHTH NERVE – HEARING

A. LOW FREQUENCY: 512 CYC/SEC. TUNING FORK

☐ Normal   ☐ Other (describe)

B. HIGH FREQUENCY: FINGER RUSTLE. WHISPER

☐ Normal   ☐ Other (describe)

57. NINTH & TENTH NERVES

58. PALATE – SYMMETRY

☐ Normal   ☐ Other (describe)

59. PALATE – ELEVATION (voluntary and involuntary)

☐ Normal   ☐ Other (describe)

60. PHONATION

☐ Normal   ☐ Other

61. ELEVENTH NERVE – STERNOCLEIDOMASTOID AND TRAPEZIUS FUNCTION

☐ Normal   ☐ Other

62. TWELFTH NERVE – TONGUE

NONE   FINDING (describe)

0   1

☐   ☐   Weakness or Paralysis

☐   ☐   Deviation on Protrusion

☐   ☐   Atrophy

☐   ☐   Fasciculation

☐   ☐   Other

63. MUSCLE MASS EXAMINATION (specify abnormality)

NONE   FINDING (describe)

0   1

☐   ☐   Atrophy

☐   ☐   Hypertrophy

☐   ☐   Hypoplasia

☐   ☐   Aplasia

☐   ☐   Other

66. MUSCLE POWER (localize and grade weakness as questionable, mild, moderate or severe in comments)

☐ Normal   ☐ Other (describe)

67. MUSCLE TONE: Use the following code to grade tone.

1 Hypotonic
2 Questionable Hypotonicity
3 Normal
4 Questionable Hypertonicity
5 Hypertonic – Spastic
6 Hypertonic – Rigid
8 Other (describe)
9 Unable to Evaluate

	BILATERAL	RIGHT	LEFT
68. UPPER EXTREMITY			
69. LOWER EXTREMITY			
70. NECK FLEXORS			
71. NECK EXTENSORS			
72. TRUNK			

73. ABNORMAL MOVEMENTS (description should specify location and severity, whether present at rest and/or with voluntary movement)

NONE   FINDING   (describe)

0   1

☐   ☐   Fasciculations

☐   ☐   Myoclonus

☐   ☐   Spontaneous Tremor

☐   ☐   Intention Tremor

☐   ☐   Athetosis

☐   ☐   Chorea

☐   ☐   Dystonia

☐   ☐   Ballismus

☐   ☐   Tic

☐   ☐   Mirror Movements

☐   ☐   Other (describe)

74. COORDINATION (gross and fine motor includes finger-nose, finger-pursuit, heel-knee, rapid alternation, rapid finger movement and activities such as buttoning, writing, etc.)

NONE   FINDING   (describe)

0   1

☐   ☐   Dysmetria

☐   ☐   Ataxia

☐   ☐   Dysdiadochokinesia

☐   ☐   Awkwardness not otherwise classified

☐   ☐   Other (describe)

Figure A–9.   Pediatric-Neurologic Examination (Continued)

77. HAND PREFERENCE

78. Observed
- ☐ Variable
- ☐ Ambidextrous
- ☐ Predominantly Right
- ☐ Predominantly Left

79. Reported
- ☐ Variable
- ☐ Ambidextrous
- ☐ Predominantly Right
- ☐ Predominantly Left

80. EYE PREFERENCE
- ☐ Variable
- ☐ Predominantly Right
- ☐ Predominantly Left

81. RIGHT AND LEFT IDENTIFICATION (the child with eyes open is requested to perform the following actions:)

	PASSED 0	FAILED 1
A. Show me your right hand.	☐	☐
B. Show me your left eye.	☐	☐
C. Put your right hand on your left eye.	☐	☐
D. Put your left hand on your right ear.	☐	☐

82. FOOT PREFERENCE
- ☐ Variable
- ☐ Predominantly Right
- ☐ Predominantly Left

83. STATION (Romberg Position)
- ☐ Normal
- ☐ Unsteady, Eyes Open
- ☐ Increased Unsteadiness, Eyes Closed
- ☐ Other (describe)

84. GAIT (including heel and toe walking, hopping on one foot, running)
- ☐ Normal
- ☐ Abnormal due to Specific Neurologic Defect
- ☐ Abnormal due to Non-Specific Neurologic Defect (awkwardness)
- ☐ Abnormal due to Bone, Joint, Muscle Disease or Skin Lesion
- ☐ Other (describe)

87. REFLEXES: Use the following code for grading reflexes:

- 0 Absent
- 1 Hypoactive
- 2 Normal
- 3 Increased
- 4 Increased with Clonus
- 9 Unable to Evaluate

	BILATERAL	RIGHT	LEFT
88. BICEPS JERK			
89. TRICEPS JERK			
90. KNEE JERK			
91. ANKLE JERK			

92. SUSTAINED ANKLE CLONUS (6 or more beats)
- ☐ None
- ☐ Present Bilaterally
- ☐ Present Only on Right
- ☐ Present Only on Left

93. SUPERFICIAL ABDOMINAL REFLEX
- ☐ Present and Symmetrical
- ☐ Other (describe)

94. CREMASTERIC REFLEX (male only)
- ☐ Present and Symmetrical   ☐ Not Applicable
- ☐ Other (describe)

95. PLANTAR RESPONSES

	BILATERAL	RIGHT	LEFT
FLEXOR			
EQUIVOCAL			
EXTENSOR			
OTHER (describe)			

96. SENSATION

97. TOUCH
- ☐ Normal   ☐ Other (describe)
- ☐ Test not Indicated

Figure A–9.   Pediatric-Neurologic Examination (Continued)

100. PAIN

☐ Normal   ☐ Other (describe)
  0   9
          ☐ Test not Indicated
            9

101. POSITION SENSE

102. Passive Movement of Great Toe (minimum 5 trials)

☐ Normal   ☐ Other (describe)
  0   9

103. Location of Finger in Space

☐ Normal   ☐ Other (describe)
  0   9

104. STEREOGNOSIS (both hands — Present all objects visually prior to
      test. Allow identification verbally or by selection.)

105. FINE

☐ Normal (if normal skip to 107)   ☐ Other (describe)
  0   9

106. GROSS

☐ Normal   ☐ Other (describe)
  0   9

107. AUTONOMIC FUNCTION

108. VASOMOTOR (describe abnormality)

☐ Normal
  0
☐ Abnormal by Examination
  1
☐ Abnormal by History
  2

109. SWEATING (describe abnormality)

☐ Normal
  0
☐ Abnormal by Examination
  1
☐ Abnormal by History
  2

110. SPHINCTERS (Bladder and Rectal — describe abnormality)

☐ Normal (history)
  0
☐ Abnormal by Examination
  1
☐ Abnormal by History
  2

111. SPEECH

☐ Normal   ☐ Other (describe)
  0   9

114. MENTAL STATUS

☐ Normal   ☐ Other (describe)
  0   9

115. INTELLECTUAL STATUS

☐ Normal   ☐ Other (describe)
  0   9

116. OTHER SIGNS, REFLEXES, TESTS, ETC.

☐ No   ☐ Yes (describe)
  1   9

117. IMPRESSION

118. NEUROLOGICAL ABNORMALITIES

☐ None
  0
☐ Neurologically Suspicious but no Definite Abnormalities
  1   (describe reasons for this statement in detail)
☐ Neurologically Abnormal Child (describe fully and give reasons)
  2

119. ABNORMALITY ON VISUAL SCREENING (without referral)

☐ No   ☐ Yes (describe)
  1   9

120. NON-NEUROLOGICAL ABNORMALITIES (check all that apply)

☐ None
  0
☐ Minor Abnormalities or Deviations (describe)
  1
☐ Questionable Abnormalities (describe)
  2
☐ Definite Major Abnormalities (describe)
  3

121. UNSATISFACTORY CONDITIONS FOR EXAMINATION

☐ Absent   ☐ Present (specify)
  0   9

122. REFERRED FOR FURTHER EVALUATION

☐ No   ☐ Yes (describe)
  1   9

Figure A–9.   Pediatric-Neurologic Examination (Continued)

VISUAL ACUITY

DATE													
VISUAL R													
ACUITY L													
V.A. with R													
GLASSES L													
PASS (P) or FAIL (F)													

COLOR VISION

DATE _____	RESULT: PASS FAIL	Comments: _____

SKIN TEST FOR T.B.

DATE	READING in m.m.	RESULT: NEG. POS.	"MANTOUX": NEG. POS.
DATE	READING in m.m.	RESULT: NEG. POS.	"MANTOUX": NEG. POS.

HEARING SCREENING

DATE	Sweep (Sw) Threshold (T)	RIGHT EAR 250	500	1000	2000	4000	8000	LEFT EAR 250	500	1000	2000	4000	8000	PASS(P) FAIL(F)

Figure A–10.   Screening Tests for Vision, T.B., Hearing

PHYSICAL GROWTH – GIRLS: 2 TO 18 YEARS

NAME:_____DATE OF BIRTH_____

NCHS PERCENTILES*

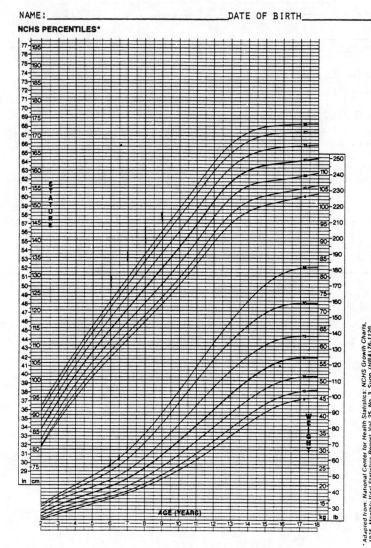

Figure A–11.   Growth Chart

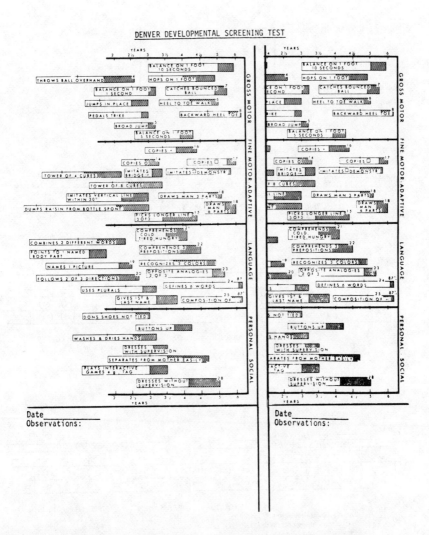

Figure A–12. Denver Developmental Screening Test

DENTAL SCREENING			DENTAL SCREENING			DENTAL SCREENING		
Date _____			Date _____			Date _____		
Teeth Missing	No	Yes	Teeth Missing	No	Yes	Teeth Missing	No	Yes
Caries	No	Yes	Caries	No	Yes	Caries	No	Yes
Abnormal Gums	No	Yes	Abnormal Gums	No	Yes	Abnormal Gums	No	Yes
SCREENING RESULT: PASS FAIL			SCREENING RESULT: PASS FAIL			SCREENING RESULT: PASS FAIL		

DENTAL EXAMINATION

DIRECTIONS FOR USE OF TOOTH CHART

FOR EACH EXAMINATION A POSITIVE ENTRY MUST BE MADE FOR EACH TOOTH. 20 ENTRIES FOR DECIDUOUS TEETH, AND 32 FOR PERMANENT TEETH. USE RED PEN OR PENCIL FOR ENTRIES OF DEFECTS FOUND IN CURRENT EXAMINATION, AND BLUE PENCIL TO INDICATE ANY PREVIOUS FILLINGS. A TOOTH IS CONSIDERED UNERUPTED WHEN NO PORTION OF IT IS THROUGH THE GUMS. PLACE A LETTER OR LETTERS (SEE CODE) IN THE BLOCK BESIDE THE CIRCLE TO DESCRIBE THE CONDITION OF THE TOOTH. FOR THOSE MARKED WITH EITHER d OR D AND f OR F, MAKE A SPOT OR SPOTS IN THE CIRCLE TO INDICATE THE SURFACE WHICH SHOWS EVIDENCE OF CARIES, FILLINGS, OR BOTH.

CODE FOR CHART AND SUMMARY

CONDITION OF TOOTH	DECID	PERM
NORMAL	n	N
DECAYED—REQUIRES FILLING	d	D
EXTRACTION NECESSARY	e	E
FILLED PREVIOUSLY	f	F
MISSING	m	M
UNERUPTED	u	U

DATE _____

RIGHT SIDE OF MOUTH									LEFT SIDE OF MOUTH							
		E	D	C	B	A	DECID.	A	B	C	D	E				
8	7	6	5	4	3	2	1 PERM.	1	2	3	4	5	6	7	8	

UPPER   LOWER

	DECIDUOUS	PERMANENT	MOUTH HYGIENE
Decayed requiring filling	(d) _____	(D) _____	Clean _____
Extraction - done or required	(e) _____	(M) _____	Fair _____
Previously filled _____	(f) _____	(F) _____	Poor _____
TOTAL	(d+e+f) _____	(D+M+F) _____	

DATE _____

RIGHT SIDE OF MOUTH									LEFT SIDE OF MOUTH							
		E	D	C	B	A	DECID.	A	B	C	D	E				
8	7	6	5	4	3	2	1 PERM.	1	2	3	4	5	6	7	8	

UPPER   LOWER

	DECIDUOUS	PERMANENT	MOUTH HYGIENE
Decayed requiring filling	(d) _____	(D) _____	Clean _____
Extraction - done or required	(e) _____	(M) _____	Fair _____
Previously filled _____	(f) _____	(F) _____	Poor _____
TOTAL	(d+e+f) _____	(D+M+F) _____	

Figure A–13.   Dental Screening & Examination

TEACHER'S HEALTH OBSERVATIONS

Name of Child _____ Date_____

Grade _____ Class _____

Name of Teacher _____

Please check items as directed. Add comments next to the item or at the end of the form.

A. *Observations of Child's Body*
Check any of the following you have noticed:
EYES:
1. Eyes crossed, in or out
2. Red, runny or itchy eyes
3. Deformity of eyes
EARS:
4. Discharge or running from ears
5. Deformity of ears
SKIN AND HAIR
6. Skin rash
7. Lack of cleanliness of skin or hair
8. Sores on skin
9. Nits in hair
10. Pale or sallow skin, or other color
11. Evidence of physical abuse or harsh punishment
12. Unusual scars
NOSE:
13. Continuous runny nose
14. Deformity of nose
CHEST:
15. Wheezing sounds in chest
BONES AND MUSCLES:
16. Deformity of spine
17. Deformity of hands, arms
18. Deformity of legs, feet
19. Deformity of head
APPEARANCE:
20. General neglected appearance
21. Appears too thin
22. Appears too fat
B. *Observations of Child's Body Functions and Symptoms*
Check any of the following which the child complains of, or demonstrates, more severely or more frequently than most classmates of same age:
MOVEMENTS:
23. Clumsiness
24. Limp or abnormal gait
25. Poor coordination
26. Poor writing or drawing
27. Convulsions, fits, or spells
28. Spells of inattention or staring into space
SPEECH:
29. Unclear speech
30. Delayed speech
31. Stammering or stuttering
VISION:
32. Poor vision
HEARING:
33. Poor hearing
NOSE:
34. Frequent nose picking or rubbing
HEAD:
35. Headaches
MOUTH:
36. Drooling
SKIN AND HEAD
37. Frequent scratching
CHEST:
38. Cough
39. Short of breath with exercises

GASTROINTESTINAL
40. Poor eater
41. Recurrent stomach aches
42. Soils self with bowel movements
URINARY:
43. Frequent urination
44. Wets pants
C. *What is your general opinion of this child's health?*
Check *one* of the following:
45. Perfectly healthy
46. Specific problem(s) as noted, but generally healthy
47. Not in good health
D. *Observations of Child's Behavior*
Check any of the following which the child demonstrates more severely or more frequently than most classmates of the same age:
48. Temper tantrums
49. Impulsive behavior
50. Explosive behavior
51. Hyperactivity or restlessness
52. Extremely quiet or withdrawn
53. Sleepy or lethargic
54. Tics or grimacing
55. Wanting too much attention
56. Contrary or stubborn
57. Selfish in sharing
58. Fighting with other children
59. Purposely destroys things
60. Masturbates
61. Nail-biting
62. Thumb-sucking
63. Frequent or prolonged absence from classroom
64. Cannot follow directions
65. Tasks incomplete
66. Uncooperative
67. Poor attention span
68. Poor verbal behavior
69. Lacks self-confidence
70. Child is not progressing in emotional development
71. Child is not progressing in intellectual development
E. *What is your general opinion of this child's behavior?*
Check *one* of the following:
72. Behavior is appropriate for age range
73. Behavior is relatively inappropriate for age range
74. Behavior definitely limiting learning abilities
F. *Observations of Child's Social Adjustment*
Check if you have noticed any problems in the following areas:
HOME:
75. Problem in child's relationships at home
76. Problem in parents' attitude to child
77. Poor parental attitude to child's problem
78. Evidence of neglect of the child
79. Evidence of physical abuse or severe punishment of the child
SCHOOL:
80. Problem in child's adjustment to school
81. Problem in child's attitude to school
82. The child's absenteeism is a problem
83. Performance is not at grade level, or is a problem
84. The child is not developing satisfactorily in school
Further Observations and Explanations of Items Checked:

Figure A–14.   Teacher's Health Observations

Right Side of Record (Problem Management)

PROBLEM - ORIENTED MEDICAL RECORD
PROBLEM LIST

NAME _____

ADDRESS _____

BIRTH DATE _____ SEX ____ RACE ____

NO.	PROBLEM	DATE S.N.P. ENTER	DATE M.D. CHECK	DATE RESOLVED	INACTIVE PROBLEMS

Figure A–15.   Problem List

PROBLEM MANAGEMENT

Progress Notes

D Data (new information)

A Assessment (does information alter the nature of the problem?)

P Plan   - D Diagnostic
            Rx Therapeutic
            PE Patient Education

Date	No.	N O T E S	Date for Action/Accomplishment

Figure A–16.   Progress Notes

Date	No.	N O T E S	Date for Action/ Accomplishment

Figure A–16.   Progress Notes (Continued)

LETTER TO PARENT REGARDING
HEALTH SERVICES FOR KINDERGARTEN STUDENTS
provided by School District

Dear Parent of Kindergarten Student:

   We, in the Division of Health Services of the School District,
congratulate you and your child on reaching the great milestone of school
entrance!

   We would like to take this opportunity to tell you of the Health
Services we offer to assist you in keeping your child as healthy as
possible, so that school is both a valuable and enjoyable experience for
your young student:

   First, the School District provides health services which are
   required by State Law, namely, school nurse service, and tests
   for vision, hearing, growth, and tuberculosis;
   Second, the School District provides for all its students additional health services not required by State Law, especially,
   immunizations, care of sick and injured children, and health
   education;
   Third, the School District provides for all its students additional health services. These additional health services have
   been shown to be of great value to parents and children, and to
   school health staff as they attempt to serve school children and
   their parents. These health services are: student's health
   history, pediatric examination, tests of development and color
   vision, dental screening, medical review of the student's classroom function, and expanded school nursing in which nurses work
   more closely with parents to bridge the gaps between School
   Health Services, the school, the family physician,and community
   health services.

   These new health services have been developed and are being
monitored by a team of professionals from the School District, the
Pennsylvania Department of Health in consultation with the Pennsylvania
Department of Education.

   In these new services the role of the traditional school nurse has
been expanded through special training to that of a School Nurse Practitioner.

   Your School Nurse Practitioner will contact you within the next few
weeks to make an appointment, at your convenience, for a conference regarding the health services your child will receive. It would be helpful if you completed the attached STUDENT'S HEALTH HISTORY befor your
conference with your School Nurse Practitioner. At this confidential
conference your School Nurse Practitioner will review the STUDENT'S
HEALTH HISTORY with you and will be able to answer your questions regarding her role, and the new health serv ices and their value to your
child.

   Should you have any question in the meantime please do no hesitate
to cll me at _____ anytime between 9:00 a.m. - 2:30 p.m.

                              Yours sincerely,

                              School Nurse Practitioner

Figure A–17. Letter to Parent

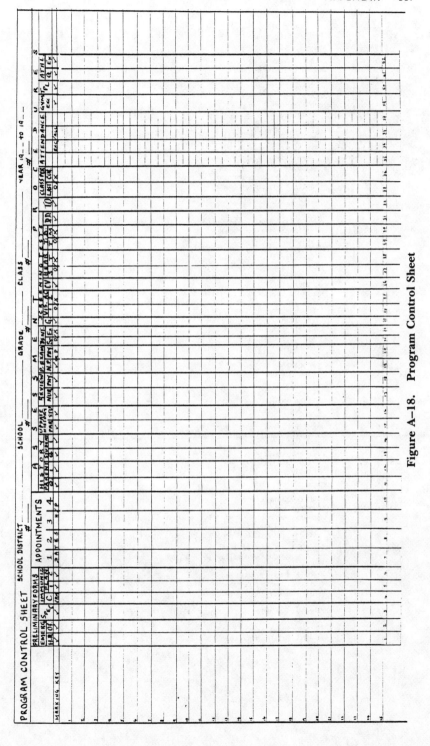

Figure A–18. Program Control Sheet

PROGRAM CONTROL SHEET

Column	Heading
1 - 6	Preliminary Forms
1, 2	Emergency Information
1	Health Room Copy
2	School Office Copy
3	Special Health Needs
4 - 6	Immunization
4	Complete
5, 6	Plan
5	Incomplete Immunization, Plan Written
6	Immunization Plan Completed
7 - 10	Appointments (with parent for review of health history)
7	1 date of 1st appointment
8	2 date of 2nd appointment
9	3 date of 3rd appointment
10	4 date of 4th appointment
	Assessment Procedures
11 - 14	Health History
11 - 12	Parent
11	Questionnaire Completed
12	Interview Completed
13 - 14	Student
13	Questionnaire Completed
14	Interview Completed
15 - 16	Update Health History Questionnaire
15	Parent
16	Student
17 - 18	Review of Health Record (after completion of Health History and most other assessment procedures)
17	Nurse
18	Physician
19 - 20	Physical Examination
19	Nurse Practitioner
20	Physician
21 - 22	Dental
21	Screening
22	Examination
23 - 31	Screening Tests
23	Growth
24 - 25	Visual Acuity
24	Screening
25	Re-test
26	Color Vision
27 - 28	Hearing (Audiologic)
27	Sweep
28	Threshold
29 - 30	Tuberculosis
29	Tine
30	Mantoux
31	Denver Developmental Screening Test
32	Teacher Observations
33 - 34	Class Performance
33	Lowest quantile (or decile) in last marking period of previous school year
34	Lowest quantile (or decile) in second marking period of current year
35 - 38	Attendance (excused days) (unexcused days)
35	First Marking Period
36	Second Marking Period
37	Third Marking Period
38	Fourth Marking Period
39	Gym Excuses (number noted at least once for past and current year)
40	Temporary Problem List in use on child's record
41 - 42	Athletic
41	Questionnaire
42	Physical Examination

INDEX